Bioethic

A Systematic Approac

Second Edit

BERNARD GERT,
Stone Profe
Intellectual and Moral Phi
Dartmouth
Adjunct Professor of Ps
Dartmouth Medica

CHARLES M. CULVER, MD.,
Professor of Medical E
Barry U

K. DANNER CLOUSER, B.D.
University Professor of Hi
Pennsylvania State University College of

OXF

UNIVERS

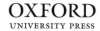

OXFORD
UNIVERSITY PRESS

Oxford University Press, Inc., publishes works that further
Oxford University's objective of excellence
in research, scholarship, and education.

Oxford   New York
Auckland   Cape Town   Dar es Salaam   Hong Kong   Karachi
Kuala Lumpur   Madrid   Melbourne   Mexico City   Nairobi
New Delhi   Shanghai   Taipei   Toronto

With offices in
Argentina   Austria   Brazil   Chile   Czech Republic   France   Greece
Guatemala   Hungary   Italy   Japan   Poland   Portugal   Singapore
South Korea   Switzerland   Thailand   Turkey   Ukraine   Vietnam

Published by Oxford University Press, Inc.
198 Madison Avenue, New York, New York 10016

www.oup.com

Oxford is a registered trademark of Oxford University Press

Library of Congress Cataloging-in-Publication Data

Gert, Bernard, 1934–
Bioethics : a systematic approach / Bernard Gert, Charles M. Culver,
K. Danner Clouser.—2nd ed.
p. cm.
Includes bibliographical references and index.
ISBN-13 978-0-19-515906-6
1. Medical ethics.   I. Culver, Charles M.   II. Clouser, K. Danner.   III. Title.
R724.G46 2006
174.2—dc22   2005050871

2   3   4   5   6   7   8   9

Printed in the United States of America
on acid-free paper

Preface

This book is an extensive revision of *Bioethics: A Return to Fundamentals*. We have changed the subtitle to *A Systematic Approach*, in order to emphasize that what distinguishes our approach to bioethics from almost all others is that it is systematic. We provide a systematic account of our common morality as a public system; we do not merely accept our thoughtful moral decisions and judgments, but show how all of these decisions and judgments can be explained in terms of a common moral system. We then apply this common moral system to the moral problems that arise in the practice of medicine. We do not make ad hoc judgments about particular cases and policies, but show that all of these judgments about cases and policies are related to and justified by this common moral system. We also show, in a systematic way, that the concept of rationality that is used to justify morality is the same concept that is used to define the critical bioethical concept of malady or disease. Further, we offer an account of the concept of death and provide an account of euthanasia that fits within the systematic account of morality and rationality that we have provided. We even show that this systematic account explains the controversy about the morality of abortion. Our approach to bioethics is fundamentally at odds with most of the current approaches to bioethics.

Our subtitle, *A Systematic Approach*, thus both describes the content of this book and speaks to a concern. The content consists of concepts, information, lines of reasoning, and theory that are basic to medical ethics. Our concern is provoked by numerous observations of the state of the field, chief among which is the tendency on the part of many to regard each area of applied ethics as an entity unto itself, that is, as independent of a general account of morality. Few, if any, systematic attempts are made to relate a general account of morality to any applied field, including the field of bioethics. Correspondingly, there is a tendency for professionals coming into the field to be trained in the culture of medical ethics, in its classic cases and standard resolutions, but with no real understanding of common morality or of its relation to the various branches of applied ethics.

Witness the spate of medical ethics anthologies being published. In the requisite sections of the books (always in the introductory or first chapter) dealing with theory, there is typically a gathering of various approaches to ethics, or moral theories, with a brief description and, sometimes, a critique of each one. But there is no systematic investigation of the different approaches or moral theories, no attempt to discover or validate the foundations of these moral theories, and no effort to attempt to relate these moral theories to the systematic solving of medical ethical problems. Indeed, typically, theory is never mentioned again in the rest of the book. Of course, knowledge of medical practices and of the realistic alternatives is essential for dealing with actual problems, but without the framework provided by a systematic account of morality, moral decisions tend to be made ad hoc.

We acknowledge that medical ethical problems often can be satisfactorily resolved on the fly, citing ad hoc rules, cases, principles, or traditions, as they come to mind. In these instances, ordinary moral understanding provides those involved with an acceptable agreed upon resolution to the problem and the citing of "proofs" or "principles" is generally nothing more than academic window dressing. However, ordinary moral understanding is often not sufficient to understand more complex and difficult cases. Whenever a case provokes disagreement among different participants, something beyond implicitly shared moral intuitions is necessary, especially when the disagreement cannot be resolved, e.g., the moral acceptability of abortion. Contrary to the standard assumptions, a systematic account of morality provides an explanation and justification of why there is often more than one morally acceptable alternative to controversial moral problems. Understanding this can promote more civil and fruitful discussion of these controversial moral problems.

Thus, in addition to its theoretical value, we believe that there is considerable practical value in discovering and validating the foundations of those moral beliefs that guide decisions and actions, and in systematically relating them to fundamental concepts and problems in medical ethics. This explains our subtitle *A Systematic Approach*. Indeed, we believe our exposition of the linkage between morality in general and its expression in medical ethics in particular is clear enough to be of conceptual help to all areas of applied ethics. It explains both why most medical decisions are uncontroversial and thus do not provoke any moral discussion, and why some moral issues in medicine are so controversial. Only an appreciation of the systematic character of moral thinking allows for some unresolvable moral disagreement without degenerating into relativism.

Most of the themes and concepts in this book were developed to some extent in our previous book *Bioethics: A Return to Fundamentals*, but we have made some significant changes in some of these topics, and have introduced some completely new topics. For example, this current book contains chapters on abortion and on "what doctors must know," subjects that were not addressed at all or only tangentially in the previous book. Also, significant changes, additions, and improvements have been made in our treatment of the concepts of consent and malady, and we have devoted an entire chapter to the concept of mental maladies. We also develop our arguments against principlism and show how the authors of principlism misunderstand our view, which undermines their criticisms of us. In the chapter on "what doctors must know," we discuss the pervasiveness of probabilistic phenomena in medicine. We give examples of several measures derived from clinical epidemiology and discuss the implications of these measures for the consent process. The chapters on death and euthanasia have been updated; the former by considering advances in technology, the latter by taking into account the Supreme Court decision concerning physician-assisted suicide. Most significant, this current book integrates all of these themes and concepts, grounding them in a systematic account of rationality and morality. The connections among bioethics, morality, rationality, and values are clearly explored, made explicit, and shown to be systematic.

To be systematic requires considering the implications that each part of the account of morality has for every other part. There must be consistency throughout the moral system. If a feature is judged to be morally relevant in one case, that same feature must be judged to be morally relevant in every other case of the same kind. Not only must there be consistency within the moral system but there must also be consistency in applying the rules, ideals, and lines of reasoning to different persons. If a violation of a moral rule is justified in one case, it must be justified in all cases with the same morally relevant features. The emphasis on consistency and coherence is in direct opposition to the ad hoc approach characteristic of much of bioethics.

We are aware that talk of a "systematic account" may connote something monolithic and presumptuous. That is unfortunate since misunderstanding of this matter has had a considerable negative impact on bioethics. Our systematic account of ethics is not monolithic; it does not claim that there is a unique right answer to every moral question. On the contrary, one of its virtues is that it provides an explanation of why some moral disagreement is unresolvable. Nor is our approach presumptuous, for it includes as morally acceptable all positions on controversial topics that have been accepted by any significant number of people. We do not reject as unacceptable any position that any impartial rational person might put forward.

Our systematic approach is distinct from all of the standard moral theories. Unlike Kantian views, we recognize the importance of consequences. Unlike consequentialist views, we emphasize that morality is a *public* system. For example, in considering whether a moral rule violation is justified, the decisive consideration is not the consequences of the particular violation in question, but the consequences of everyone knowing that this kind of violation is allowed. Breaking a moral rule in circumstances when one would not be willing for everyone to know that such violations are allowed is contrary to the impartiality required when considering violating a moral rule. That morality is a public system that applies to all rational persons explains why everyone knows what morality forbids, requires, discourages, encourages, and allows. Our recognition of this is why our account of morality does not lead to the kinds of counterexamples that have led so many in bioethics and in other areas of applied ethics to consider themselves anti–moral theory or, in what amounts to the same thing, to adopt the anthology approach to ethical theory, that is, to advocate different theories for different problems.

The appropriateness of the descriptive name "common morality" for our account of ethics will become clearer as the reader progresses through the book. Meanwhile, in this context, we wish to point out that the description of our account as "impartial rule theory" is extremely misleading. Although rules are an important aspect of our account of morality, we continually emphasize that these rules can be properly understood only as they function within the moral system. Other essential components of the moral system include moral ideals, specification of the "morally relevant features" of situations that help focus the search for the relevant facts, and an explicit two-step procedure for dealing with conflicts among rules and between rules and ideals. These features are all implicit in our ordinary moral decisions and judgments, and leaving out any of them distorts our common understanding of morality. Thus we regard "common morality" as the appropriate name for our approach.

We wish to acknowledge the help that we have received from many sources in the writing of this book. Bernard Gert continues to acknowledge the value of working with challenging Dartmouth College students, and the research environment and support offered by Dartmouth College. He also wishes to thank the Centre for Applied Philosophy and Public Ethics (an Australian Research Council–funded Special Research Centre at Charles Sturt University) for the stimulating environment at the Australian National University where he spent the summer of 2004 working on the chapter on moral disagreement. An earlier version of that chapter was published in their journal, the *Australian Journal of Professional and Applied Ethics.*

Charles Culver wishes to thank, for their encouragement and support of his scholarly efforts, Dr. Chester Evans and Dr. Doreen Parkhurst of the Barry University School of Graduate Medical Sciences. He also wishes to thank the physician assistant students of that school for their perceptive and stimulating reactions to many elements of the material contained in this book.

We wish to explicitly thank Jeffrey House of Oxford University Press for his encouragement and wise counsel during our preparation of this book. This is the third OUP book for which Jeff has served as our editorial mentor and we are enormously grateful both for his general support and his many specific suggestions about how to clarify our writing.

Unfortunately, this revision of *Bioethics: A Return to Fundamentals* has not had the benefit of one of the authors of that book. K. Danner Clouser died on August 14, 2000, at Mary Hitchcock Memorial Hospital in Lebanon, New Hampshire, at the age of seventy, almost five years after first being diagnosed with pancreatic cancer. We continue to list him as an author of this book, because much of what he wrote for that first book has remained in this one. Though that alone is not the reason for his inclusion, since both of us have learned so much from Dan that his influence on this book continues to be significant. We feel privileged to have had him as our colleague for so many years and we wish to dedicate this book to him.

Contents

Contents

Bioethics

1

Introduction

The Rationale

Background

Our goal is to provide an account of morality that is systematic and accessible and that enables the reader to understand why some of the problems of bioethics can be resolved and why there is unresolvable disagreement concerning other problems. In addition to explaining how common morality is related to general bioethics, we also explain how it clarifies some core concepts of bioethics such as paternalism and euthanasia. Although describing the system of common morality, providing its foundations, and demonstrating its usefulness are central to our work, we also provide philosophical analyses of important concepts such as death and disease. We also explain why the concept of rationality, which is central to explaining and justifying morality, is also crucial in understanding the concept of disease.

Common morality is the framework on which we build, first by explicating how morality works, then by justifying this framework by explaining why it would be favored by all persons, insofar as they use no idiosyncratic beliefs and are seeking agreement with others, as a public system for everyone. Finally we explain how, while common morality remains the same, different cultures, including subcultures like professions, can build on this framework in slightly different ways. Because everyone already knows the general features of common morality, they also know a great deal about bioethics. Common morality is the framework on which bioethics is appropriately built. That is why people are able to have sophisticated discussions about moral problems within biomedicine without ever having had a course in ethics or moral theory.

Ours is a deliberate effort to counteract the "ad hocness" that has generally characterized biomedical ethics since its birth (or rebirth) in the 1960s. It has often been pejoratively referred to as "quandary ethics" or "dilemma ethics," implying thereby that bioethics consists of puzzles that, though they may fascinate or entertain, are not amenable to systematic analysis and resolution, and hence almost any answer will, and usually does, suffice. This implies a lack of system, in that the answer to any one puzzle is unrelated to the answer to any other, and this in turn implies that there is no way to know whether the answers to two distinct dilemmas are consistent or inconsistent with each other.

The any-answer-will-suffice (or all-answers-are-unique) mind-set has been perpetuated by the way medical ethics is usually taught. We call it the "anthology" method.[1] Typically, several different ethical theories are presented with no attempt to reconcile them. Kant would say this, Mill would say that, and Rawls would say something else. The student naturally concludes that moral theory is confused, irrelevant, or totally relativistic.

Often the anthologies suggest using one theory to solve a particular kind of problem and another theory for a different kind of problem. Yet there is neither consistency among the different theories nor a clue as to which problems are to be assigned to which theory. There is certainly nothing wrong with assimilating the best from every traditional theory, but these insights must be incorporated into a comprehensive theory and not left at odds with each other. Our own theory incorporates features from all of the traditional theories. From the utilitarians we take the importance of consequences. From Kant we take the importance of impartiality. From the social contract theories we take the requirement that morality must be acceptable to all rational persons. And from natural law theories we take the requirement that morality must be known to all normal adults. Yet we blend these insights into a single coherent and comprehensive framework within which *all* moral problems can be considered.

The irrelevance of moral theory is the theme of a movement growing out of the last two decades of applied ethics. Not seeing how the abstractions and high-level generalizations of moral theory could ever take into account the particulars of moral experience, many have concluded that moral theory is irrelevant to practical moral decisions.[2] Others believe that "any single morality," especially one that is justified by a moral theory, must be wrong. They believe that such a morality must work by deduction from assumed first principles, must provide unique answers to every moral question, and consequently cannot be sensitive to different cultures and practices.[3] These critiques apply only to inadequate theories. That the critics who argue that moral theories cannot take account of all of the particulars of moral experience consider only inadequate theories makes it understandable why they reach those conclusions. However, that inadequate theories are irrelevant or worse does not mean that an adequate theory is.

We agree with much of the criticism of the standard moral theories, including other accounts of common morality.[4] Most of these moral theories are not of much use in helping one to decide what to do in particular circumstances. This is a legitimate criticism of almost all of the standard moral theories, for they often claim that they can provide a unique right answer to every moral question. Since many physicians as well as philosophers are looking for unique right answers, it is not surprising that they are disappointed when the theory fails to provide them. However, it is not a legitimate criticism of a moral theory that it does not always provide a unique right answer to every moral question. Not all moral questions have unique right answers. Our theory not only explicitly acknowledges that there are some unresolvable moral disagreements but also explains the source of these disagreements. However, it always distinguishes between morally acceptable and morally unacceptable answers. In doing ethical consultations, it is not uncommon for us to present two or more morally acceptable alternatives, and then to be told by a physician that he wants an answer to his question, not to be given a lesson in ethical theory. While we understand and sympathize with this desire to have a unique right answer, we think it important that physicians recognize that certainty can be as difficult to achieve in controversial moral matters as in complex and difficult medical situations.

Many critics of moral theory seem to share an unspoken assumption that a moral theory should be simple, that it should be statable as a memorable one-line slogan, and that it should provide a quick fix or decision procedure.[5] Although morality must be understandable to everyone who is subject to moral judgment, and all of them must be able to guide their conduct by it, morality, like grammar, need not be simple. An adequate moral theory must provide an account of morality, or the moral system, that is sufficiently complex to deal with its complicated subject matter. Even though it cannot always resolve every moral disagreement, it must always provide understanding and guidance by making clear what is responsible for that disagreement. It must also make clear what are the limits to acceptable moral disagreement. That there is not always agreement on the right answer does not mean that there is not agreement that some of the proposed answers are wrong. A complete and systematic moral theory should not provide a unique answer to every moral question—not all moral questions have such answers—but it should explain why the disagreement is unresolvable, and so promote the kind of fruitful discussion that may lead to a decision acceptable to all.

Moral System and Moral Theory

It is important not only to distinguish morality or the moral system from the moral theory that describes and justifies it but also to make this distinction correctly. The moral theory contains an explicit statement of common morality or the moral system. It is the moral system that accounts for the considered moral decisions and judgments thoughtful people commonly make. For us, the moral system comes first; the moral theory is a systematic description and justification of that moral system. Most philosophers mistakenly believe that a moral theory should generate a moral system. Whereas the moral systems that are generated by moral theories are supposed by some to provide a unique answer to every moral problem, we recognize that common morality does not provide unique answers to all moral questions. Although the moral system described by our moral theory provides a common framework for working through moral problems, it does not presuppose that this working-through process will always yield a unique correct answer.

It is because they have considered only inadequate moral theories that critics of moral theory have found moral theory unhelpful in practical circumstances. We believe that an adequate moral theory, especially an adequate description of the common moral system, is not only possible but also that it is important for doing applied and professional ethics. Inasmuch as moral theory includes a description of morality, the accuracy of that description must be continually examined by seeing if it accords with the considered moral decisions and judgments of thoughtful people. This is what is meant by saying that moral theory should be firmly based on and tested by clear moral intuitions. Thus the theory depends on and remains strongly related to moral experience. It is the philosophical analysis of this intuitive database that leads to the explicit formulation of the moral system, and this analysis of the database also explains why not all moral problems are resolvable.

Moral theory should also give an account of how the moral realm differs from the nonmoral realm. It should enable one to distinguish moral from nonmoral matters. It should give an account of the scope and boundaries of morality, for example, why there is disagreement about whether or to what degree the protection of morality gets extended to nonrational beings. It should help in distinguishing morality from many of its look-alikes, such as philosophies of life, which can significantly mislead if they are viewed as moral systems. Moral theory should identify what situations give rise to moral concern as well as what aspects of those situations are morally relevant. Identifying the facts or features of a situation that are morally relevant is crucial. Failure to even provide such a list of features, let alone defend the list, is typical of all the traditional moral theories. However, without a list of morally relevant features, a determination of the morality of an action or correctness of a moral judgment by appeal to the theory is impossible. Simply invoking a *ceteris paribus* clause, that is, saying everything else remains the same, provides no way to consistently determine if two cases are both of the same kind.

A moral theory should be able to distinguish morally acceptable from morally unacceptable solutions in particular circumstances and to help in identifying relevant factors in deciding among the morally acceptable alternatives. A moral theory should explain why there is often more than one morally acceptable alternative and why equally informed, impartial, rational persons can sometimes disagree. In these situations, when there is unresolvable disagreement, the theory should make clear precisely why the disagreement is unresolvable and what, if anything, could change so that there would be a unique morally acceptable solution to the problem. Moral theory should be unifying in the sense of conceptually holding together in a single framework all the strands of emphasis that individually form the basis for one or another traditional moral theory, such as consequences, rules, rights, and virtues. It should not only explain how a violation of a moral rule can be justified, it must also distinguish between the strength of different justifications. And finally, a moral theory should give an account of morality's universality as well as its sensitivity to cultural, professional, and local practices.

In this book we provide such a moral framework for making bioethical decisions. This framework includes an account of morality grounded in certain universal features of human beings, their fallibility, rationality, and vulnerability. It explicitly takes into account the probabilistic nature of medical practice, in particular the inherent uncertainties that are an integral part of medical diagnosis and treatment. It also includes analyses of basic concepts, such as competence, consent, death, euthanasia, malady, paternalism, and rationality, which are explicated and integrated with the moral theory. This framework is not a decision procedure for moral reasoning. It is not a conceptual machine for churning out moral conclusions. Rather, it provides a guide for determining what is and is not relevant in moral decision making; it exhibits the strengths and the limitations of moral theory; it explains why moral disagreements occur and why some cannot be resolved. We do not attempt to deal with the complete array of medical ethical problems, but we do provide an adequate, rigorous, and sound conceptual foundation for dealing with all of these problems.

Rationality and Irrationality

Although our primary concern is to provide a clear and useful account of morality, it is almost equally important to provide an account of rationality that will be of use in dealing with the actual problems that arise in medical practice. It is because the standard philosophical accounts of rationality are so far off the mark in describing the ordinary understanding of rationality, which is the understanding of rationality that applies in medicine, that the traditional accounts of morality are so inadequate. On almost all of these accounts, a positive definition of rationality is provided, and any action, desire, or belief that does not meet this definition is labeled as irrational. (Or often, because such a claim is sometimes clearly absurd, the term "nonrational" is used.) Thus, on the most popular account, a rational action is defined as one that is the most efficient means to obtaining the overall satisfaction of a person's desires; any action that does not meet this definition is labeled as irrational, or perhaps nonrational. This definition has the consequence that hardly anyone ever acts rationally. This is, by itself, sufficient to prove that the definition does not correctly capture what we ordinarily mean by describing an action as rational. However, things get even worse.

In addition to being a positive definition of rationality, the maximum satisfaction of desires account of rationality is also a formal definition. There is no specific content at all; that is, on this standard account of rationality there is no limit on the content of the desires that count toward the maximum satisfaction of desires. Thus, if killing oneself in the most painful possible way were one of a person's desires, satisfying it would count in favor of the action being rational. It should be obvious that this account of rationality does not describe the use of "rational" in ordinary life or in medicine. The account we offer is in stark contrast with this most popular philosophical account. First, we do not offer a positive definition of rational, but rather offer a definition of "irrational," and count as rational any action that is not irrational. Among other benefits of this way of defining "rational," this method allows for almost all actions of almost all people to be rational. It also makes room for the category of rationally allowed actions, those actions that it would be rational either to do or not to do. Only rationally required actions, such as stepping out of the way of a speeding truck, are irrational if not done.

As the previous example of a rationally required action indicates, we do not define an irrational action in a formal way, but rather define it in terms of content. The paradigm of an irrational action is an action that has as its intended result the agent's death, pain, disability, loss of freedom, or loss of pleasure, and the agent does not believe that anyone, including himself, will thereby avoid any of these harms or gain any benefits, such as increased consciousness, abilities, freedom, or pleasure.[6] A complete account of irrational actions would include actions without compensating benefits, in which a person *intentionally* acts in a way to significantly increase his risk of suffering any of these harms; actions in which a person *knowingly* acts in a way that will result in his suffering these harms, or significantly increases his risk of suffering them; and actions such that the agent *should know* would have this kind of result. Any action that does not fit in one of these categories counts as a rational action. This account actually picks out those actions that are regarded by all as irrational. No one performs these actions unless he is suffering from a mental disorder or is temporarily overcome by some strong emotion. It is this account of irrationality that we use in providing our account of common morality.

The Nature of Morality: An Overview

Our account of morality in chapter 2 is central to much that we do, and to the novice, it can seem complicated. Therefore, the point of the following overview is to present an easy introduction, a helpful gestalt. We want to assure readers that they already know most of what we are going to say and that we are only making this knowledge explicit and more precise. What follows is only a sketch of our view, accurate but not complete, and with only hints of arguments. Its purpose is to describe an overall framework within which to understand the details that will emerge, particularly in the next several chapters.

On Demarcating Morality

Consider for a moment what you would do if you were just setting out to describe the phenomenon of morality. Where would you look? What phenomena would you describe? How would you know what was within the moral realm and what was outside it? That is, how would you distinguish the moral from the nonmoral (as opposed to the immoral)? What is it that marks something as distinctively within the realm of morality? Though commonly claimed by philosophers, it is not the language used, for example, such words as "ought," "should," "bad," "good," "right," and "wrong." (Fewer than 10% of the uses of these terms have anything to do with morality.) The point, almost universally overlooked, is that one must already know the essential features of morality (at least in some rough, preliminary way) before he sets out to study the phenomenon of morality or else he would not know what in the world to focus upon.

This work of demarcation is an important first step for us. We argue that the existence of certain kinds of considerations, such as various rules, ideals, and procedures, constitute the clearest indication of morality at work. The specific rules we take as a component of the core of morality are those usually categorized as "moral rules." They are such rules as "do not kill," "do not deceive," "keep your promises," "do not cheat," and so on. These rules are essential components of morality. Of course, they are only part of what constitutes a system of morality, but they are absolutely crucial as part of the raw material of morality on which a moral philosopher must work. It is a philosopher's job to explicate, clarify, and organize these rules, which are such an important part of morality. More important, a philosopher must explain how these rules fit within a system, so that conflicts between the rules can either be resolved or seen to be unresolvable. As deeper understanding develops, some pre-analytically selected rules may even be excluded because they fail to meet the developing body of criteria for a moral rule. These conceptual maneuvers, accomplishing the systematization, are dictated by the underlying rationales discovered as the philosopher analyzes these moral phenomena.

We do not claim that the moral rules (whose essential role is to proscribe certain actions that commonly cause harm) are all there is to morality, or even that they are the foundation for the rest of morality. Also significant are the moral ideals, which are what many consider to be the heart of morality, because the moral ideals encourage people to prevent or relieve harm to others rather than merely to avoid causing some harm, which is what the moral rules require. Morality (that is, the common moral system) contains even more than rules and ideals. It also encompasses a list of the kinds of features of situations that are morally relevant and that must be used to describe situations that are to be subjected to moral reasoning and analysis. And, finally, morality must have a procedure for dealing with conflicts of the rules with each other and with the ideals. We have been described as having a "rule-based" morality, but that is a false and misleading description of our account of morality. A more accurate characterization is that we regard morality as a public system. It is a complex system known to all to whom it applies and it has those four main components: moral rules, moral ideals, the morally relevant features of situations, and a two-step procedure for dealing with conflicts among rules or between rules and ideals. Thus the system is not "rule based," rather rules are only one component of the system and can be properly understood only as functioning within that system.

Our demarcation of moral phenomena is a significant starting point for "doing ethics." It recognizes that morality is an ongoing human enterprise that long predates the attempts of any philosopher to understand it. It also means that the philosopher's systematic and explicit account of morality will be grounded in the ordinary practice of morality. This system of morality must not go against the firm and basic intuitions expressed in ordinary morality. In that sense, the philosopher "discovers" (or, perhaps, "uncovers") morality rather than invents it. It makes no sense to speak or think of "inventing" morality. Such a morality would have no purchase on human behavior, no authority, and no basis in the experience of human purposes, interactions, and emotions. Morality is a phenomenon that has existed from the beginning of human history, a phenomenon that we must try to understand more thoroughly. Any result of reasoning that goes against basic moral intuitions throws great suspicion on that line of reasoning or on the theory that embodies it. Beginning, as we do, with the ordinary understanding and practice of morality ensures that our account of morality will ring true to the human experience of morality. There will be no problem of "principles" or "axioms" being so abstract or so general that their application to real problems turns out to be nearly impossible.

As indicated above, ordinary moral rules and ideals are not the only points of departure for understanding morality. There are other commonly accepted features of morality, such as that morality is rational, beneficial, impartial, and applicable to all persons who can understand it and can guide their actions accordingly, all of the time, in all times and places. This is not to say that it is universally agreed that there is a universal code of behavior that answers all questions, but only that everyone who is not a moral relativist or skeptic believes that these commonly accepted features are essential characteristics of morality.

That the system of morality must be a public system is part of the very meaning of morality. It is a public system in that it is known to all to whom it applies. It also applies to everyone impartially; that is, to say that morality requires this or encourages that is to say that it requires this or encourages that for everyone in those same morally relevant circumstances. In being systematic, one cannot be content with the commonly employed "*ceteris paribus*" clauses ("all other things being equal"), which effectively hide the problem of having to determine precisely what those other things are that have to be equal. It is crucial that what counts as "the same morally relevant circumstances" be specified. Because humans do not and cannot have complete knowledge and because they are fallible and narrowly focused on their own concerns, they need a public system to guide them. In order to avoid bias, to gain perspective beyond their own self-serving interests, and to regularize their behavior in the face of inadequate knowledge about the present and the future, this public system must apply impartially to all. Insofar as there is a God who can foresee the total consequences of all actions (and thus could unerringly choose in every instance an action that has the best consequences for all time), God would not need rules or a public system. However, this presupposes that in every situation there is one combination of consequences that are "the best consequences for all time" as well as presupposing that there is no problem with the idea of a God who knows the future completely, including all the choices that will be made, making any choices.

The Content of Morality

An important conclusion, based on our systematic and explicit account of morality (referred to above) is that the point of morality is the lessening of the amount of evil or harm suffered by those protected by morality. (We use "evil" and "harm" interchangeably.) Given the vulnerability of human beings, this requires a set of moral rules such that, the more they are unjustifiably broken, the greater will be the amount of evil or harm suffered. The evils or harms humans care about avoiding comprise a specifiable and finite list. These are harms that all rational persons want to avoid unless they have an adequate reason not to. Therefore a rational person has a strong self-interest in having others act in accord with the moral rules, namely, in order to avoid having harm caused to himself and those he cares about.

These evils (or harms) are death, pain, disability, loss of freedom, and loss of pleasure. Except for death, each of these evils or harms can be more or less serious, and so it makes no sense to claim that one kind of harm is worse than another. Some degrees of pain are so severe that they are ranked by some as worse than death but other degrees of pain are ranked by some as less than the loss of an important pleasure. Some regard death as worse than any degree of pain, and a given degree of one harm (e.g., a particular loss of freedom) is not ranked above or below a given degree of some other harm (e.g., a particular pain) in the same way by everyone. Although everyone agrees that some harms are worse than others, within rather broad limits rationality allows people to rank particular evils in different ways. This fact lies at the source of many moral disputes. The participants fail to understand that, although there is a limit on what counts as a rational ranking, there is no objective ranking of the various harms that resolves all controversies.

Each general moral rule takes the form of a prohibition; each either proscribes the causing of one of the evils on that finite list of evils on which all rational persons agree, or proscribes kinds of actions that generally increase the amount of harm. Never unjustifiably violating these moral rules is what is required by morality. Because they are (or can be put) in the form of prohibitions ("Do not kill," "Do not cheat," "Do not cause pain," etc.) they can usually be followed all the time, and followed impartially toward everyone (thus satisfying several key features of morality). Meeting these basic requirements of morality does not usually involve great dedication, inner strength, outstanding character, or noble virtues; it simply involves abstaining from unjustifiably causing harm. It is possible for all normal adults to do this, although admittedly occasions often arise in which it is very tempting to act immorally.

As we have stressed, however, the moral rules are not all there is to morality. To be sure, unjustified violation of any moral rule is prohibited for everyone, but since the moral rules are basically proscribing specific actions, one could conceivably be perfectly moral by staying home in bed. However, the aspect of morality that most people generally associate with being morally good, namely, preventing or relieving harm, especially going out of one's way to help others, making sacrifices for them, or running risks for them is what we call "following moral ideals." Acting in this way is not simply avoiding causing harms, it is positively engaging in some action to prevent or relieve such harms. On our account these kinds of actions are an essential part of morality. The precepts that encourage us to prevent or relieve those very harms that the moral rules require us not to cause, we call "moral ideals."

There are crucial conceptual differences between moral rules and moral ideals. It is praiseworthy to justifiably follow moral ideals, but punishment is inappropriate for failure to follow them, whereas it is simply expected that everyone will obey the moral rules and, generally, punishment seems appropriate for all serious unjustified violations of a moral rule. The key difference is that morality requires that the moral rules never be unjustifiably violated by anyone with regard to anyone protected by morality. The moral rules can be impartially obeyed toward everyone, all the time, but that is not true of the moral ideals. Even if one spent a significant part of her life preventing evil, it would not be humanly possible to be doing it for everyone, impartially, all the time.

There is another perspective from which to grasp the orientation of our approach to morality. This begins with the fundamental realization that there is a finite core of evils (or harms) that all rational persons would avoid unless they had an adequate reason not to. These harms, the deliberate non-avoidance of which with regard to oneself constitutes the very meaning of irrational action (as discussed in chapter 2), naturally form the basis of morality. Since morality prohibits causing these harms to each other and encourages helping each other avoid these harms, it would be irrational not to support it as a public system that should govern the behavior of all who can understand it and guide their behavior accordingly.

Traditionally, moral philosophers sought "the greatest good," believing that once that was discovered, all the rest would fall neatly into place.

From the dawn of philosophy, the question concerning the *summum bonum*, or, what is the same thing, concerning the foundation of morality, has been accounted the main problem in speculative thought....[7]

It is claimed that whatever action would bring about the greatest amount of that greatest good would be the moral act for that occasion. But there is no agreement on what that greatest good is; rationality requires that certain evils be avoided, but there is no universally agreed upon ranking of the evils, let alone any agreed upon ranking of the various goods. All rational persons agree on what the goods are (consciousness, freedom, pleasure, and abilities) insofar as they are the "opposites" of the evils. Further, no rational person would avoid these goods unless he or she had an adequate reason to do so. Nonetheless, gaining these goods is far less important than avoiding the evils. This explains why the moral system that all rational persons advocate as a public guide for the behavior of everyone focuses on the avoiding and preventing of harms. Consequently, the hard-core foundation of morality is what all rational persons agree they want to avoid (unless they have an adequate reason not to), namely those specifiable evils: death, pain, disability, loss of freedom, and loss of pleasure. Humans do not want to suffer such harms, so keeping others from causing them becomes the consensual core of morality (the moral rules) along with the encouragement to prevent or relieve those evils (the moral ideals).

It would be dangerous to urge everyone simply to "promote good," if that precept were believed to give moral authority for everyone to impose on others whatever he thinks is good. It would be giving license for universal paternalism. There is wisdom in the old expression "Don't do me any favors" as well as in the ancient medical imperative "Most important, do no harm." Common morality adopts the safer policy of urging others never to cause harms and, if and when morally justifiable, to prevent harms. The danger in adopting "Promote good" as a basic moral precept (or beneficence as a basic moral principle) is that it can encourage unjustified paternalism.

Of course, if no moral rule, especially no deception or deprivation of freedom, were violated in promoting good, doing so would be morally acceptable, and often even praiseworthy. But obeying moral rules that prohibit the causing of harms is not only a safer option but also far more important. Humans are far more certain of and concerned with what they want to avoid than with what they wish to gain. The world's great literature has often described in exquisite detail the tortures of hell, but very seldom the pleasures of heaven; for it is very easy to describe what all people want to avoid, but much harder to describe what they all want to have. Acting on moral ideals, that is, preventing evils, is more important than promoting goods. Following these ideals is not only morally praiseworthy, but unlike promoting goods, doing so may provide an adequate justification for violating a moral rule, even without the consent of the person toward whom one is violating the rule.

Particular Moral Rules

The moral rules that individually proscribe causing each of the listed evils and that proscribe certain kinds of actions known to cause those harms we call "the basic general moral rules." These are considered general because they apply to all rational persons, at all times, and in all places. What counts as causing death, pain, or disability, or as depriving of freedom or pleasure may differ in fine detail from one culture to another, but whatever the details, the causing of the basic harms to another person is always proscribed.

In order for these rules to be general, that is, applicable to all persons in all times and places, there can be no reference to anything that might not have existed in all times and places, for example, cars, legislatures, marriage, alcohol, contracts, guns, and so on. Yet many moral rules in every culture are formed around these various objects, technologies, institutions, and practices that differ from one culture to another. Those moral rules, in effect, are proscribing the causing of the same list of harms that are proscribed by the general moral rules. If a culture has both deadly chemicals and streams of pure water, it will very likely have the "particular" moral rule, "Do not pollute the streams." If a culture has family units and a society in which an education is necessary to flourish, there well might be a "particular" moral rule, "Provide your children with an education." These rules are referred to as "particular" because they are formed by a relevant basic general moral rule in conjunction with a cultural behavior that might lead to the harm in question. In our examples, the basic general moral rule "Do not kill" was conjoined with the existence of toxic chemicals and streams. And the fact that lack of an education increases the risks of children suffering harms was conjoined with the existence of family responsibilities for one's children to "provide your children with an education," a duty required by the rule "Do your duty."

The basic general moral rules provide the universal strands that unify all the various formulations of particular moral rules throughout various cultures, times, and places. That is because the harms that are proscribed by the basic general moral rules are universally recognized as harms to be avoided. Thus, particular moral rules are formulated to discourage causing those harms that might arise from behavior that involves idiosyncratic cultural institutions and practices.

Professional Ethics

One hears constantly of many "ethics"—administrative ethics, business ethics, engineering ethics, environmental ethics, legal ethics, medical ethics, military ethics, psychiatric ethics—with new ones arising all the time, for example, genetic ethics and neuroethics. Are these all different? Are the professionals in these fields each making up his or her own ethics? Is each set of ethics distinctive? It would certainly make a multiring circus of ethics if they were. Ethics would be without form or content and refer only to rules of behavior that could totally differ from one realm of activity to another. That view would be counterintuitive to our sense of ethics as well as contrary to our empirical knowledge of these various specialty ethics.

Our view of professional ethics is roughly analogous to our account of particular moral rules. In the case of medicine, for example, professional ethics would be the general moral system in combination with the various institutions, practices, and relationships indigenous to the "culture" of medicine. In interacting with the structures of medical practice, "Do not deprive of freedom" would yield the moral requirement "Obtain valid consent." Similarly, "Do not cause pain or suffering" would lead to the particular medical moral rule "Do not breach confidentiality."

Thus professional ethics should not be seen as a unique and distinctive enterprise, or even as a different kind of ethics. Ethics is one basic and universal moral framework that can take different forms in different contexts, but only in order to avoid the same harms and accomplish the same purposes. The circumstances, the concepts, the relationships, the actions, and the goals of a practice, profession, or enterprise certainly differ from one another. Nevertheless, the basic moral system will be expressed in the terms of that activity so as to avoid causing those harms acknowledged as such by all rational persons. Professional ethics has an additional and significant aspect, by our account. One of the basic general moral rules is "Do your duty," and particular duties can require not only preventing harm but also promoting good. But what constitutes one's duty in a particular profession, although crucial to the ethics of that profession, is not completely determined by the general moral framework. The determinants of that duty are considered in chapter 4, where we discuss professional ethics more extensively.

A Preview of the Book

Our intention is to provide the moral framework and the conceptual tools, including an understanding of the pervasively probabilistic nature of medicine, that are sufficient to allow those with adequate knowledge of the relevant biomedical practices and of the facts of particular cases to determine the morally acceptable alternatives open to the moral agent. We present our view of the moral enterprise (including the need for theory), a description of morality, and an account of key concepts integrally related to morality and to moral matters within medicine. To illustrate how our account of morality works, we both propose solutions to some of medicine's central ethical issues, as well as explain why some problems cannot be resolved.

Chapters 2, 3, and 4 focus on moral theory as such. Chapter 2 describes our account of the moral system as it works in its complex ways. As grammar underlies ordinary speaking, whether the speakers know it or not, so the moral system underlies ordinary moral deliberations, whether the deliberators know it or not. Our mission is to describe that moral system. As part of the moral system, chapter 2 describes the moral rules, the moral ideals, the morally relevant features, and the two-step procedure for handling moral conflicts. It also discusses such related matters as the scope of morality and why there are unresolvable moral disputes. It not only contains an explicit description of the moral system, it also contains a brief account of the justification of the moral system. The moral theory presented in chapter 2 thus provides the theoretical framework for our analysis and explains the basic concepts that we apply to the particular problems that we discuss later in the book.

Chapter 3 discusses the phenomena of moral disagreement. Although most moral disagreement is based upon disagreement on the facts, or beliefs about the consequences of an action, impartial rational persons, equally well informed about the facts and probabilities, can still sometimes disagree. We examine the four other sources of moral disagreement: differences in rankings of harms; differences in ideology; differences in interpretation of moral rules; and differences on the scope of morality, that is, on who is fully protected, or protected at all, by the moral rules. We examine the opposing views on abortion and show that none of them appreciates that there is no unique correct way to determine the scope of morality.

Chapter 4 discusses particular moral rules that apply in medicine as well as the special duties of doctors and others in the health care professions and explains how these rules and duties are related to the general moral framework. In medicine, the same morality is found, though changed in a systematic and predictable way. We explore the system underlying those different faces of morality, showing that they are part and parcel of one morality. We pay particular attention to the relationship of professional ethics to ordinary morality. The concept of duty is developed: its grounding in roles and relationships, its relation to professions, and its moral significance.

In chapter 5, in order to sharpen the distinctiveness and adequacy of our approach, we contrast it with the most popular "theory" being used in bioethics. We coined the term "principlism" to describe that approach.[8] We gave it the name of "principlism" because it simply appeals to certain "principles" such as those of autonomy, beneficence, nonmaleficence, and justice, without these principles being embedded in any system. Principlism's popularity and familiarity make it a convenient vehicle through which to make crucial points concerning moral theory. It is instructive to see in what way principlism is flawed; it enables us to highlight important features necessary for an adequate account of morality.

Subsequent chapters present analyses of those concepts, such as disease and death, that are fundamental for dealing with the moral problems of biomedicine and that are relevant to understanding the nature of medical practice. Chapter 6 presents our concept of "malady," which is an explication of the common concept of disease. Maladies include more than diseases—for example, allergies and injuries are also included—but it builds on and does not distort the ordinary concept of disease. We have finally recognized that in denying that abnormality is ever a sufficient condition for a condition to be a malady, we do not need to deny that it is a necessary condition. This recognition results in a revised account of malady, such that pregnancy is no longer a malady. Chapter 7 deals with the special problems involved in clarifying the nature of mental maladies. Chapter 8 deals with the kinds of information doctors need to know, including the probabilistic nature of medical practice. Chapter 9 deals with competence, its task-specific nature, and its relationship to rationality, irrationality, and the emotions. It also discusses coercion and deals with the kinds of information doctors need to tell their patients, including, but not limited to, the essential elements of valid consent.

Chapter 10, the chapter on paternalism and its justification, illustrates how our general account of morality provides the clearest account of this extremely important concept in medicine. Paternalism, in our view, is a rich, crucial, and helpful concept. As a syndrome label, it assists in pulling together what were previously thought to be disparate signs and symptoms, thereby enabling them to be seen as an organized, identifiable process. So the concept of paternalism leads one to see many facets of the doctor-patient relationship in a morally fruitful way. The concept of paternalism helps one to focus on the true moral issues involved. Having narrowed in on the fundamental moral issues, one knows more precisely what actions need to be morally justified, and why they need justification. Paternalistic behavior always needs to be justified because it always involves violating a moral rule. Because we regard the procedure for justifying a violation of a moral rule to be essential in moral reasoning, we discuss that procedure in detail in the context of paternalistic behavior. That also provides the occasion for us to contrast how the utilitarians, deontologists, casuists, and virtue theorists would deal with this "essential in moral reasoning" and how they fall short on such a fundamental moral maneuver.

Chapter 11 deals with the definition of death, and, in light of some new considerations, arrives at a more basic and encompassing definition than what we and others have previously offered. It enables us to reach reconciliation with certain other accounts of death. Chapter 12 discusses euthanasia. This discussion, like our discussion of other concepts, utilizes many of the insights, maneuvers, and distinctions that are embedded in our account of morality. We focus on the moral relevance of the various means of "helping to die," and of withdrawing food and fluids in particular. We also stress the important difference between patient refusals, which generally must be respected, and patient requests, which need not be. We also discuss the Supreme Court decision concerning whether states can prohibit physician-assisted suicide.

The thrust of our book is to demonstrate the unity, adequacy, and necessity of theory for understanding and resolving some of the moral problems of biomedicine. The concepts, the maneuvers, the distinctions, and the exceptions should all be consistent with and unified through theory. The fact that equally informed, impartial, and rational persons sometimes disagree also must be accounted for by moral theory. Theory, in other words, should give a unified account of all the bits and pieces of moral experience. We realize that such claims about theory are controversial, but our intention in this book is to make good on those very claims.

Taking moral theory seriously does not conflict with the seriousness with which we take common morality; on the contrary, it is because we take common morality so seriously that we think it important to make it explicit and to provide an explicit justification for it. Nor does taking moral theory seriously conflict with our belief in the natural ability of human beings to deliberate insightfully and successfully about moral problems. On the contrary, our moral theory rests upon these foundations. We intend for this book to be an encouragement for people to have more trust in their basic moral intuitions. It is ironic that it can be so difficult to supply the grounds for that encouragement. As we said, moral theory needs to be complex to account for the complexity of morality, but morality need not be any more difficult than speaking and understanding one's native language. Complexity is not the same as difficulty.

Notes

1. There are many examples of the anthology method. Most do not even seem aware that they are offering several theories and leaving the reader in a quandary over what to make of such a variety. Every anthology concludes that all we can do is look for insights from each of the various theories, but they provide no clues as to which insight to apply when, or which insight outweighs which.

2. See Clarke and Simpson (1989).

3. See Brand-Ballard (2003) and Turner (2003).

4. See Beauchamp (2003).

5. We have in mind those myriad of articles, usually in medical journals and usually dealing with practical moral problems, which all too often give a passing, obligatory nod to a phrase of a moral theory that the authors seem to believe justifies whatever conclusions they have reached. The phrase might simply be "the justice principle"—not stating it or arguing for it, but simply mentioning it as though its name alone furnished sufficient backing for the author's position. Often it is the "autonomy principle" that is named as the "theory" that proves the author's conclusion. Sometimes it is slightly more elaborate, for example, "the greatest good for the greatest number," or "Always treat a human being as an end in himself and never as a means." At best, these are overly simplistic slogans, but they are frequently presented by authors as a sophisticated theoretical validation of the points they are making. See Gert (1989).

6. We are talking about the most common use of "irrational action," a "personally irrational action." There is also a philosophical use of "irrational action," sometimes called an "objectively irrational action," in which an action has these harmful consequences for the agent without compensating benefits for anyone, independent of the agent's beliefs or of what he should know.

7. Mill, (1863), 1.

8. See Clouser and Gert (1990).

2

Morality

We are aware that many people believe there is no substantial agreement on moral matters. We are also aware that there is even less agreement on the adequacy of any account of morality. We believe that these views are due to the understandable but mistaken concentration on such controversial moral issues as abortion and euthanasia, without realizing that such controversial matters form only a very small part of those matters on which people make moral decisions and judgments. Indeed, most moral matters are so uncontroversial that people do not even make any conscious decision concerning them. The uncontroversial nature of these matters is made clear by almost everyone's lack of hesitancy in making negative moral judgments about those who harm others simply because they do not like them. There is the same lack of hesitancy in making moral judgments condemning unjustified deception, breaking promises, cheating, disobeying the law, and not doing one's duty. Morality, as we understand it, applies only to a person's behavior toward others; it does not apply to behavior that affects only the agent. It is not immoral to deceive yourself or to break a promise to yourself, nor is it immoral to cheat at solitaire. Harming yourself without an adequate reason is not immoral, it is irrational.

An explicit, clear, and comprehensive account of morality helps to make clear the uncontroversial nature of many medical decisions. Such an account also helps in understanding some of the controversial moral problems that arise in the practice of medicine. Our account provides a common framework on which all of the disputing parties can agree, thus making clear what is responsible for the

21

disagreement, and what might be done to manage that disagreement. It is intended to be an account of the moral system that is already implicitly used by thoughtful people when dealing with everyday moral problems. The point of making the moral system explicit is to make it helpful to these people when they are confronted with new, difficult, or controversial moral problems.[1]

Those who deny the possibility of a comprehensive account of morality may, in actuality, merely be denying what we also deny, namely, that a systematic account of morality provides an answer to every moral problem. Common morality does not provide a unique solution to every moral problem. Readers should not expect that every moral problem will have a single best solution, that is, one that all equally informed, impartial, rational persons will prefer to every other solution. Although in many cases common morality does provide a unique answer, most of these cases are not interesting. Only in a very few situations does an explicit account of morality settle what initially seemed to be a controversial matter, for example, some aspects of euthanasia (see chapter 12). Most controversial cases do not have a unique answer, but even in these cases an explicit account of morality is often quite useful. Common morality places significant limits on legitimate moral disagreement, that is, it always provides a method for distinguishing between morally acceptable answers and morally unacceptable answers. That there is not always agreement on the best solution does not mean that there is not agreement on the boundaries of what is morally acceptable.

Most people, including most philosophers and physicians, tend to be interested more in what is controversial than in what is uncontroversial. It is routine to start with a very prominent example of unresolvable moral disagreement (e.g., abortion), and then treat it as if it were typical of the kinds of issues on which people make moral judgments. The fact that moral disagreement on some issues is compatible with complete agreement on most other issues seems to be almost universally overlooked. Many philosophers seem to hold that if equally informed, impartial, rational persons can disagree on some moral matters, they can disagree on all of them. Thus many philosophers hold either that there is no unique right answer to any moral question or that there is a unique right answer to every moral question. The unexciting but correct view is that some moral questions have unique right answers and some do not. The matters on which there is moral agreement far outnumber the matters on which there is moral disagreement, although we admit that the areas of moral disagreement are more interesting to discuss.

Common Morality

The existence of a common morality is demonstrated by the widespread agreement on most moral matters. Everyone agrees that such actions as killing, causing pain or disability, and depriving of freedom or pleasure are immoral unless there is an adequate justification for doing them. Similarly, everyone agrees that deceiving, breaking a promise, cheating, breaking the law, and neglecting one's duties also need justification in order not to be immoral. No one has any real doubts about this. People do disagree about the scope of morality, for example, whether nonhuman animals or embryos are protected by morality; however, everyone agrees that moral agents, that is, those whose actions are themselves subject to moral judgment, are protected. Thus, doubt about whether killing nonhuman animals or embryos needs to be justified does not lead to any doubt that killing moral agents needs justification. Similarly, people disagree about what counts as an adequate moral justification for some particular act of killing or deceiving and on some features of an adequate justification, but everyone agrees that what counts as an adequate justification for one person must be an adequate justification for anyone else in the same situation, that is, when all of the morally relevant features of the two situations are the same. This is part of what is meant by saying that morality requires impartiality.

Everyone also agrees that some people, for example, the severely mentally retarded, should not be subject to moral judgment if they do not even know what kinds of behavior morality prohibits (e.g., cheating), requires (e.g., keeping promises), discourages (e.g., doing nothing to help those in need), encourages (e.g., relieving someone's pain), and allows (e.g., deciding which pair of socks to wear). Although it is difficult even for philosophers to provide an explicit, precise, and comprehensive account of morality, most cases are clear enough that everyone knows whether or not some particular act is morally acceptable. No one engages in a moral discussion of questions like "Is it morally acceptable to deceive patients in order to get them to participate in an experimental treatment that has no hope of benefiting them but that one happens to be curious about?" because everyone knows that such deception is not justified. Although the prevalence of hypocrisy makes clear that people do not always behave in the way that morality requires or encourages, it also confirms that all people know the general kinds of behavior that morality does require and encourage. That everyone who is subject to moral judgment knows what kinds of acts morality prohibits, requires, discourages, encourages, and allows, is part of what is meant by saying that morality is a public system.

Morality as a Public System

A public system is a system that has the following two characteristics: (1) All persons to whom it applies (i.e., those whose behavior is to be guided and judged by that system) understand it (i.e., know what behavior the system prohibits, requires, discourages, encourages, and allows); and (2) It is not irrational for any of these persons to accept being guided and judged by that system. The clearest example of a public system is a game. A game has an inherent goal and a set of rules that form a system that is understood by all of the players. It is not irrational for all players to use the goal and the rules of the game to guide their own behavior and to judge the behavior of other players by them. Although a game is a public system, it applies only to those playing the game. Morality is a public system that applies to all moral agents; all people are subject to morality simply by virtue of being rational persons who are responsible for their actions. That people are required to act morally regardless of any personal ends they might have may explain Kant's claim that the demands of morality are categorical, not hypothetical.

In order for all rational persons to know what morality prohibits, requires, discourages, encourages, and allows, knowledge of morality cannot involve beliefs that are not held by all rational persons. Only facts or beliefs that are known to all moral agents can be necessary in order to know what kinds of actions morality prohibits, requires, and so forth. Thus, no facts or beliefs discovered by modern science can be necessary, for none of these facts or beliefs is known by all moral agents. The same is true of any religious belief, for no particular religious belief is held by all rational persons. Only those beliefs that it would be irrational for any moral agent not to hold are essential for knowledge of morality. We call such beliefs *rationally required* beliefs. Beliefs that it would be irrational for any moral agent to hold, we call *rationally prohibited* beliefs. Beliefs that are neither rationally required nor rationally prohibited, we call *rationally allowed* beliefs.

Rationally required beliefs include general factual beliefs such as: all moral agents are vulnerable, they can be killed, caused pain, be disabled, and be deprived of freedom or pleasure by other people. Moral agents also have limited knowledge and are fallible. Having these beliefs is necessary in order to be a moral agent. On the other hand, no *rationally allowed* beliefs can be part of the moral system, even though some rationally allowed beliefs, for example, beliefs about the facts of the particular case, are often necessary for making particular moral decisions or moral judgments. In addition to the rationally required *general* beliefs, there are rationally required *personal* beliefs. These are beliefs that *all* moral agents have about themselves, for example, beliefs that they themselves are vulnerable, that is, they can be killed and caused pain, and so forth, and are fallible. These rationally required personal beliefs differ from the rationally allowed personal beliefs only in that the latter beliefs are not true of all moral agents and hence are not known to all.[2] Even though personal beliefs about one's race, gender, religion, abilities, etc., are as certain to the agent as the rationally required personal beliefs, morality cannot be based on them, because not all moral agents know these rationally allowed personal beliefs about others.

Although morality is a public system that is known by all those who are held responsible for their actions, it is not a simple system. A useful analogy is the grammatical system used by all speakers of a language. (People are speakers of a language if they can understand and can be understood by other speakers of the language.) Almost no speaker can explicitly describe this system, for example, when the subjunctive tense should be used, yet they all know it in the sense that they use it when speaking and in interpreting the speech of others. If there is a conflict between the way speakers use the language and an explicit account of the grammatical system, the speakers always win. It would be a mistake to accept any description of a grammatical system that rules out speaking in a way that these speakers know is commonly regarded as acceptable or allows speaking in a way that they know is commonly regarded as completely unacceptable.

A *moral theory* is an attempt to make explicit, explain, and, if possible, justify morality. By morality we mean the *moral system* that people use, not necessarily consciously, in deciding how to act when confronting moral problems and in making their moral judgments. An adequate moral theory must present an account of morality that uses concepts or principles that are understood by everyone who is subject to moral judgment.[3] Although we realize that most moral decisions do not explicitly employ any account of morality, we hope that the account of morality that we present will accomplish three tasks: (1) reassure health care professionals who have made correct decisions, but who still feel uneasy because they cannot make their moral reasoning explicit; (2) provide a framework that can be used for understanding disputes among health care professionals or between health care professionals and patients, making clear why there may be no unique best solution; and (3) provide a framework for explicitly dealing with those rare cases in which health care professionals do not know what to do.

We also hope this account of morality will be used to teach those entering the health care professions that the moral framework that is used in medicine is the same moral framework that they have always used. Although doctors, nurses, and other health care professionals have some special duties that cannot be deduced from common morality, these duties cannot be incompatible with it either. The difficult moral problems that health care professionals commonly face require knowledge of both common morality and of the specific duties and ideals of those who are professionals in the health care field. These specific duties and ideals may sometimes seem to conflict with the requirements of common morality, but a proper understanding of both confirms that the moral system provides a method for dealing with those conflicts in the same way that it deals with other conflicts within common morality (see chapter 4).

Most moral theories, for example, those of Kant and Mill, no matter how complex they are themselves, unfortunately present overly simple accounts of morality.[4] Indeed, many philosophers seem to regard their moral theories as generating a new and improved morality, rather than as describing and justifying our common morality. Some philosophers seem to value simplicity more than agreement with commonly accepted moral judgments. This may be because normally they do not use the systems generated by their theories to help resolve specific moral problems, although almost all of them hold that every moral problem has a unique right answer. These philosophers seem as if they would rather put forward theories that lead to obviously counterintuitive moral judgments than to admit that morality is too complex to be accounted for by their theories.

In reaction to this oversimplification of morality, many in applied ethics, particularly medical ethics, claim to be anti–moral theory. They quite rightly regard various overly simple accounts of morality as worse than useless. Unfortunately, they seem to accept the false claim that an ethical theory must provide an overly simple account of morality. One of the legitimate attractions of early versions of principlism (see chapter 5) was that it correctly denied that there is a unique solution to every moral problem. However, with their adoption of the method of specification, it is no longer clear that Beauchamp and Childress, the major proponents of principlism, still hold this view. Unfortunately, Beauchamp and Childress still seem unable to understand that morality can be a single unified system that provides a framework for dealing with all moral problems and yet not provide a unique solution to every moral problem.[5] The anti-theory view sometimes leads those in bioethics to accept the incorrect and damaging view that all moral reasoning is ad hoc or completely relative to the situation. Casuistry is often taken as if it were anti-theory and did not presuppose a common moral system for which casuistry was a method of interpretation and application.

Mistaken Accounts of Morality

Careful reflection on what are universally acknowledged to be moral rules, such as "Do not kill" and "Do not cheat," makes clear that morality is best conceived as a guide to behavior that rational persons put forward to govern the behavior of others toward themselves and those for whom they are concerned, whether or not they plan to follow that guide themselves. Many philosophical accounts of morality, however, present morality as if it were primarily a personal matter. The dominant philosophical view of morality now, and perhaps as far back as Socrates, seems to be that morality is primarily intended to provide a guide for the individual person who adopts it.[6] In order to reconcile this personal-guide view of morality with the acknowledged view that morality applies to everyone, many philosophers have tried to prove that all rational persons would put forward the same guide to conduct for others as they adopt for themselves.

Regarding morality as providing a personal guide also results in a far wider account of morality than is appropriate, as if any judgment about how a person ought to act (e.g., that he ought to brush his teeth twice a day) is part of a moral guide. Morality is about how one ought to act, but that is not a definition of morality; rather, it is a claim that morality is primarily about actions. It corrects another widespread but mistaken philosophical view that morality is primarily about what is the best state of affairs. From the moral point of view, the only reason for one wanting to know what is the best state of affairs is because one realizes these affairs may have some bearing on what actions ought to be done. Sometimes, of course, these affairs will not have any bearing on these actions, as that state of affairs cannot be brought about. It is dangerous to view morality as being concerned with the best state of affairs since, oftentimes, what is regarded as the best state of affairs can be brought about only in a morally unacceptable way, for example, by deceiving patients in order to get them to consent to a beneficial treatment. Of course, whether or not one's behavior counts as morally unacceptable will sometimes be determined by the end to be achieved, for example, saving a patient's life may justify deception. These kinds of problems are discussed in more detail in the chapter on paternalism and its justification.

Rationality and Morality

Everyone agrees that if a certain way of acting is irrational, that is, not even rationally allowed, no one ought to act in that way. But just because an action is rationally allowed does not mean that everyone agrees that one ought to act in that way. On the contrary, it is often rationally allowed, that is, not irrational, to act immorally. That an action is rationally allowed does not entail that one ought to act that way. However, everyone agrees that no one ever ought to act irrationally. An adequate moral theory must provide an account of rationality that explains why it has this kind of force.[7]

Although everyone agrees that they ought never act irrationally, people often do act irrationally. Acting on one's emotions is usually acting rationally, but people sometimes act on their emotions without considering that their actions will have harmful consequences for themselves. Sometimes even when they do consider these consequences, their emotions impel them to act irrationally. People who have a mental disorder, for example, a phobia, often act irrationally. But regardless of how they actually act, people acknowledge that they should not act irrationally. An adequate account of rationality must be such that it explains why, even though people do sometimes act irrationally, no one thinks that he ought to act irrationally.

Rationality is very intimately related to harms and benefits. Everyone agrees that unless a person has an adequate reason for doing so, it would be irrational to avoid any benefit or not to avoid any harm for herself or those for whom she cares. Our account of rationality, although it accurately describes the way in which the concept of rationality is ordinarily used, differs radically from the accounts normally provided by philosophers in two important ways. First, it makes irrationality rather than rationality the basic concept; second, it defines irrationality by means of a list rather than a formula. In the objective sense of an irrational action, a person correctly appraises an action as irrational when she correctly believes (1) it will cause, or significantly increase the probability of, the agent's suffering (avoidable) death, pain, disability, loss of freedom, or loss of pleasure, and (2) there is no objectively adequate reason for the action.[8] Any intentional action that is not irrational is rational.

The close relationship between irrationality and harm is made explicit by this definition, for this list also defines what counts as a basic harm or an evil. Everything that anyone counts as a harm or an evil, for example, thwarted desires, maladies, and punishments, necessarily involves at least a significant increase in the probability of (avoidable) death, pain, disability, loss of freedom, or a loss of pleasure. However, complete agreement on what the basic harms are is compatible with considerable disagreement on the ranking of these harms. Especially since all of the harms except death have degrees, and even death occurs at very different ages, there can be no agreement that any one of these harms is always worse than the others. Some people rank dying several months earlier as worse than a specified amount of pain and suffering while other people rank that same amount of pain and suffering as worse. Thus, it is rationally allowed for most terminally ill patients either to refuse death-delaying treatments or to consent to them.

Our experience on ethics committees is that most moral disagreements (e.g., whether or not to treat an incompetent patient), are based on disagreements about the facts of the case (e.g., on how painful the treatment will be and how long it will relieve the painful symptoms of the patient's disease). Differences in the rankings of the harms account for most of the remaining disagreements, for example, how much pain and suffering is it worth to prevent a patient from dying? Often the factual disagreements about prognoses are so closely combined with different rankings of the harms involved that they cannot be disentangled. Further complicating the matter, the probability of suffering any of the harms can vary from insignificantly small to almost certain, and people can differ in the way that they rank a given probability of one harm against a different probability of another harm.

Disagreement about involuntary commitment of people with mental disorders that make them dangerous to themselves often involves two kinds of disagreement. The first is a disagreement about what percent of these people would commit suicide if not committed. Even if there is agreement that one in twenty patients would commit suicide if not committed, there may still be disagreement about the rankings of the probabilities involved, such as whether a 5% risk of death within one week for one person compensates for the certainty of three to five days of a very serious loss of freedom and a significant probability, say

30%, of long-term mental suffering, secondary to that loss of freedom, for nineteen persons. Actual cases usually involve much more uncertainty about outcomes as well as the rankings of more harms.[9] Considerable disagreement on what counts as the lesser evil or greater harm in any particular case is compatible with complete agreement on what counts as a harm or evil.

A decision that involves an increase in the probability of oneself suffering some harm will be irrational unless one has an adequate reason for that decision. Thus, not only what counts as a reason but also what makes a reason adequate must be clarified. Objective reasons for acting are facts that can make some otherwise objectively irrational action rational.[10] We are aware that "a reason" refers not only to what we call objective reasons and personal reasons but also to beliefs that explain a person's actions, whether the belief is rational or not. We do not use "a reason" to refer to beliefs that explain a person's action; that is what we call "a motive." We use "a reason" to refer only to objective and personal reasons. Although most beliefs that are personal reasons are also mo- tives for most people, some reasons such as a belief that a person unknown to the agent will benefit from his action may never serve as a motive for some agents. But this belief is a personal reason for all persons in an appropriate situation, whether or not it serves as a motive for them, and the corresponding fact is an objective reason.

Objective reasons for acting are facts that the action will avoid, prevent, or significantly decrease the probability of anyone suffering (avoidable) death, pain, disability, loss of freedom, or loss of pleasure, or will cause, or significantly increase the probability of, anyone gaining consciousness, or obtaining more ability, freedom, or pleasure.[11] What was said about evils or harms in the last paragraph also holds for the goods or benefits mentioned in this definition of a reason. Everything that people count as a benefit or a good, for example, health, love, and friends, is related to one or more of the items on this list or to the absence of one or more of the items on the list of harms. Complete agreement on what counts as a good is compatible with considerable disagreement on whether one good is better than another, or whether gaining a given good or benefit adequately compensates for suffering a given harm or evil.

An adequate objective reason for acting is a fact that a significant number of otherwise rational persons regard as compensating for the harm suffered by the agent.[12] People count as otherwise rational if they almost never knowingly act so as to suffer any harm without an adequate reason. No rankings that are held by any significant religious, national, or cultural group count as irrational. The ranking by Jehovah's Witnesses of the harms that would be suffered in an afterlife as worse than dying decades earlier than one would if one accepted a transfusion is not an irrational ranking. Similarly, psychiatrists do not regard any beliefs held by any significant religious, national, or cultural group as delusions or irrational beliefs. The belief by Jehovah's Witnesses that accepting blood transfusions will have bad consequences for their afterlife is not regarded as an irrational belief or delusion. Any rationally allowed belief that is a personal reason counts as an adequate personal reason for an action if any significant group regards it as an adequate personal reason for that action. Irrationality would not be the fundamental normative concept if there were not complete agreement (among all those whose views are taken seriously) that no one ever ought to act irrationally. This view of irrationality requires that no actions count as irrational unless there is almost universal agreement that they not be done.

Counting any action that is not irrational as rational results in two categories of rational actions: those that are *rationally required* and those that are merely *rationally allowed*. If no religious beliefs are involved, an example of a rationally required action, that is, an action that would be irrational not to do, would be an otherwise healthy person taking a proven and safe antibiotic for a life-threatening infection. However, refusing a death-delaying treatment for a painful terminal disease, even if no religious beliefs are involved, will only be rationally allowed, that is, will not be irrational either to do or not to do. These two categories share no common feature except that they are both not irrational. This account of rationality has the desired result that everyone who is regarded as rational always wants himself and his friends to act rationally. Certainly, on this account of rationality, no one would ever want himself or anyone for whom he is concerned to act irrationally.

Although an action counts as rational when it is rationally allowed for a person to act in that way, it may be *unreasonable* for a particular person to act in that way, given her particular rankings of the harms and benefits involved. It is only when the intended consequences of an action are solely or primarily with regard to the agent, as in deciding which of two incompatible medical treatments to adopt, that there is a clear sense to the notion of an unreasonable action. In this context, an unreasonable action is a rationally allowed action that is chosen even though it conflicts with the rankings of harms and benefits of the person choosing. For example, it may be rationally allowed to choose either of two alternative treatments, both equally effective, but with a different mix of harms and benefits. Suppose, however, that the first treatment involves the risk of a harm that the patient ranks as very serious, for example, impotence, whereas the second involves the risk of causing allergies to certain kinds of foods, which the patient has no particular desire to eat. Unless he has an adequate reason, it would be unreasonable for that patient to choose the first alternative. For another patient with different rankings, one who liked the foods to which the treatment might cause an allergy and who had no interest in sexual activity, it would be unreasonable to choose the second treatment.

Although this account of rationality may sound obvious, it is in conflict with the most common account of rationality, where rationality is limited to an instrumental role. A rational action is often defined as one that maximizes the satisfaction of all of one's desires, but without putting any limit on the content of those desires.[13] This definition results in an irrational action being defined as any action that is inconsistent with such maximization.[14] Unless desires for any of the harms on the list are ruled out, however, it turns out that people would not always want those for whom they are concerned to act rationally. Consider a young person who becomes extremely depressed and desires to kill himself. No one concerned with him would encourage him to satisfy that desire even if doing so would maximize the satisfaction of his present desires. Rather, everyone concerned with him would encourage him to seek psychiatric help. They would all hope that he would be cured of his depression and then come to see that he has no adequate reason to kill himself.[15] The fact that rationality has a definite content and is not limited to a purely instrumental role conflicts with most philosophical accounts of rational actions, as well as those offered by most of the social sciences, including economics.[16]

Some may claim that both of these accounts of rationality are misconceived. Following Hume, they may claim that the basic account of rationality is not primarily related to actions at all, but rather to obtaining true beliefs. Scientific rationality consists of using those scientific methods best suited for discovering truth. Scientific rationality is related to belief, but rationality related to belief cannot be taken as the fundamental sense of rationality. The account of rationality as avoiding harms is more basic than that of rationality related to belief or of reasoning correctly. Scientific rationality cannot explain why it is irrational not to avoid suffering avoidable harms when no one benefits in any way. The avoiding-harm account of rationality does explain why it is rational to reason correctly and to discover new truth, namely, because doing so helps people to avoid harms and to gain benefits.[17]

The avoiding-harm account of rationality makes clear that in a conflict between morality and self-interest, it is not irrational to act in either way. It is neither irrational to act contrary to one's own best interests in order to act morally, nor is it irrational to act immorally if it is in one's own best interest to do so. It may even be rationally allowed to act contrary to both self-interest and morality, if, for example, friends, family, or colleagues benefit. Indeed, altruistic immorality is the cause of far more serious evil than morality done for self-interest. Just consider all those who sacrifice their own interests but act immorally in service of their country or religion.

Morality and self-interest do not always oppose each other; indeed, they are usually quite compatible. Many people, including some physicians and scientists, mistakenly believe that they cannot be acting immorally if they act to benefit others and contrary to their own self-interest. They do not recognize that they are acting immorally in helping to cover up the mistakes of their colleagues because they believe that since they, themselves, have nothing to gain and are even putting themselves at risk, they must be acting morally. Those who hold a virtue theory of ethics have difficulty in explaining why self-sacrifice for others is sometimes immoral. The phenomenon of sincere but unjustified paternalism makes clear that altruism and morality are not the same.

Although some philosophers have tried to prove that it is irrational to act immorally, this conflicts with the ordinary understanding of the matter. Everyone agrees, for example, that if a physician is certain that he will not be discovered, it may not be irrational, that is, it may be rationally allowed, for him to deceive a patient about a mistake that he has made, even if this is acting immorally. Although we, like everyone else, favor people acting morally, in this book we are not attempting to provide motivation for acting morally. That motivation usually comes from the way one has been brought up. But even having the appropriate motivation is not adequate without a proper understanding of morality. Providing that understanding of morality is one of the primary goals of this book. Having a concern for others must be tempered by the realization that it is arrogant to think that morality does not apply to oneself and one's colleagues in the same way that it applies to everyone else.

Morality is a public system. And with regard to obeying the moral rules it requires impartiality with regard to all moral agents, that is, those who are held morally responsible for their actions. It is morally unacceptable to violate a moral rule if one could not publicly allow that violation, that is, be willing for everyone to know that they are allowed to violate that moral rule when all of the morally relevant features are the same. Failure to appreciate the significance of impartiality leads to altruistic immorality, sacrificing one's own interests for family, friends, or colleagues, when one would not be willing for everyone to know that they are allowed to act in that way. It can also lead to misguided loyalty to one's nation, religion, or any other group. The failure to understand what moral impartiality requires is also responsible for many instances of unjustified paternalism.

Impartiality

Impartiality is a more complex concept than is generally recognized. Even many dictionaries mistakenly define it simply as not favoring one more than another and regard impartiality as equivalent to fairness, as if one could not impartially enforce laws that one knew to be unfair. Impartiality does not, by itself, guarantee moral behavior if one is impartial with regard to an inappropriate group or in an inappropriate respect. In fact, it cannot even be determined if A is impartial until the group with regard to which A is impartial and the respect in which A is impartial are specified. The following analysis of the basic concept of impartiality confirms that to understand fully what it means to say that a person is impartial involves knowing both the group with regard to which her impartiality is being judged and the respect in which her actions are supposed to be impartial with regard to that group. A is impartial in respect R with regard to group G if and only if A's actions in respect R are not influenced at all by which members of G benefit or are harmed by these actions.

It is also not generally understood that morality does not always require impartiality. Morality requires impartiality only when one is considering violating a moral rule. It does not require impartiality when deciding which people to help, for example, which charity to give to. One reason that most philosophical accounts of morality are correctly regarded as having little practical value is because they do not recognize that morality requires impartiality only in very limited circumstances, namely, when considering violating a moral rule. Even John Stuart Mill remarks that a person is more likely to be censured than praised for not favoring family and friends when there is no duty to act impartially.

Just as an adequate general account of impartiality must relate impartiality to some group, for example, a father being impartial with regard to his own children, so an adequate account of the impartiality required by morality must relate it to some group. People differ concerning who is included in the group with regard to which morality requires impartiality. The minimal group toward which morality requires impartiality consists of all moral agents and former moral agents who are still persons (incompetent but not permanently unconscious patients). This group is the minimal group because all rational persons would favor impartial obedience to the moral rules, for example, "Do not kill" and "Do not deceive," with regard to a group including at least all of these people. Further, in the United States and the rest of the industrialized world, almost everyone would include in the group toward whom the moral rules require impartiality, all children, including infants who will become moral agents. However, the claim that moral rules require impartiality with regard to any more extended group quickly becomes controversial.

Many hold that the impartially protected group should include only moral agents, former moral agents, and children who will become moral agents, while many others hold that this group should include all potential moral agents, even nonsentient ones, such as an embryo from the time of conception. Still others hold that this group should include all sentient beings, that is, all beings who can feel pleasure or pain, whether potential moral agents or not, for example, horses and pigs. Since fully informed rational persons disagree about who is included in the group toward which morality requires impartiality, there is no way to resolve the issue philosophically. This is why discussions of abortion and animal rights are so emotionally charged and often involve violence. There are no conclusive arguments for any of these competing views, which is why the morality of abortion is an unresolvable issue. We examine this issue in more detail in the following chapter. Morality, however, does set limits to the morally allowable ways of settling unresolvable moral disagreements. These ways cannot involve violence or other unjustified violations of the moral rules, but must be settled peacefully. One of the often neglected functions of a moral theory is to determine what counts as a genuinely unresolvable moral disagreement. Once this is determined, one of the proper functions of a democratic government is to settle these genuinely unresolvable moral disagreements by peaceful means.

As noted, the respect in which one must be impartial toward the minimal group (or any larger group) is when considering violating a moral rule, for example, killing or deceiving. Since all of the moral rules can be regarded as prohibitions, it is fairly easy to obey them impartially. Impartiality is not required in following the moral ideals, for example, relieving pain and suffering, for it is humanly impossible to follow the ideals impartially even with regard to the minimal group toward which morality requires impartiality. One of the more obvious flaws of many forms of consequentialism, such as utilitarianism, is that it makes no distinction between moral rules and ideals and so seems to require impartiality in all of one's actions. Failure to understand that morality requires impartiality only with respect to obeying the moral rules has even caused some to deny that morality requires impartiality.[18] The kind of impartiality required by morality involves allowing a violation of a moral rule with regard to one member of the protected group (e.g., a stranger), only when the same kind of violation would be allowed with regard to everyone else in the group (e.g., a friend).

Acting in an impartial manner with respect to the moral rules is analogous to a referee impartially officiating a basketball game, except that a moral agent is part of the group toward which he is required to be impartial. The referee judges all participants impartially if he makes the same decision regardless of which player or team is benefited or harmed by that decision. All impartial referees need not prefer the same style of basketball; one referee might prefer a game with less bodily contact, hence calling somewhat more fouls, while another may prefer a more physical game, hence calling fewer fouls. Impartiality allows these differences as long as the referee does not favor any particular team or player over any other. Holding that there is a unique correct way to call fouls, as many philosophers are inclined to do, illustrates the kind of unrealistic thinking that makes most people regard philosophy as having no practical value. Just as calling fouls impartially allows for differences, moral impartiality allows for differences in the ranking of various harms and benefits as long as one would be willing to make these rankings public and one does not favor any particular person or group, including oneself or one's friends, over any others when one decides to violate a moral rule or judges whether a violation is justified.

Common Morality as a Justified Moral System

To justify morality is to provide a strong argument that morality is the kind of public system that, given that rational persons use only beliefs that all of them share, namely, rationally required beliefs, and that they are trying to reach agreement with other rational persons, all rational persons would endorse as a guide for everyone to follow. There is no way to guarantee that all rational persons will agree unless they use only beliefs that all of them share, namely, rationally required beliefs. This limitation to rationally required beliefs is not an arbitrary limitation. Morality is a public system that applies to all rational persons, thus it can involve only those factual beliefs that are shared by all rational persons. Both morality itself and the justification of morality can make use of only rationally required beliefs with regard to the moral framework that is shared by all moral guides. Morally acceptable societal guides, however, can also use beliefs that are shared by all those to whom that system applies, for example, members of that society.[19]

Further, particular moral decisions and judgments depend not only on knowledge of the moral system but also on beliefs about the particular situation. As noted above, our experience on ethics committees and in doing ethics consultations has been that most actual moral disagreements are based on disagreements about the facts of the case, especially disagreements about prognoses. However, we have noted that particular moral decisions and judgments may also depend on how different harms and benefits are ranked. A decision about whether to withhold a genetic diagnosis from a patient, for example, of Huntington's disease, involves a belief about the *magnitude* of the risk of telling, such as the probability of the information leading him to kill himself or to suffer a severe lengthy depression, and the *ranking* of that degree of risk of death or depression against the certain loss of freedom to act on the information that results from that information not being provided. Equally informed, impartial, rational persons may differ not only in their beliefs about the degree of risk but also in their rankings of the harms involved, and either of these differences may result in their disagreeing on what morally ought to be done.

Common morality, which is the framework for all justified moral systems, applies to vulnerable and fallible people. Its goal is to lessen the amount of harm suffered by those protected by it. It must recognize and accommodate the fallibility of people and the need for the system to be understood by everyone to whom it applies. It includes: (1) *rules* prohibiting acting in ways that cause, or significantly increase the probability of causing, any of the five harms that all rational persons want to avoid; (2) *ideals* encouraging the prevention or relief of any of these harms; and (3) a procedure for determining when it is justified to violate a moral rule. Although it is useful to provide a clear, comprehensive, and explicit account of the justified moral system that is common morality, it is not useful, but rather dangerous, to claim to provide a system that can be applied mechanically to arrive at the correct solution to a moral problem. Not all moral problems have unique correct solutions. Common morality only provides a framework for dealing with moral problems in a way that is acceptable to all impartial rational persons; it does not provide a unique right answer to every moral question. In what follows we make explicit the details of the common moral system. No one will find anything surprising in our explication.

The Moral Rules

The first five moral rules prohibit directly causing the five harms.

(1) *Do not kill* (includes causing permanent loss of consciousness).

(2) *Do not cause pain* (includes causing mental pain, e.g., sadness and anxiety).

(3) *Do not disable* (more precisely, do not cause loss of physical, mental, or volitional abilities).

(4) *Do not deprive of freedom* (includes freedom from being acted upon as well as depriving one of the opportunity to act).

(5) *Do not deprive of pleasure* (includes sources of pleasure).

The second five moral rules include those rules that, when not followed in particular cases, usually but not always cause harm, and always result in harm being suffered when they are not generally followed.

(6) *Do not deceive* (includes more than lying).

(7) *Keep your promise* (equivalent to "Do not break your promise").

(8) *Do not cheat* (primarily involves violating rules of a voluntary activity, e.g., a game).

(9) *Obey the law* (equivalent to "Do not break the law").

(10) *Do your duty* (equivalent to "Do not neglect your duty").

The term "duty" is being used in its everyday sense to refer to what is required by special circumstances or by one's role in society—primarily one's job or special situation—not as philosophers customarily use it, which is to say, simply as a synonym for "what one morally ought to do."[20]

What Counts as a Violation of a Moral Rule?

As mentioned earlier, people often differ in their interpretation about what counts as breaking the rule. Not every action that results in someone suffering a harm or an evil counts as breaking one of the first five rules. It is often important to distinguish between an action that is a justified violation of a moral rule and one that is not even a violation of a rule at all. A scientist who discovers that another scientist's apparently important new discovery was plagiarized may know that reporting this will result in harm to the plagiarist. Reporting her findings, however, is not a violation of any rule against causing harm. Almost no one would say that it is, but determining whether or not it is depends upon the practices and conventions of the society. (See chapter 4 for further discussion.)

On the other hand, a doctor who receives valid consent from a patient and then causes pain to that patient (gives an immunization injection) in order to prevent greater pain in the future (contracting influenza) is breaking the rule against causing pain, even though this violation is strongly justified. Now consider a physician who responds to a couple's question and informs them that their fetus has some serious genetic problem, such as cystic fibrosis, when she knows that this will result in their suffering considerable grief. If she has verified the information and told them in an appropriately considerate way, then many would say that she did not break the rule against causing pain and her action requires no justification. It seems plausible to say that it is the facts about their fetus's condition that caused the pain. Indeed, not responding truthfully to their question would be an unjustified violation of the rule against deception. On this interpretation, the physician is acting like the scientist reporting a mistake by another scientist. However, one might interpret the situation to be like the doctor justifiably breaking the rule against causing pain with the valid consent of the patient. But if the doctor does not tell that truth in as kind and gentle a fashion as she can, then this second interpretation seems more accurate and the violation of the rule may not even be justified. It is part of the duty of doctors not to cause more suffering than necessary when giving information about any serious malady.

It is quite clear that lying, namely, making a false statement with the intent to deceive, counts as a violation of the rule prohibiting deception, as does any other action that is intentionally done in order to deceive others. But it is not always clear when withholding information counts as deception because it is not always clear what one has a duty to tell. Thus, it is not always clear that one needs a justification for withholding some information, (e.g., that the husband of the woman whose fetus is being tested did not father that fetus) because it is not clear that the physician has a duty to tell this information. One might say that there is no duty to tell the husband that he is not the father unless the physician has agreed to disclose this information at the outset. Perhaps the best way to avoid this difficult situation is to make clear prior to doing the genetic testing that information of this kind will not be disclosed.

In scientific research, what counts as deceptive is determined in large part by the conventions and practices of the field or area of research. If it is a standard scientific practice to smooth curves depicting data or not to report unsuccessful experiments, then doing so is not deceptive, even if some people, especially those who are not expected to read the reports, are deceived. However, when a practice results in many people being deceived, especially if it is known they will read the results, it is a deceptive practice even if it is a common practice within the field or area, for example, releasing to the public press a premature and overly optimistic account of a "cure." This creates false hope for many of those suffering from the related malady. Recognition that your action is deceptive is important, for then you realize that without an adequate justification, your action is immoral.

Justifying Violations of the Moral Rules

Almost everyone agrees that the moral rules have justified exceptions; most agree that even killing is justified in self-defense. Further, there is widespread agreement on several features that all justified exceptions have. The first of these involves impartiality. Everyone agrees that all justified violations of the rules are such that if they are justified for any person, they are justified for every person when all of the morally relevant features are the same. The major value of overly simple slogans like the Golden Rule, "Do unto others as you would have them do unto you," and Kant's categorical imperative, "Act only on that maxim that you could will to be a universal law," are as devices to persuade people to act impartially when they are contemplating violating a moral rule. However, given that these slogans are often misleading, a better way to achieve impartiality is to consider whether one would be prepared for everyone to know that this kind of violation is allowed.

The next feature on which there is almost complete agreement is that it must be rational to favor everyone being allowed to violate the rule in these circumstances. Suppose that someone suffering from a mental disorder both wants to inflict pain on others and wants pain inflicted on himself. He is in favor of any person who wants others to cause pain to himself, being allowed to cause pain to others, whether or not they want pain inflicted on themselves. This is not sufficient to justify that kind of violation. No impartial rational person would favor allowing anyone who wants pain caused to himself to cause pain to everyone else, whether or not these others want pain caused to themselves. The result of allowing that kind of violation would be an increase in the amount of pain suffered with no benefit to anyone. That would be clearly irrational.

Finally, there is general agreement that a violation is justified only if it is rational to favor that violation even if everyone knows that this kind of violation is allowed. A violation is not justified simply if it would be rational to favor allowing everyone to violate the rule in the same circumstances when almost no one knows that it is allowed to violate the rule in those circumstances. What counts as the same kind of violation, or the same circumstances, is determined by the morally relevant features of the situation. We discuss these features in the next section, but here is a simple example. It might be rational to favor allowing a physician to deceive a patient about his diagnosis if that patient were likely to be upset by knowing the truth, when almost no one knows that this kind of deception is allowed. In order to make this kind of deception justified, however, it has to be rational to favor allowing this kind of deception when everyone knows that deception is allowed in these circumstances. Only the requirement that the violation be publicly allowed guarantees the kind of impartiality required by morality. (See chapter 10 for further discussion.)

Not everyone agrees about which violations satisfy these three conditions, but there is general agreement that no violation is justified unless it satisfies all three of these conditions. Recognizing the significant agreement concerning justified violations of the moral rules, while acknowledging that people can sometimes disagree, results in all impartial rational persons accepting the following attitude toward violations of the moral rules: Everyone is always to obey the rule unless an impartial rational person can advocate that violating it be publicly allowed. Anyone who violates the rule when no impartial rational person can advocate that such a violation be publicly allowed may be punished. The "unless clause" only means that when an impartial rational person can advocate that such a violation be publicly allowed, there may be disagreement among impartial rational persons about whether or not the rule should be obeyed. It does not mean that they agree it should not be obeyed.

Morally Relevant Features

In deciding whether an impartial rational person can advocate that a violation of a moral rule be publicly allowed, the kind of violation must be described using only morally relevant features. Since the morally relevant features are part of the moral system, they must be understood by all moral agents. This means that any description of the violation must be such that it can be reformulated in a way that all moral agents can understand. Limiting the way in which a violation must be described makes it easier for people to discover that their decision or judgment is biased by some consideration that is not morally relevant. All of the morally relevant features that we have discovered so far are answers to the following questions. It is possible that other morally relevant features will be discovered, but we think that we have discovered the major features. Of course, in any actual situation, it is the particular facts of the situation that determine the answers to these questions, but all of these answers can be given in a way that can be understood by all moral agents.

(1) What moral rules would be violated?

(2) What harms would be (a) avoided (not caused), (b) prevented, and (c) caused? (This means foreseeable harms and includes probabilities as well as kind and extent.)

(3) What are the relevant beliefs and desires of the people toward whom the rule is being violated? (This explains why physicians must provide adequate information about treatment and obtain their patients' consent before treating.)

(4) Does one have a relationship with the person(s) toward whom the rule is being violated such that one sometimes has a duty to violate moral rules with regard to the person(s) without his consent? (This explains why a parent or guardian may be morally allowed to make a decision about treatment that the health care team is not morally allowed to make.)

(5) What benefits would be caused? (This means foreseeable benefits and also includes probabilities, as well as kind and extent.)

(6) Is an unjustified or weakly justified violation of a moral rule being prevented? (This is usually not relevant in medical contexts, and applies more to police work and national security.)

(7) Is an unjustified or weakly justified violation of a moral rule being punished? (This is not relevant in medical contexts, and applies more to the legal system.)

(8) Are there any alternative actions that would be preferable?[21]

(9) Is the violation being done intentionally or only knowingly?[22]

(10) Is it an emergency situation in which a person most likely did not plan to be?[23]

It may be worthwhile to illustrate this general account of the morally relevant features by using standard medical situations.

(1) Among the moral rules that might be violated are those against causing pain, depriving of freedom, deceiving (including withholding information), breaking promises (e.g., of confidentiality), and even killing.

(2) The harms that might be prevented or avoided by deceiving are the anxiety suffered by the patient and a 25% increased risk of a heart attack. The harm caused might be the loss of freedom to make decisions based on the facts. In another example, the harm that might be prevented by refusing to abide by a patient's decision to stop life-sustaining treatment would be the patient's death; the harms caused would be suffering and the loss of freedom.

(3) In medical situations, the relevant beliefs and desires are normally those that lead a competent patient to validly consent to, or refuse, a suggested treatment, for example, beliefs about the consequences of accepting and refusing treatment, and desires or aversions to those consequences.[24]

(4) Except in emergency situations, doctors do not normally have a relationship with the patients that requires doctors to break moral rules with regard to patients without patients' consent. Parents and guardians do have such a relationship. This explains why guardians must be appointed if it is regarded as medically necessary to treat a patient without his consent.

(5) Benefits are limited to the conferring of positive goods. The prevention or relief of harms is included in feature 2. Although preventing harm certainly can be considered a benefit, it allows for a clearer analysis to distinguish conferring positive goods from preventing harms. Normally, medical situations are concerned only with the prevention or relief of harms, but cosmetic plastic surgery for someone who is not disfigured would be an example of providing benefits. Unlike the preventing of harms, this can almost never be done without the valid consent of the person who is to be benefited.

(6) Preventing the violation of a moral rule does not normally apply in medical situations, but it can occur when a doctor considers violating confidentiality

in order to prevent an AIDS patient from having unprotected sex with his wife who is unaware of his HIV positive status.

(7) Punishment should never be relevant in a medical situation.

(8) This feature is perhaps the most overlooked. Many actions that would be morally acceptable if there were not a better alternative become morally unacceptable if there is a better way. Persuading a husband to tell his wife that he is HIV positive is a better alternative than the doctor simply violating confidentiality by telling her himself, even though, in cases where the husband is not persuaded, it may be morally acceptable for the doctor to tell her himself.

(9) It is uncontroversially morally acceptable to provide adequate pain medication to a terminally ill patient even though one knows that this medication may hasten his death. It is, at least, controversial to provide pain medication in order to hasten the patient's death.

(10) It may be morally acceptable to overrule a patient's refusal of life-preserving treatment in an emergency situation when it is not morally acceptable to overrule the same refusal in a non-emergency situation.

When considering the harms being avoided (not caused), prevented, and caused, and the benefits being promoted, one must consider not only the kind of benefits or harms involved, one must also consider their seriousness, duration, and probability. If more than one person is affected, one must consider not only how many people will be affected but also the distribution of the harms and benefits. Two violations that do not differ in any of their morally relevant features count as the same kind of violation. Anyone who claims to be acting or judging as an impartial rational person who holds that one of the two violations is justified must hold that the other also is justified. This simply follows from morality requiring impartiality when considering a violation of a moral rule.

However, two people, both fully informed, impartial, and rational, who agree that two actions count as the same kind of violation, need not always agree on whether or not to advocate that this kind of violation be publicly allowed. They may rank the benefits and harms involved differently or they may differ in their estimate of the consequences of publicly allowing that kind of violation. For example, two persons may agree on the increase in the probability that a post-stroke patient will discontinue his physical therapy if his therapist does not harass him. They may also agree on the amount of pain that harassment will cause and on the amount of disability that will result if the therapy is discontinued. But they may disagree in their rankings of the pain caused by harassment, and the probability of the increase in disability that results from discontinuing therapy. They may also disagree about the consequences of publicly allowing that kind of violation, one holding that everyone knowing that this kind of violation is allowed will result in a very large increase in the amount of pain caused by harassment, and the other holding that it will result in only a small increase, which will be more than justified by the extra amount of disability lessened.

To act or judge as an impartial rational person is to estimate what effect this kind of violation—one with all of the same morally relevant features—would have if publicly allowed. If all informed, impartial, rational persons would estimate that less harm would be suffered if this kind of violation were publicly allowed, then all impartial rational persons would advocate that this kind of violation be publicly allowed, and the violation would be strongly justified. If all informed, impartial, rational persons would estimate that more harm would be suffered, then no impartial, rational person would advocate that this kind of violation be publicly allowed and the violation is unjustified. However, impartial rational persons, even if equally informed, may disagree in their estimate of whether more or less harm will result from this kind of violation being publicly allowed. When there is such disagreement, even if all parties are rational and impartial, they will disagree on whether or not to advocate that this kind of violation be publicly allowed and the violation counts as weakly justified.

Disagreements about whether the same kind of violation being publicly allowed will result in more or less harm stem from two distinct sources. The first source is a difference in the rankings of the various kinds of harms. If someone ranks a specified amount of pain and suffering as worse than a specified amount of loss of freedom, and someone else ranks them in the opposite way, then, although they agree that a given action is the same kind of violation, they may disagree on whether or not to advocate that this kind of violation be publicly allowed. The second source is differences in estimates of how much harm would result from everyone knowing that a given kind of violation is allowed, even when there seems to be no difference in the rankings of the different kinds of harms. These differences may stem from differences in beliefs about human nature or about the nature of human societies. For example, there may be different views on how many people would violate the rule against deceiving in these circumstances if they knew such a violation was allowed, or what effect this number of violations would have upon the society. Insofar as these differences cannot be settled by any universally agreed upon empirical method, they are best regarded as ideological.

The disagreement about whether physicians should assist the suicides of terminally ill patients is an example of such a dispute. People disagree about whether publicly allowing physician-assisted suicide will result in more bad consequences (e.g., significantly more people dying sooner than they really want to) than good consequences (e.g., many more people being relieved of pain and suffering). However, it is quite likely that most ideological differences also involve differences in the rankings of different kinds of harms, for example, whether the suffering prevented by physician-assisted suicide ranks higher or lower than the earlier deaths that might be caused by it. This issue will be discussed in more detail in chapter 12 on euthanasia.

Moral Ideals

In contrast with the moral rules, which prohibit doing those kinds of actions that cause people to suffer some harm or increase the risk of their suffering some harm, the moral ideals encourage one to do those kinds of actions that lessen the amount of harm suffered (including providing goods for those who are deprived) or decrease the risk of people suffering harm. As long as a person is not violating a moral rule, common morality encourages following any moral ideal. In particular circumstances, it may be worthwhile to talk of specific moral ideals, for example, that there are five specific moral ideals involved in preventing harm, one for each of the five harms. Physicians seem primarily devoted to the moral ideals of preventing death, pain, and disability. Genetic counselors may have as their primary ideal preventing the loss of freedom of their clients. Particular moral ideals that involve preventing unjustified violations of the moral rules can also be specified. Providing a proper understanding of morality in order to prevent unjustified violations of the moral rules may also count as following a moral ideal.

It is not important to decide how specific to make the moral ideals since, normally, following any moral ideal is praiseworthy. It is, however, important to distinguish moral ideals from other ideals, for, except in very special circumstances, only moral ideals can justify violating a moral rule with regard to someone without her consent. Utilitarian ideals, which involve promoting goods such as abilities and pleasure, for those who are not deprived, do not justify individuals in violating moral rules without consent.[25] Those who train athletes, engage in historical or scientific research, or create delicious new recipes are following utilitarian ideals. Religious ideals involve promoting activities, spirituality, traits of character, and so forth, which are idiosyncratic to a particular religion or group of religions. Personal ideals involve promoting some traits of character (e.g., ambition) that are idiosyncratic to particular persons, but about whose value people disagree.

The moral ideals differ from the moral rules in that only for the latter is there a possibility of their being impartially obeyed all of the time. No one can impartially follow moral ideals all of the time. Indeed, it is humanly impossible simply to follow them all of the time, because everyone needs to sleep sometimes. Of course, everyone favors people following the moral ideals, but most do not favor everyone following them as much as possible. Except for some extreme consequentialist philosophers, people believe that everyone is entitled to spend some time relaxing and having fun. It is only one's failure to obey a moral rule that always needs an excuse or justification. None of this should be surprising at all. Everyone counts certain kinds of actions as immoral (e.g., killing, causing pain, deceiving, and breaking promises), unless doing that kind of act can be justified. Everyone also agrees that acting to relieve pain and suffering is encouraged by morality, but doing so is not required unless one has a duty to do so. This distinction between moral rules and moral ideals should not be taken as simply an alternative formulation of the common distinction between negative and positive duties, for it is a moral rule that one keep one's promise and do one's duty, and keeping one's promise or doing one's duty may require positive action.[26]

That two moral rules can conflict, for example, doing one's duty may require causing pain, makes it clear that it would be a mistake to conclude that one should always avoid breaking a moral rule. Sometimes breaking one of these rules is so strongly justified that not only is there nothing immoral about breaking it, it would be immoral not to break the rule. A physician who, with the rational informed consent of a competent patient, performs some painful procedure in order to prevent much more serious pain or death, breaks the moral rule against causing pain, but is not doing anything that is immoral in the slightest. In fact, refusing to do the necessary painful procedure, given the conditions specified, would itself be a violation of her duty as a doctor and thus would need some stronger justification in order not to be immoral. It can be strongly justified to break a moral rule even when there is no conflict between moral rules. Sometimes acting on a moral ideal (e.g., stopping to help an accident victim) may involve breaking a moral rule (e.g., breaking a promise to meet someone at the movies), and yet everyone would publicly allow breaking the rule. It is clear, therefore, that to say that someone has broken a moral rule is not, by itself, to say that anything morally unacceptable has been done; it is only to say that some justification is needed. Normally, most medically indicated treatments that involve causing harm to the patient, including most medical operations, are completely morally unproblematic because valid consent has been given.

Applying Morality to a Particular Case

Sometimes there seems to be an unresolvable difference when a careful examination of the issue shows that there is actually a correct answer. For example, a physician may claim that deceiving a patient about a diagnosis, such as multiple sclerosis, to avoid causing a specified degree of anxiety and other mental suffering is justified. He may claim that withholding these unpleasant findings in this case will result in less overall harm being suffered than if he did not deceive. He may claim that this patient does not deal well with bad news and also is unlikely to find out about the deception. Thus, he may claim that his deception, at least for a limited time, actually results in his patient suffering less harm than if he were told the truth.

Another physician, however, may claim that this deception is not justified, no matter how difficult it will be for the person to accept the facts now or how confident the physician is that the deception will not be discovered. The latter may hold that this deception will actually increase the amount of harm suffered because the patient will be deprived of the opportunity to make decisions based upon the facts, and that if he does find out about the deception he will not only have less faith in statements made by the physician, he will also have less faith in statements made by other health care providers, thus increasing his anxiety and suffering. This is a genuine empirical dispute about whether withholding bad news from this patient is likely to increase or decrease the amount of harm he suffers. Which of these hypotheses about the actual effects of deception in this particular case is correct, we do not know, but if one is concerned with the moral justifiability of such deception, the consequences of the particular case are not decisive.

The morally decisive question is "What would be the consequences if this kind of deception were publicly allowed?" The former physician has not taken into account that a justifiable violation against deception must be one that is publicly allowed, that is, one that everyone knows is allowed. Once the physician realizes that everyone knows that it is allowable to deceive in certain circumstances, for example, to withhold bad news in order to avoid anxiety and other mental suffering, then the loss of trust involved will obviously have a worse result than if everyone knew that such deception was not allowed. It is only by concentrating on the results of one's own deception, without recognizing that morally allowed violations for oneself must be such that everyone knows that they are morally allowed for everyone, that one could be led to think that such deception was justified. Consciously holding that it is morally allowable for you to deceive others in this way when you would not want everyone to know that everyone is morally allowed to deceive others in the same circumstances is what is meant by arrogance. It is arrogating exceptions to the moral rules for yourself that you would not want everyone to know are allowed for all. This arrogance is clearly incompatible with the kind of impartiality that morality requires with regard to obeying the moral rules.

This does not mean that it is never morally justified to deceive patients. Sometimes the consequences of being told the truth may be so serious, such as a significant increase in the chances of a fatal heart attack, that a physician would be willing to publicly allow everyone to deceive in this kind of case, at least for a period of time. Only when a physician would publicly allow deception is what is called "therapeutic privilege" appropriately used. What is important is that you must think of your decision as if it were setting a public policy, one that everyone could act on when the morally relevant features were the same. Indeed, actually formulating a public policy is probably the best way to deal with controversial cases.

The Importance of Having Public Policies

Should physicians inform parents of young teenagers (age thirteen to fifteen) if their children are sexually active or taking drugs? We do not have the answer to this question, for there are good arguments both in favor of informing parents and against informing them. However, having an explicit public policy stating that parents will be informed, or that they will not, is preferable to not having any public policy at all. In the absence of any public policy, whether parents will be informed is a matter of chance, based solely on which doctor happens to examine their child, and perhaps even on how that doctor happens to feel that day. Further, neither parents nor children know what to expect. If parents are not told, they can justifiably complain that they should have been told, so that they would have been able to talk with their children and help them with their problem. If parents are told, the children can justifiably complain that their confidentiality has been violated and that if they had known that their parents would be informed, they would never have confided in the doctor.

Not having a public policy makes it impossible for either parents or children to give informed valid consent. Both are deprived of the opportunity to make an important decision because neither knows the consequences of the teenager being examined. Further, it is quite likely that both believe what they want to believe—parents, that they will be informed, and children, that their parents will not be informed. Neither group will have any evidence for their belief. This means that it is quite likely that someone will feel betrayed by what actually happens. If there is a public policy, then both parents and children will know what is going to happen, so that neither will be misled. If the policy is that parents will be notified, then children will know that their confidentiality is limited and can decide what they are prepared to tell the doctor. If the policy is that parents will not be notified, then parents will know that they cannot count on the physician to inform them of any problems and that they must seek to find out about any problems directly from their child. But even if the policy is that parents will not be notified, that does not prohibit doctors from trying to persuade the child to talk to his parents.

Further, the policy does not have to be and should not be stated in some simple way that prohibits a physician from exercising her judgment in a particular case, contrary to the general policy. Thus, if the general policy is not to inform, it should have exceptions in several cases, such as those that threaten the child's life. If the policy is to inform, it should also have exceptions, such as in cases where the child provides evidence that informing his parents would have serious negative consequences. A public policy is an informal public system and, like morality itself, allows for cases in which people can disagree about what should be done. It would be worse than naive to think that one could formulate an acceptable public policy that would never allow the physician to exercise his considered judgment. The point of having a public policy is not to eliminate judgment but to provide a context so that everyone involved has a better idea of what to expect.

Another advantage of having a public policy is that it needs to be preceded by discussion among all those involved. Once it is agreed that it is better to have some public policy rather than none, all of those involved must cooperate to formulate such a policy. This discussion is quite likely to result in everyone becoming better informed and learning about alternatives and arguments that they had not considered. Discussing all the details of a public policy is quite likely to result in better decisions, for everyone will now be aware of the complexities of the issue. Indeed, many may become aware for the first time that what they have been doing is not the same as what others have been doing. They also may become aware of consequences that had previously escaped their attention.

Perhaps, most important, the discussion should make everyone aware that fully informed rational persons can disagree, even on moral matters, without anyone being mistaken. That one can compromise one's position without any loss of moral integrity is a valuable lesson. Having a public policy, rather than each person making her own judgment, has sufficient value that an impartial person should see that having a stated public policy outweighs the fact that this policy may limit her freedom to make her own judgment. Being guided by a public policy that one has contributed to and about which one can claim it is not irrational for anyone to follow is a wonderful preparation for the kind of moral reasoning that is required for all moral problems. Indeed, if the public policy is in accord with the common moral system, it always will involve the kind of moral reasoning that we have been trying to make explicit in this chapter.

Notes

1. A more extended account of morality, and of the moral theory that justifies it is contained in Gert (2005). A shorter version is contained in Gert (2004).

2. Perhaps one would need only the single personal belief, "I am a moral agent," and then all of the other rationally required personal beliefs could be inferred from the rationally required general beliefs.

3. For example, although the principle of respecting autonomy has become exceedingly popular in bioethics, autonomy is an extremely difficult concept that is not clearly understood by philosophers, let alone by those patients to whom it is applied. (See chapters 5 and 10 for a further critique of autonomy.)

4. For example, none of them provide anything that is even comparable to the list of morally relevant features discussed below.

5. Beauchamp and Childress (2001): "No framework of guidelines could reasonably anticipate the full range of conflicts; and the impartial rule system [their name for our view] does no more to settle the problem then our system does" (389). This quote strongly suggests that Beauchamp and Childress continue to misdescribe and misunderstand our account of morality.

6. This is Plato's and Aristotle's view and also seems to be Kant's. It is explicitly the view of R. M. Hare in all of his earlier books. It is held by all those who hold that the question, "Why be moral?" is either answered by referring to the benefits to the person who asks the question, or who regard the question as nonsensical. Those who do not view morality in this way are those for whom morality and political theory are regarded as very closely related, for example, Hobbes, the utilitarians, and Rawls.

7. We are aware that the terms "rational" and "irrational" are sometimes used in a way that a person might favor acting irrationally, for example, when "irrational" means "spontaneous." However, philosophers as diverse as Plato, Hobbes, and Kant agree that no one ever ought to act irrationally. We are attempting to provide the descriptive content of the concept of objective rationality that is compatible with its fundamental normative character. There is a closely related concept of personal rationality where the action is being appraised from the point of view of the agent. But because a person might advocate that a friend do an act that is personally irrational if he has additional information that the action is not objectively irrational, it is the objective sense of irrationality that is the basic normative sense. Unless we specify differently, when we use the terms "rational" and "irrational," we are using these terms in their objective sense.

8. The parallel personal sense of an irrational action is: a person correctly appraises an action as personally irrational when she correctly believes (1) that the agent knows or expects, or should know or expect, that his action will cause or significantly increase the probability that he will suffer any of the harms, and (2) the agent believes that there is no objectively adequate reason for the action, or if he does believe there is an objectively adequate reason, this belief does not motivate him.

9. See Culver (2004) and chapter 10.

10. Personal reasons for acting are rational beliefs that can make some otherwise personally irrational actions rational. Only a belief that is seen to be inconsistent with one's other beliefs by almost everyone with similar knowledge and intelligence is an irrational belief. Psychiatrists regard such beliefs as delusions. Irrational beliefs do not count as personal reasons, for they can never make it personally rational to do an otherwise personally irrational action.

11. Personal reasons are rational beliefs with the same content.

12. An adequate personal reason is a rational belief with the same content.

13. See Gert (1990a) for examples of philosophers who hold this view.

14. This is no minor definitional squabble. Accepting such a definition of an irrational action makes it impossible for irrationality to play its role as the fundamental normative concept.

15. See Gert (1990b).

16. See Gert (1990a, 1993).

17. See Clouser and Gert (1986).

18. See Gert (1996).

19. See chapter 4 for further discussion of this issue.

20. See Gert (2005), chapter 8 for a fuller discussion of duty.

21. This involves trying to find out if there are any alternative actions such that they would either not involve a violation of a moral rule, or that the violations would differ in some morally relevant features especially, but not limited to, the amount of evil caused, avoided, or prevented.

22. Although one does not usually decide whether or not to commit a violation intentionally or only knowingly, sometimes that is possible. For violations that are alike in all of their other morally relevant features, a person might not publicly allow a violation that was done intentionally, but might publicly allow a violation that was not done intentionally, even though it was done knowingly. For example, many people would publicly allow nurses to administer sufficient morphine to terminally ill patients to relieve their pain even though everyone knows it may hasten the death of some patients. However, even with no other morally relevant changes in the situation, they would not allow nurses to administer morphine with the intention of hastening the death of a patient. This

distinction explains what seems correct in the views of those who endorse the doctrine of double effect. Such a distinction may also account for what many regard as a morally significant difference between lying and other forms of deception, especially some instances of withholding information. Lying is always intentional deception. Although withholding information is sometimes intentionally deceptive, it is sometimes only knowingly deceptive. Nonetheless, it is important to remember that most violations that are morally unacceptable when done intentionally are also morally unacceptable when done only knowingly.

23. We are talking about the kind of emergency situation that is sufficiently rare that, except for those professionally involved with emergencies, a person is not likely to plan or prepare for being in. This is a feature that is necessary to account for the fact that certain kinds of emergency situations seem to change the moral judgments that many would make even when all of the other morally relevant features are the same. For example, in an emergency when large numbers of people have been seriously injured, doctors are morally allowed to abandon patients who have a very small chance of survival in order to take care of those with a better chance, in order that more people will survive. However, in the ordinary practice of medicine doctors are not morally allowed to abandon their patients with poor prognoses in order to treat those with better prognoses. Patients' knowledge that they could be abandoned by their doctor in common non-emergency situations would cause so much anxiety that it would outweigh the benefits that might be gained by publicly allowing doctors to do so.

24. In situations when physicians are considering acting paternalistically toward a patient, it is important to consider whether the patient's relevant desires are irrational and whether his beliefs are irrational or would be if he had a higher level of intelligence or knowledge. It is also important to consider whether the implied rankings of the benefits and harms involved in the decision, based on these irrational desires or defective beliefs, is irrational. In his article "Gert's Moral Theory and Its Application to Bioethics Cases" (*Kennedy Institute of Ethics Journal*, 16(1), March, 2006), Carson Strong pointed out that we should have made the rationality or irrationality of the decision and the rationality or irrationality of the (implied or explicit) ranking of harms and benefits an explicit part of morally relevant feature 3. We think that he was correct.

25. Utilitarian ideals may sometimes justify governments in violating moral rules, but that is due to morally relevant feature four, that governments have special relationships with their citizens. See chapter 12 of Gert (2005) for a more detailed discussion of this issue.

26. As we discuss in more detail in the following chapter, there is a common misuse of the term "duty" such that all of the moral rules are taken as describing duties, rather than duties arising from specific roles and circumstances.

3

Moral Disagreement

Introduction

Why anyone would think that all equally informed, rational persons would agree on the answer to every moral question when they do not even agree about who is the best hitter in the history of baseball, or about a host of other simple matters, is an interesting question. Of course, all equally informed, rational persons agree on the answers to most moral questions, but most moral questions are not controversial. They are so uncontroversial that they are not even discussed. It is as if there is not even any question to be answered. "Is it morally acceptable to deceive or harm a person simply because you do not like him?" is not a question any moral agent seriously asks. Even though it is seldom explicitly stated, it seems to be a common philosophical view that either all moral questions have correct answers or that none of them do. Philosophers do not seem to like the correct view that some moral questions have unique correct answers and others do not. It is the mistaken view that because most moral questions have correct answers that all of them must have correct answers that leads philosophers to think that they can resolve the question of abortion.

A moral theory should provide an explicit description of common morality. It should justify this morality or show why it is not justified. A moral theory should not attempt to resolve every moral problem, as if all equally informed, rational persons must agree on the answer to every moral question. Rather, it must explain both why there is moral agreement about the answers to the overwhelming majority of questions, and why there is moral disagreement concerning the answers to a small but important number of questions. The overwhelming agreement on most moral matters is obscured by the fact that there is very little discussion of these matters and a great deal of discussion about the small number of controversial issues. But the fact that there is agreement on the answers to most moral questions is no reason to believe that there are unique correct answers to every moral question. However, it is not sufficient to simply claim that no moral theory can resolve every moral problem, it is necessary to explain why a particular controversial problem, such as abortion, is unresolvable.

If any of the standard moral theories provided more than a schema of a guide to conduct, it would be clear that they provide little support for the view that there are unique correct answers to every moral question. However, most of the standard moral theories (e.g., consequentialism, Kantian theories, and contractarianism) do offer simple slogans that strongly suggest that there must always be universal agreement among equally informed, impartial, rational persons. Thus, it is not surprising that, despite overwhelming evidence to the contrary, most philosophers continue to hold that there is a correct answer to the question about the moral acceptability of abortion, as well as to other controversial moral issues.

Moral Realism

We call the philosophical position that empirical facts about the world, not hypotheticals about the attitudes of suitably situated rational persons, completely determine the answer to every moral question *moral realism*. According to this view, these empirical facts determine whether an act is morally right, morally wrong, or morally indifferent.[1] On this view, moral disagreements, like scientific disagreements, are always disagreements about these empirical facts. This position is used to support the view that there is a unique correct answer to every moral question. Insofar as people are equally informed, impartial, and rational, they will agree in their moral decisions, evaluations, and judgments.

In most instances, talking about morality requiring impartiality with respect to obeying the moral rules creates no problems, for most instances only involve other moral agents, and there is complete agreement that morality requires impartiality with regard to all moral agents with respect to obeying the moral rules. But in discussions about the scope of morality, some, such as Peter Singer, have claimed that morality requires impartiality with regard to all beings who have interests and that this includes all sentient beings.[2] Singer not only claims that morality requires that the interests of all sentient beings be treated impartially when considering the violation of a moral rule but also that morality requires that all interests be treated equally, whether or not any violation of a moral rule is involved. No argument is offered for the claim that morality requires that all interests be treated equally; it is simply stated as if this were a universally accepted claim. However, as pointed out in the previous chapter, morality only requires impartiality when considering violating a moral rule, for it is humanly impossible to act impartially with respect to even all moral agents in any respect more than this. Furthermore, one cannot even understand talk about impartiality unless the group with regard to which one must be impartial is specified. How this group is to be specified is an issue on which equally informed, rational persons disagree. Bentham, the spiritual father of Singer, claims that morality requires impartiality with regard to any being that can feel pain, while Kant holds that morality requires impartiality only with regard to rational beings. It is the thesis of this chapter that not all equally informed, rational beings will accept either of these claims.[3]

Classical utilitarians are the paradigm of moral realists. If they are interpreted as hedonistic act consequentialists, then they hold that an act is right if it results in as great a balance of pleasure over pain (happiness over unhappiness) for everyone affected by the act as by any alternative. All other acts are wrong. If two acts would result in the same balance of pleasure over pain overall, it is morally indifferent as to which act is performed. Modifications of this view can take into account the distribution of the pleasure and pain, but on this or any other modification, given the facts, the theory comes up with a unique answer, right, wrong, or morally indifferent.

Of course, there are serious problems in taking a utilitarian theory seriously, that is, in using it as a guide for your behavior. There is no uniquely acceptable procedure for weighing and comparing either pleasures or pains. Even more serious, there is no uniquely acceptable procedure for weighing pleasures against pains, or for deciding between a larger number of people experiencing a pain of less intensity and a smaller number experiencing a pain of greater intensity. The problems are even more daunting for those versions of consequentialism that do not limit the relevant consequences to pleasure and pain (happiness and un-happiness), but also include ability, freedom, and consciousness as goods, and death, disability, and loss of freedom as evils. In light of these problems, many consequentialists no longer claim that consequentialism provides a practical moral guide to conduct, but claim only to be providing a purely theoretical moral theory. They claim only that the relevant consequences of an action and of all of the alternative actions provide a theoretical criterion for determining whether that act was right, wrong, or indifferent. (They mistakenly take these to be equivalent to morally right, morally wrong, or morally indifferent.) Of course, this does not solve any of the problems involved in ranking different pleasures (goods) and pains (evils), how to rank pleasures (goods) against pains (evils), or how to balance intensity versus extent, but it removes their practical signifi-cance. Now it is simply a theoretical problem that there is no agreement con-cerning the ranking of pleasures (goods) or pains (evils), how to rank pleasures (goods) against pains (evils), or how to balance intensity versus extent. None of this seems to bother those who hold that, at least theoretically, there must be a unique correct answer to every moral question.

Moral Constructivism

Moral realism is not the only source of support for the claim that there is a unique correct answer to every moral question. This claim is also supported by some versions of what we call *moral constructivism.* This is the view that hypothetical statements about the answers that would be given by suitably qualified and situated rational persons provide the correct answers to all moral problems and questions. Those who think that the unique correct answer to a moral question is the answer that would be given by all rational persons *if* they were in some situation such as John Rawls's original position, and were under its veil of ignorance, hold a version of moral constructivism that supports the claim that there is a unique correct answer to every moral question.

All moral constructivists who hold that all suitably qualified and situated rational persons always agree must also hold that there is a unique correct answer to every moral question.[4] However, a moral constructivist need not hold that all suitably qualified and situated rational persons always agree. Indeed, it is our contention that on any plausible account of suitably qualified and situated rational persons, they will not always agree. Unfortunately, like Rawls, most of those who hold some version of moral constructivism either assume or claim that such rational beings do always agree. Strict Kantians, who can be viewed as moral constructivists, also hold that rational persons, insofar as they are not influenced by nonrational considerations, always agree. This is because, insofar as they are solely rational beings, they have no desires that differentiate them from one another and so they have no basis for disagreeing.

It is in order to eliminate any disagreement that Rawls introduces "the original position" as the suitable situation in which qualified rational persons make their moral decisions and judgments. This original position not only eliminates all knowledge and beliefs not shared by all but also any personal characteristics on the basis of which rational persons could disagree. Although Rawls agrees with Kant that all suitably qualified and situated rational persons agree, Rawls derives this agreement primarily from the suitable situation in which rational persons must make their moral decisions and judgments, whereas Kant derives it primarily from the nature of rational persons. The claim that all suitably qualified and situated rational persons presented with the same facts always agree in their moral judgments and decisions eliminates any difference between moral constructivism and moral realism with regard to both positions' support for the claim that there is always a unique correct answer to every moral question.[5]

Other philosophers, such as intuitionists, may seem to hold that not all moral questions have unique correct answers. Sir David Ross claims that more than consequences are relevant to moral decisions and judgments, and that sometimes there are several conflicting prima facie duties or rules involved. However, Ross and others who admit that there are sometimes several conflicting prima facie duties or rules still hold that there must be some way to resolve these conflicts. Ross holds that the conflict is resolved by appealing to the moral intuitions of the right people. He has no doubt that the moral intuitions of these people will never conflict. Social contract theorists also recognize that the rules that result from the social contract might sometimes conflict, but they also generally simply assume that there will be agreement on the way to resolve this conflict. Most moral constructivists, like all moral realists, regard holding the position that any moral disagreements are unresolvable as succumbing to skepticism or relativism. The view that most moral questions might have unique correct answers, even though some moral questions do not, is not even considered as a serious proposal.

An Example of One Kind of Unresolvable Moral Disagreement

The plausibility of holding that there are unique correct solutions to every moral problem stems from a failure to consider the wide variety of moral problems. If all moral problems that are considered have the form "Should I do X?" it seems plausible to hold that the answer must be either "Yes" or "No." Of course, even with questions formulated in this way, it is sometimes the case that two equally informed, impartial, rational persons will disagree on the answer and there will be no way to resolve the disagreement. However, for some questions, unless the facts are quite different from what is generally accepted, it is not even plausible to claim that there is a unique correct answer. Consider the question about the appropriate speed limit for cars and trucks traveling on interstate highways. This is not a question with a yes or no answer; even if the alternatives are limited to five-mile or five-kilometer intervals, it requires picking the right speed limit from among several alternatives.

Setting speed limits is an important moral problem. Imposing any speed limit deprives many people of some freedom, and the lower the speed limit, the more freedom is taken away. Now suppose that we are considering the speed limit for interstate highways and that the alternatives are sixty, sixty-five, and seventy miles per hour, and that there is a correlation between a higher speed limit and some increase in the number of serious accidents. If people dispute this correlation between lower speed limits and a smaller number of accidents, holding that it is greater uniformity of speed that results in a smaller number of accidents, then the situation is different. If it were shown that limits of seventy miles per hour result in greater uniformity of speed and that this results in fewer accidents and fewer injuries and deaths than either a sixty or sixty-five miles per hour speed limit, there would be a unique right answer to the question about what the speed limit should be. The seventy miles per hour speed limit deprives people of less freedom than the lower limits and also results in the smallest amount of injury and death. If this were the case there would be a unique right answer to a controversial moral problem. Unfortunately, this does not seem to be the case.

Studies seem to show that among the alternatives listed, the lower the speed limit, the lower the number of accidents, and correspondingly the lower the number of injuries and death due to accidents. This means that there probably is not a unique right answer to the question about what the speed limit should be. Given this correlation, with a higher speed limit resulting in a greater number of accidents, there is a classic confrontation between freedom and welfare. A lower speed limit deprives of freedom, and has other economic costs associated with it, but it results in fewer accidents. Fewer accidents result in fewer injuries and deaths, as well as less property loss. However, oversimplifying in a way that is standard for philosophers, we shall consider the increased loss of freedom to be the only cost of a lower speed limit and the increased number of deaths to be the only cost of a higher speed limit. This oversimplification allows us to pose the simple question, "How many deaths avoided is worth the loss of freedom for millions of people to go five miles per hour faster?"

Suppose that the evidence shows that given our three alternative speed limits, for every five miles the speed limit is increased there is an increase of five deaths in the country per year. Is there a unique right answer to the question as to the appropriate speed limit? Suppose that for every five miles the speed limit is increased there is an increase of fifty deaths per year. Does this result in a unique right answer to the question as to the appropriate speed limit? Theoretically, some increase in the number of deaths will be large enough that it would result in all equally informed, rational persons agreeing to the lowest speed limit, that is, in a unique right answer. It is not clear that, theoretically, any increase in the number of deaths is small enough that it would result in all equally informed, rational persons agreeing on a highest speed limit, for some people claim that life is infinitely precious. It is quite clear that at some level of increase in the number of lives lost with an increase of five miles in the speed limit, equally informed, rational persons will disagree about the appropriate speed limit. This disagreement occurs despite the fact that everyone agrees that accidental deaths are to be avoided, because they also agree that deprivations of freedom are to be avoided. It is the conflict that causes the disagreement.

Of course someone might claim that there is a unique correct answer to the question of how a small loss of freedom for millions should be weighed against the loss of a few lives, but there is no reason to believe that any answer would be accepted by all equally informed, impartial, rational persons. It might be claimed that any rational person would choose a certain loss of a small amount of freedom in order to avoid even an extremely small chance of being killed. Some claim that all rational persons, not knowing any facts that would bias their decision, would always pick a strategy that minimizes their own chances of suffering the greatest harms over a strategy that provides the best overall balance of goods over evils. This is the kind of maximin strategy that John Rawls puts forward in *A Theory of Justice* in order to guide the choice of basic principles to be adopted for forming a society. Although this is a plausible strategy, it is not the only plausible strategy.[6] There is no unique answer to the question about the proper way to rank the various evils or weigh them against each other and against some goods. Equally informed, impartial, rational persons could choose several different alternatives in deciding on the speed limit.

If we are considering rational persons, there is complete agreement on the basic harms or evils, death, pain, disability, loss of freedom, and loss of pleasure. There is even complete agreement on some of the rankings of these harms that would count as irrational. It would be irrational to die in order to avoid the pain involved in having a tooth filled. Although there is no precise way to say how great the pain must be for it to be rational for a person to prefer to die rather than suffer that pain, in most real cases it is clear whether it is rational to choose to die. For people suffering from terminal maladies, it is often rational for them either to choose to die earlier to avoid the continuing pain that their illness involves or to choose to live as long as possible, even though this results in continuing pain. This personal decision may not be a moral decision, for it may not involve any other person besides the person making the decision. But if their choosing to die earlier requires other people to help, then it may become a moral matter.

It is clearly a moral matter whether to legalize physician-assisted suicide. Suppose the evidence supports the view that legalizing physician-assisted suicide does result in many people experiencing significantly less unwanted pain and suffering, but that it also results in slightly more people dying earlier than they really want to die. How many unwanted earlier deaths are too many in order to prevent how much pain and suffering for how many people? Is there a unique right answer, no matter how many unwanted earlier deaths there are and how many people avoid how much pain and suffering? However, this is a situation in which, because of an overlooked alternative, the amount of pain and suffering avoided by legalizing physician-assisted suicide is considerably less than that claimed by most proponents of legalization. Refusal of foods and fluids, as well as refusal of life-prolonging medical treatments, is already available to those for whom physician-assisted suicide would be available. Publicizing these alternatives and educating people that refusing food and fluids can result in a death that involves as little pain as legalized physician-assisted suicide means that legalizing physician-assisted suicide prevents far less pain and suffering than is claimed for it.[7]

Another example of a moral disagreement that results from a different ranking of the basic evils is disagreement about the strictness of the standards for commitment to a mental hospital, particularly with regard to patients who are regarded as being at risk for suicide. In some states there is a continual change in the commitment laws, as those who place a higher value on freedom, such as members of the American Civil Liberties Union (ACLU), battle with those who place a higher value on avoiding death, such as members of various state psychiatric associations. Many psychiatrists rank a fairly small risk of death for a few as more important than the certain loss of freedom for many and so often are prepared to cause more loss of freedom to prevent death than are most members of the ACLU. Closely linked to this disagreement about the rankings of the evils or harms is a disagreement about the consequences of everyone knowing that a given kind of violation of a moral rule (e.g., depriving a person of freedom for several days) is allowed in these circumstances. Many members of the ACLU hold that a law making it easier to commit a person is more likely to be abused than a state psychiatric association believes. A disagreement about the consequences of everyone knowing that a given kind of violation is allowed is sometimes based on a view of human nature that is not subject to empirical confirmation or disconfirmation. Then it is an ideological disagreement and often leads to unresolvable moral disagreement. Although extreme views of human nature may, in fact, be subject to disconfirmation, moderate pessimistic views and moderate optimistic ones probably are not. These different kinds of views of human nature may be the source of some unresolvable moral disagreements between political conservatives and liberals.

Although most moral theories assume that there is a unique correct answer to every moral question, democratic political theory takes it for granted that, within limits, equally informed, rational persons can disagree about what laws should be enacted. Those who, like Plato, hold that there is a unique correct answer to every moral question do not advocate democracy, but rather a philosopher king. If there is such a unique correct answer to every moral question, then because political decisions are moral decisions, it does seem as if the best strategy would be to pick that person or group of persons who is most likely to know the correct answer to be the person or group that makes the political decisions. However, if there is often no unique correct answer to some moral questions, then it is most appropriate to have each person participate, either directly or through a representative, in making that decision. The realization that there is no unique correct answer to every moral question provides strong support of a democratic political process. Admitting that there is no unique correct answer to every moral question, although often regarded as a defect in a moral theory, may actually be a significant virtue.

Other Sources of Unresolvable Moral Disagreement

The unresolvable moral disagreements that have been discussed in the previous sections stem from two sources. The first source is a different ranking of the basic evils of death, pain, disability, loss of freedom, and loss of pleasure. The second source is a difference in the estimates of the consequences of everyone knowing that they are allowed to violate a moral rule in the circumstances under consideration. This second source, which is usually not subject to empirical verification, arises from ideological differences about human nature and society. It may be closely related to the first source, as it is likely that those who have a more optimistic view of human nature value freedom higher than those who have a more pessimistic view.

A third source of unresolvable moral disagreement is a disagreement about the interpretation of a moral rule. Do some polite expressions like "So pleased to see you" count as deceiving if you are not pleased to see the person? Does wearing a wig, coloring your hair, or wearing makeup count as deceiving? Does dressing or talking in a way that one knows will upset many people count as violating the rule against causing pain or unpleasant feelings? More important, when do acts of discontinuing life-preserving treatment count as killing? The answers to these questions often turn on the conventions that have been adopted by the society. When these conventions are clear, some of these questions may have clear unique answers. However, in some cases, the situation has not arisen before so there is no settled convention, or the conventions of the society are in flux and there is no unique interpretation accepted by all equally informed, qualified, rational persons. In these cases there may be unresolvable moral disagreement.

The fourth source of moral disagreement concerns the scope of morality or about who is protected by the moral rules. This disagreement is not only about who is in the group fully protected by the moral rules, it is also about whether any of those not in this group are protected at all, and if so, how much. People disagree about whether fetuses or higher mammals are in the fully protected group, not protected at all, or protected to some degree, though not as much as moral agents are protected. They also disagree about whether the stage of development of the fetus or the level of intelligence of the higher mammal determines whether it should be fully protected, partially protected, or not protected at all. Obviously, this source of disagreement is the one that is most relevant to moral disagreement about abortion, but it is important to note that our claim that there are unresolvable moral disagreements is not an ad hoc response to the controversy concerning abortion. Not only are there other sources of unresolvable moral disagreement in addition to differences about the scope of morality, the scope of morality leads not only to disagreements about abortion but also about the treatment of animals.

However, the most common cause of moral disagreement is disagreement about the facts; it is even the most common source of unresolvable moral disagreement. Indeed, this source of unresolvable moral disagreement may be far greater than all of the other sources of unresolvable moral disagreement combined. However, because it does not give rise to any philosophical problems, it is not much discussed by philosophers. Those involved in real moral discussions, for example, those who serve on ethics committees in hospitals, know that disagreements about the facts, including disagreements about prognoses, cause almost all of the disagreement concerning what morally ought to be done. Agreement on all the facts generally results in the end of any controversy about what to do. However, often, agreement on the facts cannot be reached and so the controversy remains unresolved. We are concerned with four sources of moral disagreement that do not involve disagreement about the facts, because these are the sources that are denied or neglected by many, including philosophers. They are: (1) differences in the rankings of the harms (evils) and benefits (goods); (2) ideological differences about human nature, in particular about what would happen if everyone knew that a certain kind of violation were allowed; (3) differences about the interpretation of a moral rule, for example, what counts as killing or deceiving; and (4) differences about the scope of morality, that is, about who is fully protected, who is protected but not fully, and who is not protected at all.

Morality as an Informal Public System

Although morality always distinguishes between the set of morally acceptable answers and those that are morally unacceptable, it does not provide a unique answer to every question. One of the tasks of a moral theory is to explain why sometimes, even when there is complete agreement on the facts, genuine moral disagreement cannot be eliminated. But the theory must also explain why all moral disagreement has legitimate limits. It is very easy, as noted above, to overlook that unresolvable moral disagreement on some important issues (e.g., abortion) is compatible with total agreement in the overwhelming number of cases on which moral judgments are made. This agreement is based on agreement about the nature of morality, that it is a public system with the goal of reducing the amount of harm suffered by those protected by it. Everyone agrees that morality prohibits some kinds of actions (e.g., killing and breaking promises), and encourages certain kinds of actions (e.g., relieving pain). But it is acknowledged that it is sometimes morally justified to do a prohibited kind of action even when it does not conflict with another prohibition, for example, when it conflicts with what is morally encouraged. Breaking a trivial promise in order to aid an injured person is regarded by all as morally acceptable.

Sometimes, however, people disagree about whether a particular act counts as a prohibited kind of action like killing or deceiving.[8] People sometimes disagree on when not feeding counts as killing, or when not telling counts as deceiving. Although these disagreements in interpretation are occasionally unresolvable, if it is agreed that an action is of a certain kind (e.g., killing or deceiving), all impartial rational persons agree that it needs moral justification. Further, everyone agrees that intentionally killing or deceiving needs moral justification. Similarly, everyone agrees that actions of a certain kind (e.g., relieving pain and suffering) should be encouraged unless they involve doing a prohibited kind of action. As stated in the previous chapter, prohibitions of the former kinds of actions we call moral rules; encouragement of the latter kind we call moral ideals.

The most divisive and significant kind of moral disagreement concerns the scope of morality, that is, who should be included in the group toward which morality requires impartial treatment. This unresolvable disagreement about who is impartially protected by morality leads to the great controversies concerning abortion and the treatment of animals. Some maintain that morality is only, or primarily, concerned with the suffering of harm by moral agents, while others maintain that the death and pain of those who are not moral agents is as important, or almost as important, as the harms suffered by moral agents.[9] All agree that morality prohibits killing moral agents, but there is considerable disagreement about whether it also prohibits killing fetuses and, at least, the higher animals such as monkeys and dolphins. However, even if fetuses and animals are not included in the group impartially protected by morality, they might still have some protection. Killing them or causing them pain might require some justification, even if it does not require as strong a justification as killing or causing pain to moral agents. We discuss this issue in great detail later in this chapter when we discuss two of the most cited attempts to solve the issue of abortion.

Another source of unresolvable disagreement in moral judgment is due to differences in the rankings of harms (evils), including differences in how one ranks probabilities of harms. The disagreements about the proper speed limit is a disagreement of this kind. Indeed, many political disagreements seem to be about this kind of difference in rankings and can be regarded as a conflict between freedom and welfare (e.g., how strict the regulations concerning pollution should be). However, the difference in rankings can also be between death and pain, which is one important issue involved in the euthanasia debate. The presence of these kinds of unresolvable moral disagreements must be reflected in an adequate account of morality.

Although morality is a public system, one that all rational persons know and understand and that it is not irrational for any of them to follow, we have now shown that this does not mean that there are no unresolvable moral disagreements. Morality is an informal public system, that is, a system that has no authoritative judges or procedures that always determine the correct answer. A formal system such as law, or a formal public system such as a game of a professional sport, does have ways of arriving at a unique correct answer within that system, by granting final authority to judges, referees, or umpires. But most games, including sports, are informal public systems. When people get together to play a game of cards or backyard basketball, they are involved in an informal public system. For the game even to get started, there must be overwhelming agreement on most aspects of the game, although disagreements can arise that have no agreed upon way to be resolved. These unresolvable disagreements are either resolved in an ad hoc fashion (e.g., flipping a coin or asking a passerby), or are not resolved at all (e.g., the game is disbanded).

Morality, like all informal public systems, presupposes overwhelming agreement on most matters that are likely to arise. However, like all informal public systems, it has no established procedures or authorities that can resolve every moral disagreement. There is no equivalent in morality to the United States Supreme Court in deciding legal disputes, or the pope in deciding some religious matters for Roman Catholics. When there is no unique right answer within morality and a decision has to be made, the decision is often made in an ad hoc fashion (e.g., people may ask a friend for advice). If the moral disagreement is on some important social issue (e.g., abortion), the problem is transferred from the moral system to the political or legal system. Abortion is an unresolvable moral question. Since it has to be decided whether or not abortions are to be allowed and in what circumstances, the question is transferred to the legal and political system. They resolve the question on a practical level, but they do not resolve the moral question, as is shown by the continuing intense moral debate on the matter.

Failure to appreciate that morality is an informal public system has caused considerable confusion when talking about public policies, not only with regard to health care but also in many other areas. It is assumed that if morality does not directly provide a solution to the problem, it can always provide an indirect solution by means of an appropriate voting procedure. It is sometime mistakenly said that a just solution, by which we understand a morally acceptable solution, is one that is arrived at by a democratic voting procedure. The justness or moral acceptability of a solution to a problem cannot be determined by any voting procedure, for a majority can vote to unjustifiably deprive members of a minority group of some freedom. The moral acceptability of a solution is determined by the moral system; all that the voting procedure does is to determine which solution will be adopted. This democratic voting procedure may be the morally best way to determine which morally acceptable solution will be adopted, but it does not *make* that solution either morally acceptable or the morally best solution.

Justice

Justice has become a very important topic in medicine, partly because of the realization that the necessity for changing the allocation of health care has, and will have, a dramatic effect on the practice of medicine. Everyone agrees that the present allocation of health care in the United States is not just, but there is considerable disagreement on what is necessary to make it just. In this section we shall only talk about justice with regard to the actions of government. A government that acts in a morally acceptable way acts justly. But what is required for a government to act in a morally acceptable way? A full answer to this question would require a whole book in political theory; we shall not try to provide even an outline of an answer. We think, however, that showing the relationship between our account of morality and some issues of justice in health care may help in achieving a better understanding of these issues. The recognition that morality is an informal public system suggests the most important point; it is extremely unlikely that there is a unique right answer to how the government should act with regard to the allocation of health care. There is so much disagreement on the factual matters that it may almost be secondary to point out that there is also disagreement in the ranking of the harms and benefits involved, and also significant ideological disagreements about human nature.

Since we have no special expertise with regard to the economic and political facts, and do not wish to enter into any ideological disputes about human nature, we shall limit our discussion to what we take to be fairly uncontroversial points. One of the primary responsibilities if not *the* primary responsibility of government is to lessen the amount of harm suffered by its citizens. Diseases, injuries, and so forth, all of which we classify as maladies (see chapter 6), are some of the primary sources of harm. Thus, it is one of the duties of government to lessen the harm caused by maladies. If the costs of doing so are similar, it would be far better to prevent maladies than to treat them once they have occurred, for prevention will result in far less harm being suffered. Thus, if the costs are similar, it is far better to engage in preventive medicine, primarily public health measures, than to spend the same amount of money to cure or treat maladies after they occur.[10] If it costs less to prevent a specified number of maladies than to cure a smaller number of those same maladies, it becomes clearly irrational for any impartial person not to prefer prevention. Thus, spending a given amount of money to cure a specified number of maladies when that same amount could be used to prevent a far great number of equally serious maladies is clearly unjust.

The previous paragraph assumes that the government is spending some money to prevent the harms caused by maladies. We think it is appropriate for it to do so, but there may be some controversy on this matter. Any money the government spends must be collected from its citizens. Some may want to claim that taking money from its citizens deprives them of freedom and that this loss of freedom is so significant that preventing the harms caused by maladies does not justify causing this massive loss of freedom. We do not think many would agree with this ranking. Indeed, when considering some public health measures (e.g., vaccinations for children or ensuring a safe water supply), we know of no one who accepts this ranking. However, we accept that after a certain amount of money is spent on health care, including public health, it is appropriate to question whether more ought to be spent. And there are also questions, without uniquely correct moral answers, about how much ought to be spent on health care compared with education, public defense, the criminal justice system, and so on.

Assuming a fixed amount of government spending on health care, what would count as a morally acceptable way of spending that money, that is, what would count as a just health care delivery system? A formal but not very useful answer to that question is whatever system a fully informed, impartial rational person could advocate adopting. What kind of system could such a person advocate adopting? The answer to this is somewhat more informative: any system that such a person could regard as resulting in a lesser amount of harm being suffered due to maladies than any alternative. If no fully informed person could regard a particular health care delivery system as resulting in a lesser amount of harm being suffered than an alternative, then such a system cannot be regarded as just. The present health care delivery system is not regarded by anyone as resulting in a lesser amount of harm being suffered, which explains why no one regards the present health care delivery system as just.

Note that this account of a just health care delivery system says nothing about equality or about providing the most aid to those who are worst off. This is not because equality and aiding the worst off are irrelevant. Rather, it is because, insofar as they are relevant, they are included within the more encompassing goal of lessening the amount of harm suffered. Unlike the utilitarian account of justice, which has a goal of increasing the amount of net benefits, and so would allow massive inequality, the moral goal of lessening the amount of harm suffered sets strict limits on inequality. It also necessarily results in great concern for those who are worst off, for they are suffering greater harm than others, and so relieving their suffering will almost always be included in the overarching goal of lessening harm. The goal of justice does not, however, require that the government spend a given amount of money in order to aid one thousand who are worst off if that same amount of money will prevent more harm for one hundred thousand who are not suffering as much. It is not required that the government spend a given amount of money on treating one thousand children with a serious genetic malady rather than spending that same amount on preventing one hundred thousand children from suffering some lesser malady. It is also not required that they not spend the money on the one thousand who are worst off, for impartial rational persons can disagree on which alternative most lessens the amount of harm suffered. But, keeping the cost the same, if the number of the worst off becomes smaller and the number who can be prevented from suffering some significant but lesser disease becomes greater, it is quite likely that a point will be reached where it will be unjust to spend that amount of money on the worst off.

A government that acts in a morally acceptable way acts justly, and there is usually more than one morally acceptable way for a government to act. Thus, it is very likely that there will not be a unique right answer to the question of how health care should be allocated. Even if there is agreement that the goal of a health care allocation is to minimize the amount of harm suffered due to maladies, there will be unresolvable disagreement about what counts as the lesser amount of harm suffered. Some may claim that what is most important is minimizing the suffering of the worst off, those suffering great harm, whereas others may maintain that it is irrelevant whose suffering is minimized as long as the total amount of harm suffered is minimized. Since there is no agreed upon way to weigh and balance different evils, there is no way to resolve any plausible disagreement. Further, even if there were agreement on a more specific goal, there would still be disagreement about the best way to achieve that goal. For example, can the government do it? And if so, how best can it regulate and constrain medical practice to achieve that goal? But, even with all of this disagreement, there is universal agreement that the present allocation of health care is not just.[11]

Moral Disagreement Concerning Abortion

Abortion is not only a controversial issue, it is such an important topic that in discussing it, philosophers and others bring to bear all of the arguments, intuitions, and theories that they think will persuade others to adopt the position that they favor. Abortion is almost never discussed as an example that shows the inadequacy of some standard views about morality or about the proper role of moral theories. However, that is what we now intend to do. Rather than arguing for any one of the standard positions we hope to show that all of the standard positions concerning abortion are morally acceptable. Our primary purpose is theoretical. We intend to show that no arguments provide conclusive support either for the view that abortion is prima facie morally wrong or for the view that it is morally wrong to legally prohibit abortion.

We are using abortion as an example of an unresolvable moral issue. Holding that you have the unique correct solution to this problem and that all other answers are mistaken is an example of moral arrogance. If you believe that any fully informed impartial rational person would agree with you, you must hold that anyone who disagrees is not fully informed, not impartial, or not rational. This does not lead to civil and fruitful discussion. Accepting that a fully informed impartial rational person can disagree with you concerning the moral status of abortion does not mean that you should cease to try to persuade others to adopt your own views, or that you should cease to try to have the government and the courts support your position, but it limits the morally acceptable ways of doing this.

Common morality does not provide a unique answer to questions about abortion. Neither the claim that women almost never ought not to have an abortion nor the claim that women ought to be allowed to have abortions at any time are in conflict with common morality. Of course, many people on both sides of the abortion issue claim that common morality supports their position, but most of them recognize that some people who are full moral agents—that is, they know what kinds of actions morality prohibits, requires, discourages, encourages, and allows—hold an opposing view. Unlike the attitudes that people take with regard to most moral judgments (e.g., that it is morally wrong to lie, cheat, or steal), those who make moral judgments concerning abortion realize that they need to provide arguments to support their judgments. Many also believe that they need to show that those who make opposing judgments are mistaken.

Those who hold that judgments about abortion are personal, meaning by this that it is inappropriate to make moral judgments about abortion, are also mistaken. Abortion is not like homosexual behavior in that respect. People who think that homosexual behavior is a moral matter are mistaken; it is solely a personal or religious matter. There is no plausible interpretation of any justified moral rule such that homosexual behavior violates that rule. However, it is not a mistake to regard abortion as a moral matter, even though it is also a personal and religious matter. The moral rule prohibiting killing can be interpreted either as prohibiting abortion or as not applying to it. Those who hold that there is no correct answer about abortion need not be ethical relativists. Although accepting common morality entails accepting that it provides answers to most moral questions, it also requires accepting that it usually does not provide unique correct answers to controversial moral questions. People who understand common morality realize that the abortion issue is one of these controversial moral questions for which there is no unique answer.

It is appropriate to present arguments both for and against the moral acceptability of abortion. It is even appropriate to try to use a moral theory to persuade opponents to change their moral judgments about abortion. However, abortion is an issue that shows the futility of offering philosophical arguments, or any kind of moral theory, in order to resolve a genuinely controversial moral issue. The facts about abortion have been known for quite some time, and none of the arguments, either pro or con, have persuaded most of those on the other side to change their position. Neither side can support its claim that common morality conflicts with the position of the other side. No moral theory that correctly describes common morality can provide conclusive support to either side of the abortion debate. Only moral theories that attempt to revise or supplant common morality claim to decisively support one or the other side of the debate. However, most people's judgments about abortion are more firmly held than their views about the correctness of any revisionist moral theory. If such a moral theory results in a judgment about abortion that conflicts with their own judgment concerning abortion, they will reject that moral theory. If there were a correct moral theory that actually did resolve the moral issues concerning

abortion, then the preceding comments would be of little philosophical significance. They would simply be another set of comments deploring the intellectual
integrity of most people. However, any moral theory that resolves the abortion
question would thereby show itself to be incorrect.

The source of unresolvable moral disagreement that is involved in the moral
controversy concerning abortion is primarily a disagreement about who is in the
group that is fully protected, or protected at all, by morality or the moral rules.[12]
All rational persons agree that all those who are morally responsible for their
actions are fully protected by morality, but disagreement arises about whether
morality fully protects any beings other than those who are moral agents. Given
that moral agents know that they may cease to be moral agents and still remain
conscious persons, there is universal agreement that former moral agents who
are still conscious are fully protected. Moral agents and former moral agents
who are still conscious constitute the group that everyone agrees is fully protected. In most societies, and in all technologically advanced societies, infants
and children who have the potential to become full moral agents are also regarded as being fully protected. Any enlargement of the group beyond this is
subject to significant disagreement. People disagree about whether fetuses are
fully protected and they also disagree about whether some animals, especially
those mammals like chimpanzees and dolphins that seem to have a mental life
that is close to that of human beings, are fully protected.

People disagree not only about whether fetuses are fully protected but also
whether they are protected at all. Disagreements about the degree of protection
that fetuses have range from none at all to fully protected, and almost every
point in between. Some hold that fetuses are protected but not fully protected,
that is, they have no doubt that if it is a choice between the life of the pregnant
woman and the fetus, the woman wins, but they also hold that fetuses are sufficiently protected so that it is immoral to have an abortion unless not having one
would impose a serious hardship on or endanger the pregnant woman. On this
view, it is immoral to have an abortion if it is only an inconvenience for the
woman to remain pregnant. Others hold that the fetus is protected as much as
any moral agent, including the pregnant woman, so that unless not having an
abortion is certain to result in the death of the woman, having an abortion is
clearly immoral. At the opposite extreme, some hold that the fetus is not protected at all, so that it is not immoral for a woman to have an abortion simply
because she doesn't want to be pregnant at this time because it would spoil a
vacation trip.

To make matters even more complex, different people hold that it is morally
significant how developed the fetus is. Some hold that at the very early stage,
when the term "embryo" is more appropriate than "fetus," the newly fertilized
egg is not protected at all. However, the same people might hold that when the
fetus is close to full term, it is fully protected. Different people hold that full

protection comes at different times of development, some holding that it comes with viability, others when the brain has developed sufficiently to allow for consciousness. There is also disagreement about the time before which the fetus has no protection at all. When all of this disagreement about the importance of the time of development is added to the disagreement about whether the fetus at any stage of development is fully protected or not protected at all, it is clear that the claim that there is a unique correct answer is extremely doubtful.

The Views of Don Marquis and Mary Anne Warren

It is impossible to examine all of the arguments in favor of the various views concerning abortion, so we shall concentrate on two articles, one claiming to show that abortion is always prima facie immoral, and the other claiming to show that abortion is never immoral and should therefore always be legally allowed. We have picked these two articles for several reasons. Both of them are widely anthologized and many regard them as providing the strongest arguments for the positions they support. Both of them assume a philosophical view about moral theories that is widely used and assumed. It would be philosophically significant to show that this widely accepted philosophical view is mistaken. This significance would extend far beyond these two articles, indeed beyond the subject of abortion; in fact, beyond bioethics more generally conceived. The two articles are "Why Abortion Is Immoral" by Don Marquis and "On the Moral and Legal Status of Abortion" by Mary Anne Warren.[13] We shall refer to other articles only insofar as they provide further evidence of the kinds of mistakes with which we are concerned.

Don Marquis ends his article with this paragraph.

Finally, this analysis can be viewed as resolving a standard problem—indeed, *the* standard problem—concerning the ethics of abortion. Clearly, it is wrong to kill adult human beings. Clearly, it is not wrong to end the life of some arbitrarily chosen single human cell. Fetuses seem to be like arbitrarily chosen single human cells in some respects and like adult human beings in other respects. The problem of the ethics of abortion is the problem of determining the fetal property that settles this moral controversy. The thesis of this essay is that the problem of abortion, so understood, is solvable. (39)

The following are the final sentences of Mary Anne Warren's 1982 postscript to her article.

It is a philosopher's task to criticize mistaken beliefs which stand in the way of moral understanding, even when—perhaps especially when—those beliefs are popular and widespread. The belief that moral strictures against killing should apply equally to all genetically human entities, and *only* to genetically human entities, is such an error. The overcoming of this error will undoubtedly require long and often painful struggle; but it must be done. (73–74)

Both Marquis and Warren hold that there is a unique correct answer to the question of the moral status of abortion. Marquis says, "This essay sets out an argument that purports to show, as well as any argument in ethics can show, that abortion is, except possibly in rare cases, seriously immoral, that it is in the same category as killing an innocent adult human being." Marquis admits that his argument is based on a major assumption. He states, "Many of the most insightful and careful writers on the ethics of abortion—such as Joel Feinberg, Michael Tooley, Mary Anne Warren, H. Tristam Englehardt Jr., L. W. Sumner, John T. Noonan Jr., and Philip Devine—believe that whether or not abortion is morally permissible stands or falls on whether or not a fetus is the sort of being whose life it is seriously wrong to end. The argument of this essay will assume but not argue, that they are correct" (24) .

Mary Anne Warren confirms that she belongs in the group that Marquis characterizes by the following remark. "It is possible to show that, on the basis of intuitions which we may expect even the opponents of abortion to share, a fetus is not a person, and hence not the sort of entity to which it is proper to ascribe full human rights" (59). It is clear that Marquis and Warren, as well as most other writers on the problem of abortion, share the common assumption that facts about the fetus, "whether or not a fetus is the sort of being whose life it is seriously wrong to end" or whether or not a fetus is "the sort of entity to which it is proper to ascribe full human rights" determine the moral status of abortion.[14] This is an example of the larger assumption that, even for this controversial moral issue, there is a unique correct solution.

Don Marquis claims that this disagreement is the result of people not realizing what characteristic is responsible for the fact that it is morally wrong to kill moral agents, or as he says, people like us. According to Marquis, what makes killing us wrong is that it deprives us of our futures. He contends, correctly, that killing normal fetuses, including embryos once twinning is no longer possible, also deprives them of a future like ours. Although Marquis admits that it is also wrong to kill people who do not have a future like ours, if they do not want to be killed, he claims that having a future like ours is sufficient to make killing someone at least prima facie morally wrong. Marquis claims to have discovered that the characteristic that makes killing moral agents wrong is that it deprives them of a certain kind of future, and correctly points out that killing fetuses or even embryos has the same characteristic. Thus, for Marquis, it is irrelevant what other characteristics fetuses have; whether they are persons, or potential persons, or even whether they are conscious, if they are normal fetuses, abortion deprives them of a future like ours.

Mary Ann Warren claims that the disagreement about the morality of abortion is due to confusion between persons in the morally relevant sense, and persons in the biological sense. She claims that morality protects only persons in the morally relevant sense, not persons in the biological sense. Those having all of the characteristics of persons that Warren lists as morally relevant turn out to be moral agents, those beings who are held responsible for their action. Everyone agrees that it is wrong to kill moral agents, those who are themselves required to obey the moral rules. But Warren is prepared to admit some beings that do not have all these characteristics may still count as persons or belong to the moral community.

Warren presents a list of five characteristics: (1) consciousness, (2) reasoning, (3) self-motivated activity, (4) the capacity to communicate (linguistically), and (5) self-concepts and self-awareness. Someone having all five, as all moral agents do, is clearly a person and within the moral community. She is willing to admit that "(1) and (2) alone may be sufficient for personhood," but she insists that a being who has none of these characteristics cannot be part of the moral community. She claims correctly that early fetuses have none of these characteristics, and that even late fetuses have only one, which she does not consider sufficient.[15]

Although both Marquis and Warren agree that it is morally wrong to kill moral agents, they disagree on why it is morally wrong to do so. Marquis says that it is morally wrong because killing deprives these persons of a future like ours. Warren says that it is morally wrong because moral agents are persons and belong to the moral community. In a certain sense, both of them are correct. But the way in which they put their claims suggests that it follows directly from the facts they cite, that it is morally wrong to kill moral agents. The conclusion that it is morally wrong to kill moral agents is correct, however this conclusion does not simply follow from the facts cited by either author. Morality is not some straightforward empirical feature of the world such that, given some facts, a moral conclusion always follows with no intervening steps. When these intervening steps are put in, it becomes clear that the conclusions about abortion that both of them draw do not follow directly from the facts that they cite.

These intervening steps involve recognition that morality is a public system governing the behavior of all moral agents, that is endorsed by all moral agents who use only those beliefs that are shared by all moral agents, and who seek agreement with these other moral agents. Moral agents recognize that they are vulnerable and fallible, and so put forward a system of rules, ideals, and procedures for deciding when a moral rule is justifiably broken, that requires people not to harm others and encourages them to help others in need. This public system has other features in addition to the rules and ideals and the two-step procedure, but for present purposes, we shall be concerned only with the rules. Why do the rules have the content they do? How are the rules to be interpreted? Most relevant to the topic at hand, who are the rules supposed to protect?

As long as their futures do not involve prolonged pain and suffering, no moral agent wants to be deprived of her future. Marquis correctly assumes that people regard being deprived of their future as one of the worst things that can happen to them. According to Marquis this important fact explains why being deprived of their futures is sufficient to make killing people like us, prima facie wrong and also explains why the rule against killing is a very important, if not the most important, moral rule. Warren correctly assumes that moral agents want to protect *themselves*, so it is not surprising that the moral rules protect moral agents from being killed. Marquis is correct in explaining why moral agents regard killing as morally wrong, and Warren is correct in explaining why moral agents agree that morality protects moral agents from being killed.

However, Marquis neglects to consider whom the moral agents want to protect from being deprived of a future like ours. He simply takes it to be a fact that being deprived of a future like ours is a feature that, on its own, makes killing wrong, just as being deprived of oxygen for a given amount of time is a feature that, on its own, makes a person dead. But this is a misleading way of looking at the matter. Being deprived of a future like ours makes killing wrong because of the nature of moral agents. Common morality contains a moral rule against killing because all moral agents want to be protected from being deprived of their futures. But they need not be against all killing, or depriving of futures like ours; all that they must agree on is that no moral agents be killed or deprived of their futures. Common morality does not provide a unique answer to the question, "Who should be protected from being deprived of a future like ours?" Marquis treats "depriving of a future like ours" as a fact that makes killing wrong independent of the agreement of moral agents. But moral agents need not agree that the public system that is common morality contain a rule against killing that protects all beings that have a future like ours from being deprived of it. Once it is clear that moral agents need only agree that moral agents be protected, it is clear that the moral controversy about abortion has not been settled, but only seemed to be settled.

Warren recognizes that the moral rules fully protect all moral agents but, with no argument, also claims that they fully protect those beings who have the characteristics such as consciousness and reasoning that make them very like moral agents. She also claims, in her postscript, that morality protects to some degree, but not with the same protection as it provides to moral agents, those beings that are like, but not very like, moral agents. Warren does not explicitly support her view by noting that moral agents put forward the rule against killing in order to protect moral agents, and those very like moral agents, from being killed. Nor does she explain why some moral agents take the moral rules to protect, even if not fully, beings that resemble moral agents in what moral agents would take to be their important features. It may seem too obvious to her to point out explicitly that moral agents are more likely to be concerned with beings with characteristics that resemble their own. However, Warren's claims have force only because all moral agents want to protect moral agents from being killed and many moral agents also want to protect, although not necessarily fully, beings that resemble moral agents in their important features. She does not seem to recognize that some moral agents may be concerned with, and hence want to protect, beings that presently have none of the important characteristics of a person, if those beings would have all of these features at some future time. Some moral agents may even want to fully protect these beings.

Once one realizes that some moral agents may want future moral agents to be protected as much as present moral agents are protected, it is clear that Warren has provided no argument for her claim that nonpersons are not fully protected, or not protected at all, by the moral rules. Like Marquis, Warren simply makes some claim about the group of beings protected by morality, as if all moral agents agree on this matter. But it is quite obvious that they do not all agree. Although some moral agents want morality to protect only moral agents, other moral agents want morality to protect beings that presently have none of the characteristics of a person, but will have them, if they are not killed.[16] Hence, Warren, like Marquis, has provided no argument to which all moral agents must agree. Moral agents differ from one another about the scope of morality. They differ not only about who is fully protected by morality but also about who is protected at all. The only point on which all moral agents agree is that the minimal group that is fully protected by the moral rules includes all moral agents and former moral agents who are still conscious. That this is the only point of agreement makes it clear that there is no unique right answer to the question about the morality of abortion.

Warren also seems to be making another mistaken claim, namely, that if people legitimately disagree about whether an act is immoral, that act ought not to be legally prohibited. Put in that extreme form, it should be clear that the claim is mistaken, for it would entail that there could be no laws about morally controversial subjects. Some people hold that dolphins and the higher primates are fully protected by the moral rules, but most people do not. Very few hold that other nonhuman animals are fully protected by the moral rules, but many hold that they are protected to some degree. However, many also hold that morality does not protect animals at all. This disagreement about the scope of morality does not entail that there should be no laws prohibiting cruelty to animals. Disagreement about whether embryos and fetuses are fully protected, or protected at all by morality, does not entail that there should be no laws prohibiting abortion, either entirely, or at some stage of pregnancy.

It is true that every increase in the size of the group fully protected by morality, or protected at all, decreases the freedom of moral agents. No enlargement of the scope of morality is cost free. Although the freedom to catch dolphins is more important to those who fish, everyone's freedom is equally decreased by including dolphins in the group protected by morality. However, including fetuses in the group that is fully protected restricts the freedom of only one group of moral agents: pregnant women. Everyone other than the pregnant woman is already prohibited from harming a fetus that the pregnant woman does not want harmed. Harming a fetus of a pregnant woman who does not want her fetus harmed counts as harming the woman, and because she is a moral agent, that is already prohibited. Given that enlargements of the group that is impartially protected are due to moral agents being concerned about this kind of being, it is somewhat odd to enlarge the group by protecting the fetus from that person who is most intimately related to the fetus. One might think that if a pregnant woman does not want her fetus protected, people who are not related to that fetus at all should not restrict her freedom. She is clearly a moral agent and the fetus clearly is not.

However, just as some moral agents want animals to be at least partially protected by the moral rules, some moral agents want beings that will become moral agents, or to use Marquis's phrase, will have futures like ours, to be in the fully protected group. This is not an irrational position. It is not irrational to favor a variation of the moral system that values the life of a being who would become a moral agent as much as the freedom of someone who is already a moral agent. It is also not irrational to favor a variation of the moral system that values even the trivial freedom of a moral agent more than the life of a being that is not a moral agent. Common morality allows for the fully protected group to include fetuses, or for it to be limited to moral agents, former moral agents, and children who can interact with moral agents. Within limits, common morality allows the scope of morality to be determined by the concerns of moral agents as long as these concerns are possible using only beliefs shared by all moral agents. Beliefs not shared by all moral agents cannot be used as reasons for determining the scope of morality. Therefore, neither religious beliefs nor scientific beliefs can count as moral reasons for the fetus to be included in or excluded from the fully protected group.

Everyone agrees that all moral agents are in the fully protected group. Not everyone agrees about whether fetuses, no matter at what stage of development, should be included in this group. Marquis claims that all beings with a future like ours belong in the fully protected group. Mary Anne Warren holds not only that no fetuses belong in the fully protected group, she claims that early fetuses are not protected by morality at all. But equally informed, impartial, rational persons do not agree about whether fetuses belong in the fully protected group, or in a group that is protected at all. There is no unknown fact that, were it discovered, would resolve this disagreement. No biological discovery about an embryo or fetus will make them into moral agents. Also, no biological discovery will make it irrational for a moral agent to want to include fetuses in the fully protected group. Thus, we have a classic unresolvable moral problem. There is not even any conclusive moral argument for legally allowing each pregnant woman to make a decision with regard to her own fetus.

It may thus seem that moral theory is useless in dealing with the problem of abortion. However, that is not true. It is with regard to unresolvable moral problems that a moral theory that provides an accurate account of common morality is most useful. Showing that a problem is unresolvable should promote moral humility or tolerance in people on both sides of the issue. It should make clear that the position a person takes on this issue does not make her uninformed, irrational, or not impartial with regard to the group to which morality requires impartiality. There is no conclusive argument that the group with regard to which morality requires impartiality should be any larger than present and former moral agents or that it should not be larger. The problem of abortion also shows the need for a political or legal solution to unresolvable moral problems. It allows each side to use all morally acceptable means to persuade the courts or the legislature to adopt its position. But, and this may be the most significant point, it prohibits either side from using morally unacceptable means to achieve its goal.

With regard to abortion, it is important to realize that no one is in favor of abortions in the sense that they hold that there should be as many abortions as possible. That is, no one thinks that women should get pregnant in order to have abortions. Indeed, everyone thinks that the fewer the number of abortions, the better, if that can be done without placing any restrictions on the freedom of pregnant women. The obvious method for reducing the number of abortions without placing any restrictions on the freedom of pregnant women is to reduce the number of unwanted pregnancies. Thus, it would seem that, on moral grounds, everyone would agree to a program that reduces the number of unwanted pregnancies if that program did not itself violate any moral rules or cause serious harm.

Neither sex education nor providing birth control devices violates any moral rule. Therefore, if either of these, or some combination of them, is shown to significantly reduce the number of unwanted pregnancies, then unless it can be shown that doing these things causes serious harm, all impartial rational persons would agree that they should be done. Contraception is not a moral issue. The only arguments against contraception are religious, not moral. Thus, recognition that abortion is an unresolvable moral issue should lead those on both sides of the issue to favor any morally acceptable means for reducing the number of unwanted pregnancies, including both sex education and providing birth control devices, if they are shown to be effective and without serious harmful consequences.

We realize that our account of the abortion controversy will not satisfy those on either side of the issue. We disagree with those who claim that neither embryos nor fetuses at any stage of development are part of the moral community and that, therefore, abortion is a personal rather than a moral issue and that this means there should be no legal restrictions on abortion. We recognize that abortion is a moral issue and therefore one about which it would be appropriate to have a law. We do not, however, claim that there should be any laws restricting abortion, only that whether there should be any such laws is a matter that is properly decided by the political system. We also disagree with those who claim that embryos and fetuses at any stage of development are full members of the moral community and, therefore, must be accorded the full protection of the moral rules. We do not, however, claim that they should not be accorded the full protection, only that whether they should be so protected is a matter to be decided by the political system. We have shown that moral agents do not agree about whether embryos and fetuses at any stage of development are members of the moral community, or whether they should be fully or partly protected by the moral system.

Our plea for moral humility or tolerance does not place any restriction on the morally acceptable means that either side can use to have its position adopted by its society. But we expect that no one on either side of the abortion debate will accept our argument. We do not take this to show any weakness in our argument, but rather the truth of Hobbes's view that if our interests were as affected by geometry as they are by morality, there would be no more agreement in geometry than there is in morality.

Notes

1. This way of putting the matter presupposes a certain kind of utilitarian or consequentialist view that there is no important distinction between actions related to a moral rule and those related to a moral ideal. Those holding this view deny that there are any actions that are not morally wrong not to do, but are morally good to do. They also deny that some acts are morally bad, but not morally wrong. Our argument against moral realism is also an argument against more sophisticated accounts of morality, but it is simpler to concentrate on the most common kind of moral realism, which is this kind of consequentialist view.

2. Singer (1993).

3. It might be thought that the group toward which people should act impartially is that group that would be picked by fully informed impartial rational persons. But this assumes that we can talk about an impartial person without specifying the group with regard to which he is supposed to be impartial. This assumption is false.

4. Rawls (1971) took it to be one of the great strengths of consequentialism that it supplied a unique correct answer to every moral question and this is one reason why he requires that the attitudes of suitably qualified and situated rational persons have to be identical in the "original position."

5. Rawls recognizes that sometimes different moral requirements seem to conflict, and although he does not offer any way of resolving the conflict, he simply assumes that there must be a resolution. See Rawls, ibid., 341.

6. This strategy also results in adopting policies that provide the greatest benefits for the worst off, even if far more people would be benefited by helping those who are not so badly off. This is not a position that is held by many in the field of health care. Sweden has a policy of not resuscitating neonates weighing less than 750 grams, even though 1% of these infants might develop into normal children, because the overall cost of such a

policy is so great that far greater overall harm could be prevented by spending that money on other aspects of health care.

7. Many discussions of legalizing physician-assisted suicide ignore the alternative of patient refusal of life-prolonging treatment, including refusal of food and fluids. The Philosopher's Brief to the Supreme Court was an embarrassment because it neglected to mention this option. For further discussion of this topic see Bernat, et al. (1993).

8. There are clear paradigms or prototypes of killing (e.g., stabbing or shooting a person), but other cases are not so clear. This topic is very important in the discussion of euthanasia and is discussed in more detail in chapter 12.

9. Kant seems to hold that morality is only concerned with protecting moral agents, whereas Bentham clearly holds that morality protects all those who can suffer.

10. However, because preventive measures often involve many people who do not need them, the costs of prevention per person benefited may sometimes be significantly greater than the costs of treatment.

11. In the world's richest nation, no one can provide a sound argument with the conclusion that it is morally acceptable to have millions of children with little or no access to even minimally acceptable pediatric care.

12. There is also a problem about what is meant by "abortion." Some take abortion to mean "aborting the pregnancy," that is, removing the embryo or fetus from the woman without any concern about the effect on the embryo or fetus. Heather Gert in her article "Viability" and Judith Jarvis Thomson in her article "A Defense of Abortion" (both in Feinberg and Dwyer [1997]) both consider abortion in this sense. Thus, neither of them regards abortion as intentional killing. However, even on this interpretation, abortion almost always involves intentionally doing something that is known will result in the death of the embryo or fetus. If the embryo or fetus is considered to have any protection from the moral rules, then understanding abortion either as terminating pregnancy knowing that the fetus will die, or as intentionally killing the fetus, will both count as violating the rule against killing.

13. Both are contained in Feinberg and Dwyer (1997) 24–39 and 59–74. All page references are to this book.

14. Thomson (1997) argues that the status of the fetus does not completely determine the moral status of abortion, but she does not dispute that there is a unique correct answer to the question.

15. She has a problem with this view, for it seems to result in the conclusion that there is nothing wrong with infanticide. However, she claims "neonates are so very close to being persons that to kill them requires a very strong moral justification—as does the killing of dolphins, whales, chimpanzees, and other highly personlike creatures" ("Postscript on Infanticide, February 26, 1982," 71). This remarkable concession creates problems for the kind of moral realism that she seems to be espousing in her original article.

16. Former moral agents who are still conscious have the full protection of the moral rules even though they may not have more than one of the characteristics that Warren lists as essential for being a person. This difference between former moral agents and potential moral agents can be explained only by regarding common morality as if it were based on the agreement of moral agents concerned about protecting themselves if they lose the characteristics of a moral agent, but still remain conscious.

4

Particular Moral Rules and Special Duties

In the preceding chapters we described the basic structure of morality and showed that common morality cannot resolve all moral disagreements. In this chapter we show how this basic moral framework is related to everyday moral practices and to professional ethics. Morality at its core is a universal system of conduct that is manifested variously in different societies and segments within societies. There are moral codes in business, in various health professions, in sports, in law, in government, in the many different occupations, and so on. Properly understood, these are all expressions of the common morality incumbent on all rational persons, outcroppings of the same underlying rock formation. How this is so and what gives particular moral rules and special duties their different forms is the focus of this chapter. In everyday life it is these outcroppings that are mostly confronted, so it is important to demonstrate how these manifestations are grounded in a common morality. Otherwise these multitudinous pockets of "moral practices" are seen as just so many diverse, unrelated, free-floating enterprises with rules, customs, and practices peculiar to themselves. Revealing their close ties with the basic structure of common morality constitutes a major argument against such a disconnected view of moral conduct.

Moral Theory and the Moral System

In chapter 2 we provided a systematic account of morality, beginning with the moral decisions and judgments that thoughtful people make, and then describing the moral system that underlies those decisions and judgments. In chapter 3 we showed that some controversial moral issues cannot be resolved. That common morality allows for some unresolvable moral questions is often denied not only by philosophers but also by members of the general public who claim that the answer that they favor is the only possible morally correct answer. This is one reason why morality in practice is not always clear or consistent. So at times we have had to clarify, distinguish, and sharpen in order to nurture consistency. What we have done is to describe a moral system that is free of the distortions caused by strongly felt emotions on controversial issues and also free of the aberrations and ambiguities that are inevitably introduced by local beliefs and practices (e.g., dietary prescriptions), that have been inappropriately included in the universal moral system. We then provided a rational justification of that clarified moral system. Our justification of common morality as a public system that applies to all rational persons is based on our analysis of the concepts of impartiality, rationality, morality, and on some universal features of human nature. This aspect of our theory is what is most often referred to as our moral theory, but we regard our explicit description of common morality as an essential feature of our theory. In short, we first describe the moral system as it functions in ordinary life, and then we show that it is a valid, rationally justified, moral system that has universal application.

It is important to emphasize that we start with morality as it is and has been practiced. We are not inventing a new morality nor are we deriving morality from some abstract theory or principles. We analyze ordinary morality in order to uncover the conceptual structure that underlies it. We neither modify the old structure nor create a new one; rather, we clarify and make explicit the common moral system in order to show that most of our considered moral decisions and judgments are consistent. Our moral theory includes our explicit account of the common moral system and the rational justification of that system. That justification shows why, under the conditions we specify, rational persons who know they are fallible (have limited knowledge) and vulnerable advocate that common morality be adopted as a public system that applies to all rational persons.[1]

Particular Moral Rules and Duties

In chapter 2 we showed that the *general* moral rules were integrally connected with human nature and with rationality. Rationality requires all persons to avoid certain harms unless they have an adequate reason not to. These harms are those that the first five moral rules prohibit people from causing to others ("Do not kill," "Do not cause pain," Do not disable," etc.). The second five rules prohibit people from doing those things that usually result in someone suffering those harms ("Do not deceive," "Do not break promises," "Do not cheat," etc.). In short, all rational persons want to avoid suffering harm and part of the moral system, the moral rules, directs everyone to behave in ways that avoid causing harm to others.

Another part, the moral ideals, encourages everyone to prevent or relieve the harms that others might suffer or are suffering. It is therefore no surprise that all rational persons espouse morality as a public system to be followed by everyone. Furthermore, the very close relation of morality to some universal features of human nature, especially fallibility, limited knowledge, rationality, and the vulnerability to being harmed by others, means that these general moral rules would be endorsed by all rational people in all times and in all places.

Yet it is clear that the particular moral rules and duties with which people work in myriad settings, scattered widely in time and place, are far more diverse and context-sensitive than these general moral ideals and the ten general moral rules. What follows is our explanation of how these more specific, particular moral rules and special duties are related to the general moral rules and ideals that we have described. Examples of these myriad particular moral rules and duties are "Do not drink and drive," "Do not commit adultery," "Keep confidences," "Obtain informed consent." Our account provides an analysis of these widespread particular rules and special duties, showing how they are related to the common moral framework. Making these particular moral rules and special duties explicit allows us to acknowledge the socially relative nature of some moral rules and duties without thereby denying our view about the universal nature of the common moral framework. However, except for their dependence on knowledge that may not extend beyond a particular society or profession and whatever follows from those circumstances, there is no important theoretical difference between particular moral rules and the basic general moral rules.

As the term "duty" is normally used it always refers to a positive requirement (e.g., to obtain valid consent before treating), whereas a particular moral rule, like a general moral rule, is normally a prohibition (e.g., do not reveal confidential information about a patient). It is usually easy to see the intimate relationship of particular moral rules to the common moral system. Seeing the relationship leads to a clearer understanding about what is important for working through a moral problem that involves the violation of one of these particular moral rules. It is also often easy to see the relationship between the special duties of a profession and the common moral system. When that relationship is appreciated, we have a reliable standard against which to measure the particular rules and special duties claiming moral status. We are also able to see where, how, and to what extent cultural variables enter into moral deliberations. We may also come to understand when it is necessary to formulate new particular moral rules and duties, which is an ongoing need in society.

Looking closely at particular moral rules and special duties in a wide variety of contexts, such as in various professions, occupations, practices, and organizations, shows that many particular rules and duties are directly related to the general moral rules adapted to a special context. It is as if the beliefs, practices, customs, expectations, and traditions within various communities and subcommunities have combined with the general moral rules to produce rules and duties more specifically designed for the community, culture, or profession in question. Only the general moral rules are universal because only they involve no beliefs that are not universally held and no practices that are not universal. The rules and duties generated by blending the general moral rules with characteristics of a particular culture are not universal because they involve beliefs held by those in that culture and practices that may be limited to that particular culture or profession. Thus, particular moral rules and duties are the manifestation of the general moral rules as they are expressed within a particular culture or subculture. Later we shall focus explicitly on various professional contexts within which general moral rules and moral ideals become duties. (See table 4.1 below.)

Although "Do not kill" is a universal moral rule, people in some societies do not drink alcoholic beverages or drive automobiles, so "Do not drink and drive" cannot be a universal moral rule. But in any society where people drive vehicles and imbibe intoxicating substances, and are more likely to cause death, pain, and disability after imbibing intoxicating substances, "Do not drink and drive" is a particular moral rule. Similarly, for the institution of marriage, "Do not cheat" is the general, universal moral rule, but within a society that has a practice of marriage that requires sexual exclusivity, that general moral rule is expressed in the particular moral rule "Do not commit adultery." So particular moral rules are the expression of general moral rules in and through the nature, practices, and beliefs of a particular context. This allows common morality to be universal but still responsive to the nuances and vicissitudes of culture. Furthermore, even general moral rules can take on different interpretations in light of various beliefs, customs, and practices within society and within professions (e.g., what counts as deceptive in an audit may not count as deceptive in an advertisement). Indeed, the role of cultural context (including professional contexts) for interpreting the moral rules is very significant.

The beliefs prevalent in one culture might have the result that certain actions cause suffering, actions that in another culture cause no suffering whatsoever. Administering a blood transfusion to a devout Jehovah's Witness who has

Table 4.1

General moral rules + a cultural institution or practice ↔ a particular moral rule. For example, "Do not kill, cause pain, or disability," + the practice of drinking alcoholic beverages and the practice of driving cars ↔ "Do not drink and drive." "Do not cheat" + the Western institution of marriage ↔ "Do not commit adultery." (The institution of marriage in some cultures may not allow for this particular moral rule to be derived from the general moral rule prohibiting cheating.)

---

refused it would not only cause him lifelong anguish but also, according to him, an eternal loss of happiness in the afterlife. In his estimation, this eternal loss of happiness is a greater harm than death, and so giving that transfusion is a violation of the general moral rule "Do not cause pain," as well as the rule "Do not deprive of freedom."

Even conventions of etiquette in a culture are related to the general moral rules. In anything like normal circumstances, a gratuitous or flagrant breach of good manners that offends another person would be an instance of morally unacceptable behavior. Examples might be anything from foul language to surly behavior to extremely casual dress at a formal occasion like a funeral. Although the general moral rules relate to that which concerns all rational persons in every place and time, through features or aspects of particular cultures these general moral rules take on more particular content and interpretation. General moral rules prohibit everyone from causing pain and depriving of freedom, but it is the cultural setting that, in part, determines what is painful or offensive and what counts as depriving a person of freedom. In short, the moral rules are interpreted in light of the cultural context of beliefs and practices.

This interpretation is not a wide-open, free-for-all interpretation; the limits are rather tightly drawn. Disagreement on what counts as death, pain, disability, loss of freedom, and loss of pleasure is limited to unusual cases. Disagreement on what counts as causing these harms or on what counts as deceiving, breaking a promise, cheating, disobeying a law, or neglecting a duty is also limited. In no society can the rules be given just any interpretation one wants; every culture knows the function of these rules and finds the consequences of their unjustified violation destructive and reprehensible.

Particular Moral Ideals

As with the moral rules, there is an analogous culturally sensitive specification that takes place with respect to the moral ideals. Earlier we portrayed the particularization of the general moral rule as:

Table 4.2

General moral rule + a cultural institution or practice ↔ a particular moral rule. One would expect that the same formulation could work with respect to the particularization of the moral ideals. The parallel formulation would be: General moral ideal + a cultural institution or practice ↔ a particular moral ideal.

Recall that the moral ideals encourage positive actions to prevent or relieve harms, but following them is not morally required. A general moral ideal mentions the general categories of harms (e.g., prevent or relieve pain, or prevent disabilities); a particular moral ideal would specify a more particular harm that is to be prevented (e.g., prevent drug addiction). However, neither general moral ideals nor particular moral ideals tend to be formulated in precise ways. The general moral rules prohibit acting in ways that cause harms or significantly increase the risk of suffering harms. Formulating the rules in a precise way makes it less likely for someone to be unjustifiably punished. Because preventing harm is not morally required, there is no need for the general or specific ideals to tell one precisely what harms to prevent or relieve or precisely how to act to prevent those harms. The moral ideals encourage preventing or relieving all harms, so there is no need to pick out certain categories of harms to be prevented or relieved, or particular ways of preventing them. However, in certain contexts, particular moral ideals are expressed (e.g., "Defend freedom," "Create equal opportunity," "Relieve pain," "Work for world peace," "Feed the hungry," and "Save the whales"). Obviously whatever particular harm a society regards as serious, it encourages action to relieve or to prevent it. So the harms with which the society is most concerned strongly influence its formulation of particular moral ideals.

An interesting aspect of the moral ideals as they are expressed in different professions is that the prevention of a specific harm often becomes the duty of an individual or a group of individuals, by virtue of role, profession, occupation, or circumstance. In some circumstances everyone might even acquire a duty if a particular prevention of harm were seen as crucial to everyone. For example, in the context of the vast expanses of the western United States, where being stranded in the desert can be life threatening, there is a generally recognized duty to assist stranded motorists, providing it does not subject one to undue risk or burden.

The contextual specification of the moral ideals within professions often results in positive duties, that is, duties incumbent on individuals in that profession to take action (e.g., nurses to relieve the pain of patients). The contextual specification of the moral rules that results in prohibition of kinds of actions (e.g., doctors must not reveal confidential information about patients) is usually not referred to as a duty, but as a particular moral rule. Thus, many codified professional duties are contextual specifications of the moral ideals of preventing specific harms, rather than avoiding causing specific harms. Within the profession, these ideals become duties, and as such, doing these duties is morally required; they apply to all members of the profession just as the moral rule, "Obey the law," applies to everyone in society at large. Later in this chapter when we discuss the duties of those in the health care professions, it becomes clear that the scope of the duties in time and place are limited by the practices and purposes of the professions.

Interpretation of the Moral Rules

The influence of cultural or professional settings on the understanding of moral rules and ideals needs to be explored in more detail. In the preceding sections we provided a variety of examples of how cultural settings yield particular moral rules; in this section we show how the interpretation of moral rules may have the result that some apparently immoral behavior is not a violation of any moral rule. Some kinds of actions appear to be violations of moral rules because the actions result in someone becoming stressed, annoyed, unhappy, or misled, but further examination reveals that they are not violations. An action of this kind, which is not a violation of a moral rule although it results in someone being annoyed (e.g., wearing an orange necktie with a fuchsia shirt), does not need moral justification unless one intentionally wears this clothing primarily in order to annoy someone. Even if one knows that someone will be annoyed by what he is wearing, he violates no moral rule with respect to that person although his action results in the other person being annoyed. However, it might be following a moral ideal not to wear those clothes after discovering the other person's psychological distress.

These kinds of actions that may annoy someone else typically include one's choice of clothing, hairstyle, office decor, and so forth. They could also include lifestyles, such as whether one rides motorcycles or goes mountain climbing. In the medical context, examples of such actions would be a patient rationally deciding whether the particular burdens of his life make it not worth living, or a patient rationally deciding whether to have a less disfiguring procedure even though it decreases the probability of her long-term survival. Although these kinds of actions or decisions may cause psychological distress to others, they usually are not considered to be violations of any moral rule. What all these actions and decisions have in common is that the harm that would result from interpreting the moral rule as prohibiting such actions (e.g., taking away a person's freedom to engage in such activities or make such decisions) is greater than the harm that would result from their not being morally prohibited. The interpretation of the moral rules should be governed by the second step of the two-step procedure that is used when determining whether a particular violation of a moral rule is justified. The question that should be asked is whether everyone knowing that the rule is interpreted in one way results in less overall harm being suffered than everyone knowing that the rule is interpreted in another way.

Part of what underlies this line of reasoning is the implicit recognition that, in the above personal kinds of situations, no matter what choices one makes, someone somewhere probably will be upset, misled, or, at the very least, annoyed. It is as if humans intuitively and mutually understand that if *my* objections are sufficient to prohibit *your* choice of neckties (because your neckties are aesthetically painful to me), then *your* objections are sufficient to prohibit *my* hairstyle. Similarly, if morality prohibited your dangerous (to yourself) hobbies (because they cause me stress), then morality could prohibit my selection of friends (because they annoy you). Thus, all of these kinds of personal actions that are not intentional violations of the moral rules (that is, actions done for the purpose of causing others pain, etc.) are, under normal circumstances, not morally prohibited even if others suffer as a result. The annoyances are, on balance, considered to be lesser harms than the deprivation of freedom involved in prohibiting these actions. It is certainly a matter of mutual accommodation but it is also and especially a matter of contextual interpretation of the moral rule and of what counts as a violation.[2]

Although it is difficult to provide a universally understood description of the kind of action to which the second step of the two-step procedure should be applied, in practice there is usually no problem. For example, if a person knows he will offend someone in his office by wearing his hair in a ponytail, he can consider whether his action should even be interpreted as a violation of the moral rule proscribing the causing of pain rather than consider whether this is a justified violation of a moral rule. Essentially he is determining how he, as an impartial rational person, would judge the consequences of everyone knowing that this kind of act is interpreted as a violation of a moral rule that has to be justified. Would he judge these consequences as significantly better or significantly worse than the consequences of everyone knowing that this kind of act is not interpreted as a violation of a moral rule?

For some personal actions (e.g., hair style), it seems clear that interpreting them as "violations" would result in more harm than not interpreting them as "violations." These kinds of personal actions include (1) those involving matters so personally important, affecting primarily oneself, that each person regards making his or her own decision and not having it imposed by someone else (e.g., deciding when one's suffering outweighs the value of life) as crucial; (2) those personal actions whose effects are so variable that there may always be someone somewhere who finds it objectionable (e.g., a man wearing earrings); and (3) actions that are too trivial to worry about (e.g., using a toothpick in a public place). In all these kinds of cases, surely most rational persons would find it preferable not to interpret the moral rules so as to declare these kinds of actions as needing justification, even if some people sometimes suffer or are offended as the result of such actions.

As stated above, the justification for these interpretations of general and particular moral rules is determined by a procedure similar to the procedure for justifying moral rule violations described in chapter 2. The essence of this procedure is to describe the kind of act using morally relevant features that are universally understood, and then to calculate the balance of harms caused by regarding that kind of act as needing justification versus interpreting the relevant moral rule in such a way that the kind of act is not even regarded as a violation of a moral rule. Although it is more difficult to provide a universally understood description of a kind of act when deciding on an interpretation of a rule than when considering when a kind of violation is justified, the interpretation of moral rules is justified in the same way that violations of moral rules are justified. There are not two different standards at work.

There are several reasons why it is important to make clear that the interpretation of moral rules is not simply an arbitrary matter. Although, just as with the justification of a violation of a moral rule, there can be unresolvable disagreements concerning the appropriate interpretation of a rule, most interpretations will not be controversial. Although coming up with a universally understood description of the kind of act is difficult, it is generally understood that an act that affects others only secondarily, and whose primary effects are on the agent, does not count as a violation of a moral rule when the intention of the act is not to harm others. Realizing this explains why a large variety of actions, such as personal actions, that do result in harm for others do not, under normal conditions, count as violations of moral rules. Our moral theory explains why the interpretation of moral rules is determined by which interpretation results in a public system that results in less harm than alternative interpretations.

Highlighting the matter of rule interpretation also helps one to see that interpretations can change in different settings. The changes are not ad hoc and whimsical; they are appropriate and systematic, explained by the concept of morality as a public system. With regard to interpretations of general and particular moral rules, our theory explains why the domain of actions not covered by a moral rule can contract or expand in different groups and subgroups. Depending on the nature of the group of persons who are interacting and the intensity and frequency of their interaction, an interpretation of a moral rule may be more or less inclusive of personal actions. For example, within a family there might be a more expansive interpretation, that is, an interpretation such that more actions would need justification than is true for actions in the public at large. Thus, fewer actions might be completely up to the individual's own discretion. A style of dress, personal habits, or linguistic expressions, and so on, which, in the public at large, is interpreted as not needing justification, might well need justification within a family setting. That is because the family is living in such close quarters that small annoyances can really become major irritants for others. In that microcosm (or micro public system) the harms that result from the behavior may outweigh the harms that result from prohibiting that kind of behavior. But, of course, impartial rational persons may disagree about these different interpretations.

Similarly, within a club, a congregation, or a business office, the interpretation of moral rules might be broader, meaning that more actions need moral justification, actions that in the public at large would not be interpreted as moral rule violations. Among the reasons for the differences of interpretation are duties of certain individuals within the group. For example, a supervisor's role in keeping the office functioning efficiently may result in his regarding a worker's irritating behavior as a violation of the moral rule prohibiting causing pain, because such behavior might result in significantly more harm than would result from restraining that behavior. Also, the fact that some of these groupings have a voluntary membership indicates that the member has accepted the broader (more inclusive) interpretation and will refrain from certain behaviors that ordinarily (outside the "club" membership) are allowed by the standard interpretation of the rule.

In discussing the interpretation of moral rules it is important to remember that actions that normally are not interpreted as violations of moral rules (even though they result in irritation, discomfort, or offense) nevertheless might in unusual circumstances be considered violations. Of course, doing any action with the intention that it result in harm to another (e.g., wearing a necktie known to be offensive to a particular person in order to specifically annoy that person) is a moral rule violation. Further, using language known, or even that should be known, to be offensive to a person who is currently confined to bed and in severe pain is also regarded as a moral rule violation and is usually morally unacceptable. This kind of behavior is usually termed thoughtless or callous, and unlike most actions that are not intentional violations of moral rules, there is a low cost in avoiding this hurtful behavior and a high cost to the individuals hurt.

This crucial matter of interpretation is another area where moral disagreement can take place. Facts and the ranking of harms were previously acknowledged as sources for much moral disagreement, but there also can be genuine disagreement about how a moral rule should be interpreted in a particular context. Should it be narrowly or broadly interpreted? Is it a standard interpretation of a rule of one's profession, or is it a newer and more questionable one? Is it an interpretation significant in an ethnic subculture but not in the hospital culture in which the person finds himself?

Cautions Concerning the Interpretation of Moral Rules

Our examples have generally been instances of behavior considered acceptable by virtue of being of a special kind, namely, personal actions not intended to harm anyone, that affect others only secondarily, and whose primary effects are on the agent. However, there are many unintentional harmful personal actions that so many persons take such great offense to that they are regarded as morally unacceptable behavior. For example, public nudity or public displays of sexual intimacy are deemed offensive to so many that such behavior is interpreted as a violation of the moral rule, "Do not cause pain or suffering." People have argued for such an interpretation as a matter of taste, religion, or of the public good, but in any case the balance of harm caused and harm avoided shifts so that it seems more harm is prevented by regarding such actions as being prohibited by a moral rule than by interpreting the rule so that the action is not prohibited by it.[3]

We have been discussing actions by individuals that are usually not interpreted as violations even though sometimes they result in harm. Similarly, there are activities, practices, or policies that often result in someone being offended, upset, or disappointed even though it was never intended that any particular person be hurt in any way. A lottery has a lot of losers; a sporting event has to have losers if it is to have winners. Also, any popular event necessarily has limited capacity for spectators (so someone will be disappointed because he fails to get in), and an art show can award only a limited number of prizes (so the second-prize winner may inappropriately regard the first-prize winner as having "harmed" her by keeping her from first place). These and many other such activities are instances where, by the nature of the activity, someone inevitably suffers, though there was never any intention that any particular, identifiable individual or group suffer.

These instances of resulting harm are not interpreted as violations of moral rules because to do so would eliminate desired activities. The resulting harms are not only not intentionally caused, they may not be "caused" by any person's action at all; they are simply the natural consequences of the "rules of the game." No moral blame is attached to these practices. Viewed from the perspective of a public system, the benefits of these activities significantly outweigh any resulting harms. Of course these policies, practices, games, and social arrangements that result in someone suffering (though not intentionally) could (if in doubt) be examined from a moral point of view, that is, by seeing whether rational persons would prefer a public system that contains these activities to a public system that does not.

If, for example, the activity involved serious harm, deceit, or deprivation of freedom against a particular group, it might well be judged immoral. Boxing is an activity that sometimes comes up for this kind of moral review. Although boxers voluntarily subject themselves to the pain and risks of injury and are not supposed to try intentionally to permanently injure each other (but only to win points or render the other unable to get up before a count of ten), the fact that serious injuries often do occur can offend the sensitivities of the public sufficiently for it to consider boxing immoral. One important lesson one learns from all these examples is that there is no simple identity between a harm resulting from one's actions, on the one hand, and "causing a harm" (or breaking a moral rule) on the other. Thus, there is no simple inference from "Harm resulted from his action" to "He caused harm" or "He broke a moral rule." And given that many violations of moral rules are justified, it is even more clearly false to infer from the fact that "harm resulted from his action," that he acted immorally.

How Many Moralities?

Readers may be confused by the apparent conflict between their own awareness that there are many moral codes or "moralities" and our continuing treatment of morality as though it were one. We are, of course, aware that there are many domains with their own explicit or implicit moral codes: business ethics, environmental ethics, medical ethics, computer ethics, military ethics, government ethics, and many others. Our discussion of interpretation in this current chapter should explain, at least partially, why it appears that there are so many moralities, even though we maintain that there is but one general morality that holds for everyone in all times and places. As shown in chapter 2, morality is an informal public system that applies to all rational persons and is grounded in universal features of human nature (e.g., vulnerability, fallibility, and the rational avoidance of harm). The different interpretations of the moral rules, allowed by the informal nature of morality, explains how it seems that there are so many moralities.

Part of our task in this chapter is to show how common morality relates to all these various manifestations. It has been shown how the general moral rules, in combination with institutions, beliefs, and practices of various cultures, yield particular moral rules. That phenomenon illustrates the universality of morality, while accounting for its protean manifestations in various cultures and settings. Morality, properly understood, is culture sensitive; it is expressed through the practices, beliefs, and institutions of a culture. As we have emphasized, this does not mean that anything goes, for the general moral rules establish ranges of morally permissible and morally required actions. The various cultures provide the "shading" and nuances that result in the various harms being weighed differently, such as minimizing the importance of a generally regarded very serious harm, because of particular beliefs held by a significant number of people in the culture. For example, in some cultures there might be such a strong belief in a desirable afterlife that loss of life is ranked as less serious than any significant pain or disability. Even in a certain age group, maybe octogenarians, death may generally be more welcome than enduring significant prolonged pain.

Professional Ethics

Professional ethics is another "culture" in which the general moral rules are subject to interpretation and yield both particular moral rules and special duties. Each profession or each domain of activity has practices, understandings, and dilemmas that call for a specific fashioning of the various moral rules and ideals to deal with the particularities of its activities.

For example, in medicine the need for the physician to obtain intimate information from the patient, combined with the fact that people generally do not want intimate information about themselves to be revealed, taken in conjunction with the general moral rule not to cause pain generates the duty not to breach confidentiality. Traditionally it has been understood and expected that confidences would not be violated, and formulating the duty of confidentiality simply makes it more explicit.

Another example of medicine's particularizing of general morality is in the matter of truth telling. The general moral rule, "Do not deceive," in medicine—unlike in everyday life—may require a physician to tell the truth to his patients. However, in the context of medical practice, this broader interpretation makes it more useful as an action guide. Whereas in ordinary circumstances, one is morally required not to deceive, one is not morally required to "tell the truth."[4] Even if my neighbor would benefit from knowing that the price of a certain stock is going up, I have not deceived him by not telling him about it. But in medicine it is the physician's duty to disclose to the patient the relevant facts about the patient's medical condition, so that the physician not telling this information is interpreted as deceiving. There can be exceptions, but they must be morally justified, as must all violations of moral rules. This duty has come about by the needs and the expectations that occur within the doctor-patient relationship. Hence, in the particular circumstances of the practice of medicine, this interpretation of the general moral rule is appropriate.

Similarly, the medical duty to obtain informed consent before proceeding with therapy is derived from the general moral rule "Do not deprive of freedom" because of the context of the characteristic interactions and procedures of medicine. The very nature of the practice of medicine makes causing pain so ever present (just in order to accomplish its aims) that protections against that happening without the patient's permission must be institutionalized into medicine's moral code. Thus, the general moral rule prohibiting the deprivation of freedom is particularized for the special circumstances of medicine; it is expressed in the medical duty to obtain informed consent, which, among other things, guards against anyone being deprived of the opportunity to choose whether or not to undergo a medical or surgical procedure, especially a painful one. Essentially all modern codes of ethics for the health care professions makes obtaining valid consent an explicit duty of physicians and other health care workers.

"Do Your Duty" and Professional Ethics

Many of the duties of a profession are particular applications of the general moral rules (which are valid for all persons in all times and places) in the context of the special circumstances, practices, relationships, and purposes of the profession. Thus, the duties are far more precise with respect to the special circumstances characterizing a particular domain or profession. The goal of morality remains the same, namely, to lessen the overall evil or harm suffered by people, but now the duties are more precise with respect to and sensitive to a special realm of activity. This point might be more intuitively seen by considering the general moral rule, "Obey the law." Obviously, laws vary from place to place, depending on such matters as history, culture, and beliefs. The general moral rule that requires obeying the law requires doing or abstaining from a kind of action when this kind of action is required or prohibited by a particular law.

Similarly, the general moral rule "Do your duty" requires doing or abstaining from a kind of action when this kind of action is required or prohibited by a duty. Recall (from chapter 2) the justification of this rule as a moral rule. If not followed in general, there would be a considerable increase in the amount of harm suffered. That is because people become dependent on others doing their duty; they come to rely on these others and to make plans around them, expecting that they will do their duty. This is true of lifeguards, babysitters, college professors, firemen, insurance agents, policemen, doctors, and countless others. It is to the interest and well being of everyone that no one neglects her duty unless she has an adequate justification for doing so.

Where do these duties come from? Who decides what they are? It should be clear that duties are normally associated with roles, occupations, relationships, and the professions. The duties constitute the expectations that everyone can legitimately have of those in that role, occupation, relationship, or profession. Society has certain expectations of firemen, doctors, lifeguards, parents, and airplane pilots. How do these expectations get established?

There are many sources for role-related duties. Tradition is a major one. A group comes to provide a particular service, in a particular way, and eventually others come to count on these provisions. Thus, a tradition is born. It may be a role (e.g., of firemen) that develops over decades, even centuries. Sometimes the providers can develop expectations in the public by practice and by projection of image through advertising or group promotion. Very often the groups have a code that specifies what can be expected of them by others. Certain standards evolve so that now these become "duties" because others have come to count on these actions. Thus, there are "standards of practice" in medicine that have become duties of the profession.

Many moral disputes pivot on the vagueness of duties: everyone may agree that everyone is morally required not to neglect his duty, but not everyone agrees on precisely what those duties are. The details of duties can be vague because of a variety of factors: the tradition is not clearly established; there are various interpretations of the code; and different practices and standards of practice are followed in different parts of the country. The duties of parents and of babysitters are seldom stated in codes or contracts; it is debatable whether a sports hero has a duty to live an exemplary life (inasmuch as his or her behavior influences the young). Not infrequently these issues are settled in court (e.g., whether ophthalmologists have a duty to screen all of their patients over forty for glaucoma by measuring intraocular pressure) and the resultant court ruling then becomes another tradition relevant for interpreting duty, namely, the legal tradition. The precedents set in such cases become the "standard of care" in those particular roles or occupations.

The nature of duties is a rich topic, especially important to an understanding of bioethics. Our point in chapter 2 was to show the justification for the moral rule "Do your duty." Our point here is to show that duties grow out of various roles and relationships. The importance of duties is that they show how a general moral rule can be significantly culture sensitive. Apart from very limited duties that arise from circumstances, we do not think it appropriate to talk about universal duties; we regard duties as developing around particular roles, relationships, and practices in any "culture," whether familial, professional, occupational, or social. If there are valid expectations that others have come to count on, then it is likely that a duty exists. The duty "grew up" and became at least informally codified and is indigenous to that particular setting and culture.

Although books and articles on medical ethics frequently appeal to the "duties" and obligations of health care professionals, these appeals generally are simply ad hoc declarations. No theory is provided that explains how particular duties are derived from or dependent on common morality. Indeed, some think that particular duties in professions, especially medicine, were developed completely independently of common morality and are often in conflict with it. Others seem not to want to distinguish professional duties from the general moral rules. Both of these views are mistaken. Although there can be a conflict between a particular duty and some other moral rule, just as there can be conflicts between two moral rules or a moral rule and a moral ideal, professional duties do not generally conflict with common morality. When there is a conflict, it is to be resolved using the same two-step procedure that is used in all other cases of conflict. However, in moral disputes it is important to make the distinction between professional duties and general moral rules because some action, whether it is required by a general moral rule or only because a professional duty requires doing it, may change the way one deals with the problem. If the latter is the case, that duty might be changed, but the general moral rules do not change.

It may well be that the so-called Principles of Biomedical Ethics should be understood as simply a rough classification of duties of health care professionals at a certain level of generality. As such, the principles are a kind of generalized grouping of duties (divided into four or five categories) that have accrued to the health care professions. This classification is not based on any theory and the duties are not related to one another in any systematic way; rather, the "duties" are listed under a given principle in order to facilitate discussion of them. The context for these observations about the "principles" is provided in chapter 5 in which we present a general critique of "principlism." We will now and again refer to the concept of duty throughout the following chapters, but we never use the term "duty" to refer to a general moral requirement that is universal. We always use the term in the way that it is ordinarily used, to refer to a requirement that is based upon particular circumstances, relationships, or roles. Obviously, in a discussion of bioethics, most of the duties we discuss will be based upon the professional roles of those in the health care field. Our goal to this point has been to show how common morality bears on professional duties, and to show how these duties often are derived from common morality in conjunction with the details of the context in which these duties apply.

Other Sources of Duties

We have discussed the integral relationship of professional ethics to common morality. We have shown how the moral rules are interpreted or give rise to professional duties, thus articulating moral requirements that are much more specific to the particulars of the practice of that profession. The rules prohibiting deceiving, cheating, breaking promises, depriving of freedom, causing pain, and so forth, have interpretations that involve these professional duties. In the United States, a doctor is violating the rule "Do not deceive" when he does not tell a patient the truth about her diagnosis or prognosis, because he has a duty to provide that information. The duties of doctors result from the moral problems that typically confront those in that profession.

With that as background the next step toward viewing professional ethics will be easier to understand. Our basic distinction between moral rules and moral ideals (chapter 2) enables us to explain how the moral ideals play a role in professional ethics. Some of these moral ideals become duties that require members of the profession to go above and beyond what is required by the general moral rules. That means the profession is not content with simply not causing harm, but it commits itself, in specified circumstances, to going out of its way to prevent and to relieve harm. Some of the moral ideals express the aspirations of the profession. Whether the ideals become duties or aspirations is context sensitive; that is, it is at least partly determined by each profession's capabilities and interests. Doctors presumably do not turn away anyone in need of medical care; they treat regardless of ability to pay. Doctors always act primarily in the best interest of the patient rather than in their own interest. Doctors are dedicated to the prevention and cure of sickness and suffering. Some of these ideals have become duties, others are aspirations; which of these they become is largely set by the medical profession, though perhaps clarified and modified by law and society.

There is always some vagueness concerning the ideals. When do they cease to be accepted as simply ideals and become instead duties of the profession? In ordinary morality, the general moral ideals are characterized by their being impossible to follow toward everyone, impartially, all the time. Similarly, a profession treats its accepted ideals as goals, as something to be worked toward, as aspirations. It can hardly fulfill these ideals toward everyone, impartially, all the time. Nevertheless, some ideals do become duties, while others do not, and it is important to be aware of the difference. Those that doctors are expected to follow toward each of their patients might be considered duties. Necessarily those ideals that become duties need to have significant limitations, because it is humanly impossible to follow the general moral ideals toward all one's patients, all the time. These duties are generally limited to those that can be accomplished while in the presence of the patient: eliciting relevant information or explaining information relevant to obtaining consent for therapy. Of course there can be some dispute about how much time and effort is required of a doctor to do his or her duty and how much constitutes going above and beyond duty, and thus acting on an ideal. Many ideals or aspirations never become duties. Medicine might pledge itself to achieving health defined as total mental, physical, and social well-being, but no one holds the profession, let alone an individual physician, responsible for failing to accomplish that goal.

The admonition to physicians "Always act in the best interest of one's patients" is vague and can be interpreted so as to make it impossible to satisfy completely. If a physician goes out of town for a vacation, she is hardly acting in the best interests of her patients. There is probably always some patient who is in need of the physician's help, or who at least would do better or feel better if the physician were never away. The same holds true of the normal workday. Should a physician be on call twenty-four hours a day, forever, in order to satisfy maximally "the best interest of her patients"? Should she spend many hours with each patient? These actions cannot literally become the duty of any individual physician, though in achieving ideals, groups of physicians might make certain rational arrangements among themselves in order to fulfill the ideal of twenty-four-hour coverage for their patients, or, for that matter, for a whole town. But notice that once this achievable goal is stated and practiced, it might become a duty for this group of physicians because people reasonably come to count on it and may be harmed if that duty is neglected. But when that duty holds and when it does not, when it is clearly a duty and when it is not becomes the focus of many lawsuits. However, the unclear or disputed cases do not discount the value of the distinction between duty and ideal; indeed, they make it important to become as clear as possible about the distinction in different circumstances. Most cases are clear-cut, but there are always some instances that remain vague and can only be settled by adjudication or stipulation.

Professional Rules of Conduct

Many duties that apply to individuals by virtue of their occupation or role are not particularizations of general moral rules or ideals in the context of that profession. The "rules of conduct" for professional conduct contain a diverse collection of duties, only some of which are directly related to the general moral rules or ideals. This fact can be confusing because the different types of duties have different purposes; some serve general moral goals and some serve the special goals of the members of the profession. It is important to sort out these duties so they can be understood and evaluated in terms of their purposes, their validity, and their relationship to common morality. We have already described those that are directly based on common morality (both moral rules and moral ideals), which are expressed as duties and aspirations within the context of a particular profession. But mixed in with those duties and aspirations that are directly related to the general moral rules and ideals are at least two other types of duties: preventive and group-protective.

Particular Moral Rules—Preventive Rules

The preventive rules are those rules that prohibit behavior that, though not immoral in itself, is thought to make immoral acts more tempting and thus more likely. They serve to diminish enticement to break a moral rule. Examples of this kind of "preventive" moral rule is the rule among baseball players that they not bet on games, and the rule among lawyers that they not be mentioned as inheritors in the wills of their clients. Usually these rules are written and agreed upon by the profession itself as part of its code of ethics. However, the rules might be enforced by law if they are thought to affect the public (e.g., that physicians not refer their patients to facilities and services in which the physicians themselves have a financial interest). Notice that none of these forbidden actions are immoral in and of themselves. Rather, the existence of the forbidden practice is considered a "moral hazard" in that it has the appearance of immorality and could easily lead to real immorality.

The baseball player might be tempted to play poorly for his team in order to win the bet he had placed; the lawyer might be tempted to manipulate her way into receiving a portion of the inheritance from one of her clients; the physician might send his patient for unnecessary diagnostic services from which the physician gains financially. All these latter actions are, of course, immoral simply by virtue of the general moral rules (the rules, e.g., proscribing cheating, deceiving, causing pain, and depriving of freedom). However, the preventive moral rules are prospective in nature, designed to help avoid unjustified violations of moral rules. The preventive moral rules themselves then become part of the profession's ethical code so that, now, though doing the action they proscribe does no harm in itself, breaking that rule must be considered immoral for those members within the group, because, for those within that group, following that rule has become their duty.

Particular Moral Rules—Group-Protective Rules

The group-protective rules mixed in with the particular moral rules and the preventive moral rules in the various codes of conduct serve more to enhance or preserve the public image of the group, or to prevent some harm from being done to the group or to other members of the group. These "group-protective" rules are more like guild rules: rules that the profession regards as necessary to protect the vital interests of the profession or occupation itself, such as prohibitions against trying to lure away each other's clients. These rules are taken as more important than the exhortations to enhance or nurture the profession, for example, the exhortations to engage in some activity (group aspirations) that enhances the public image of the profession. However, when a group-protective rule is taken as harming those outside the group, society, acting through the courts, may invalidate the rule. This is what happened to the group-protective rule prohibiting doctors from advertising. Although the medical profession claimed that this was not merely a group-protective rule, but that it protected the general public from false or misleading claims, the courts decided that it deprived the general public from the information it might need to make an informed choice about its medical care. Thus, the courts invalidated these rules and forbade the profession from enforcing them. As with the particular moral rules, moral ideals, and the preventive rules, these group-protective rules become obligatory for the members of that occupation or profession and they can be censured by the profession for violating the rules.

What is the relationship of these various rules to morality? Obviously the particular moral rules and ideals are part and parcel of morality because they are contextual expressions of the general moral rules and ideals. And the preventive rules might be seen as being based on moral ideals, because they are prohibitions designed to prevent harms by requiring their members not to put themselves in the position where breaking general moral rules would be easy and tempting.

The group-protective rules, however, are not derived from common morality, although all members of the profession are required to obey them. As with all the rules in the codes, group-protective rules are duties of the members of that group. Each member of the group benefits from obedience to these mutually agreed upon rules, and members are required to fulfill them. The fact that "Do your duty" is a general moral rule is, no doubt, partially responsible for thinking of codes of conduct as moral codes. But the most that can be said about the group-protective rules is that they must be morally acceptable. They must not involve unjustified exceptions to any of the general moral rules. No matter how one thinks about this mixed bag of rules called "professional codes," "codes of ethics," or "codes of conduct," the important moral point is this: they are morally acceptable as long as they do not require unjustifiable violations of any general moral rules. *No one can have a duty to do something immoral.* So there cannot be a duty to protect a colleague in the group if that involves deceiving, cheating, or causing pain or suffering to someone outside the group.

A group or profession cannot simply construct any rules of behavior it wants and make them "duties." To be considered "duties," these rules must not only not involve unjustifiable violations of any general moral rules, they must also not be in conflict with the goal of morality: to reduce the amount of evil in the world. Notice how the preventive rules, though not proscribing immoral actions themselves, do proscribe actions that can all too easily lead to breaking a moral rule. As such they are integrally related to the moral rules, but they apply only to those who are members of the group in question. In a sense, these preventive rules could be seen as turning moral ideals into duties inasmuch as they call for some self-sacrifice (e.g., of freedom) in order to achieve a prevention of harm. A group can always take on itself a more stringent morality, that is, one that not only does not violate any of the general moral rules but also that demands more of its members than is required by the general moral rules. Even the morally acceptable group-protective rules protect other members of the profession from suffering unwanted harms, without thereby causing harm to those not in the profession; thus, even they are supportive of the general goal of morality of lessening the amount of harm in the world.

Moral Expertise

An important goal of the previous two chapters is to give confidence to general readers to engage in moral deliberation and discussion. Because there is basically only one morality, people's moral intuitions, trained and honed in everyday life, should stand them in good stead in professional ethics. All rational persons can and must participate in making moral decisions. There is no moral expertise; everyone understands morality without the need for such expertise. Of course, thinking about moral problems may improve one's moral judgments and some people have more reliable moral intuitions than others, that is, their judgments are less likely to need revision after detailed discussion. However, every normal adult can and does discuss moral issues in a meaningful way without having had a course in either ethical theory or professional ethics.

The use of the term "ethicist" or "bioethicist" is very misleading. An ethicist or bioethicist is not an authority on ethics or bioethics in the same way that a physicist is an authority on physics or a chemist on chemistry. No one should defer to an ethicist when a moral decision is called for. Nor should one allow an ethicist or "moral expert" to overrule one's own moral intuitions or to inhibit one from participating in moral deliberations. Ordinary understanding of ethics is usually sufficient, as long as one knows and appreciates the facts, purposes, understandings, and relationships of the field with whose ethics she is dealing.

Common morality itself is fairly straightforward; everyone understands what it is to harm someone, to deceive, to cheat, to neglect one's duty, and so on, and even has a good sense of when the situation is such that they would favor everyone knowing that they can violate the rule in these circumstances.

The technical language of professional ethics can sometimes obscure the real moral issues. Although technical language can allow one to make valuable distinctions and can facilitate precision, it can also incline people to think that they have resolved some moral issue when they have simply learned to apply some technical terms. It can also force one's thinking into fixed categories and consequently to obscure the complex and subtle nature of many moral problems. The nature of morality as an informal public system that applies to all rational persons conflicts with the idea of "moral experts." What passes for moral expertise is often simply facility in the use of the technical language of bioethics. The proper role of those involved in bioethics is to clarify and to make explicit what people already know. It is to remind health care professionals to use their moral understanding and not to be misled by the technical language of bioethics.

Notes

1. Although evolutionary considerations can explain why many of the features of morality have been adopted by all societies with regard to all of its members, it cannot explain why we now include all rational beings as belonging to the group protected by morality.

2. This line of reasoning is often expressed in the language of rights: "I have a right to wear my hair as long as I want, no matter what anyone thinks." See Gert (2005, 177–180).

3. See Feinberg (1985) for a detailed discussion of these matters. Of particular interest is a description of the most offensive bus ride imaginable.

4. Telling the truth is not normally required by the rule "Do not deceive," for telling the truth requires far more than simply not deceiving. For a fuller discussion of this point, see Gert (2005, 190).

5

Principlism

Introduction

Having presented our own account of common morality, together with its justification, we devote this chapter to comparing it to principlism, the most widely
used account in biomedical ethics.[1] Because the use of principlism is so pervasive, we want to highlight the significant differences between it and our systematic account in order to make certain that aspects of principlism are not
unwittingly and automatically read into our own account. Inasmuch as part of
the rationale for this book is to show the usefulness of a systematic account, we
think it appropriate to show in detail that the lack of any unifying theory in
principlism makes it far less useful in dealing with controversial issues than our
account. Since the primary practical value of an explicit account of morality is in
the help it can provide in dealing with controversial issues, showing that our
account is more valuable in this respect, should be sufficient to show its greater
overall usefulness. On a purely philosophical level, the two accounts differ quite
dramatically. We offer a detailed account of the moral system and provide a
justification for it. Principlism presents only a schema of an account of morality
and no attempt to justify it at all. In a sense, this comparison addresses the main
point of this book, that insofar as any moral theory is needed or useful, a
systematic account, such as ours, has far more value than an account such as
principlism, which is an unsystematic and ad hoc collection of independent
principles.

In arguing that our account of morality is more adequate and more useful we point out how, unlike principlism, our moral theory (1) not only explains and justifies the overwhelming agreement on moral matters but also explains and justifies the limited disagreement; (2) provides a clear, coherent, and comprehensive account of how our common morality applies to medical matters; and (3) provides an account of common morality that is easily understood, and actually provides guidance for new kinds of cases. Thus, in this chapter, we focus particularly on the advantages of our systematic account over all schematic accounts such as principlism. We concentrate on the version of principlism put forward by Beauchamp and Childress, for it is the most developed. But similar serious problems are present in all of the principlist accounts regardless of the content of their principles.

Principlism is characterized by its citing of principles that constitute the core of its account of biomedical ethics; for Beauchamp and Childress these principles are beneficence, autonomy, nonmaleficence, and justice. The account of Beauchamp and Childress is so entrenched in the minds of some bioethicists that clinical moral problems are often grouped (for conferences, papers, and books) according to which principle is deemed most relevant and necessary for resolving them. It has become fashionable and customary to cite one or another of these principles as the key for resolving a particular biomedical ethical problem. Throughout much of the medical bioethical literature, authors seem to believe that they have provided a theoretical solution to the problem being discussed when they have mentioned one or more of the principles. Thus, not only do the principles presumably lead to acceptable solutions but they are also treated by many as the ultimate grounds of appeal.

We examine principlism by looking at its undeniably leading account, that of Beauchamp and Childress, as manifested in the many editions of their book *Principles of Biomedical Ethics.*[2] Their account is the very best the position has to offer, and it is their account that has pervaded the world of biomedical ethics. For many years it has provided the conceptual framework of the Georgetown Intensive Bioethics Course, a one-week summer course that has been attended by thousands from the United States as well as from around the world. Beauchamp and Childress's book is outstanding in its insights about particular problems in bioethics and for its sensitivity to important issues and relevant subtleties. Our criticism focuses only on their account of morality and its relationship to biomedical ethics.

Comparison of Common Morality and Principlism

As we have emphasized in several previous articles on principlism, we are criticizing Beauchamp and Childress as the very best spokesmen for the principle-based approach to bioethics. However, we are concerned about the widespread popularization of principlism throughout the biomedical ethics world, where the use of principles simply masks ad hoc and unreasoned decisions and judgments. Beauchamp and Childress are very careful not to use their principles to resolve any controversial issue; they simply use the principles to focus their discussion of particular issues. It is crucial to distinguish between using principles as a guide to decision making and as a way to focus discussion of issues. Their discussions of these issues are always quite knowledgeable and often quite insightful. Our objection is to the framework they claim to be using. Even though Beauchamp and Childress have changed their theoretical account considerably over the years, their discussion of particular cases has not changed. Our concern is with the practitioners of principlism who do not realize that its point is to focus discussion and not to resolve any controversial issues. We think it is important to emphasize this point because principlism is still flourishing.

Beauchamp and Childress's 4th edition (1994) so modified their account in response to criticisms that one reviewer entitled his article "The Beginning of the End of Principlism," and said that their new claims "constitute a radical change and herald the end of 'principlism.' "[3] Beauchamp and Childress's 5th edition (2001) devotes even more space to theoretical issues, including a misguided criticism of our account. It is misguided because Beauchamp and Childress continue to regard our theory as an "impartial rule theory," although we provide an account of common morality that explains the moral decisions and judgments of ordinary, thoughtful people. Further, they label as common morality theories the purely schematic accounts of W. D. Ross and William Frankena, which, like principlism itself, consist of nothing but a set of principles or prima facie rules, with no system in which they are embedded. Like Ross and Frankena, Beauchamp and Childress have no account of the nature or role of impartiality, and no distinction between the moral rules, to which obedience is required, and moral ideals, which people are encouraged to follow. Their only account of the procedure to be used when there is a conflict between the principles is that the principles should be specified, but they do not provide even one example of how this specification works to resolve a controversial problem.

Beauchamp and Childress have conflicting views about morality. They say, "In its most familiar sense, *morality* refers to norms about right and wrong human conduct that are so widely shared that they form a stable (although usually incomplete) social consensus" (2–3). This innocuous sounding statement leads them into errors. By concentrating on right and wrong human conduct, that conduct to which the moral rules apply, and neglecting good and bad human conduct, to which the moral ideals apply, they make it seem as if morality consists of nothing but prohibitions and requirements. They then say, "All persons who are serious about living a moral life already grasp the core dimensions of morality. They know not to lie, not to steal property, to keep promises, to respect the rights of others, not to kill or cause harm to innocent persons, and the like" (3).

Their listing of the rules of morality is remarkably similar to our list of the rules of common morality. However, they then go on to say the following: "We will refer to the set of norms that all morally serious persons share as *the common morality*. The common morality contains moral norms that bind all persons in all places" (3).

They then distinguish between common morality and morality by claiming that common morality consists of "norms that all morally serious people accept as authoritative" whereas morality includes those norms that "bind only members of specific moral communities." They misleadingly used the phrase "moral ideals" to refer to those norms that "bind only members of specific moral communities," that is, to prohibitions and requirements that are not universal. The full quote goes as follows: "*Morality* consists of more than *common morality*, and we should never confuse or conflate the two. For example, morality includes *moral ideals* that individuals and groups voluntarily accept, *communal norms* that bind only members of specific moral communities, extraordinary virtues, and the like. The common morality, by contrast, comprises all and only those norms that all morally serious persons accept as authoritative" (3). Thus, according to Beauchamp and Childress, neither common morality nor morality includes what we have termed "moral ideals," those precepts that are universally regarded as morally good to act on, but which are neither prohibitions nor requirements. This restriction of common morality to the moral rules, and of morality to duties and aspirations of particular groups, excludes what we call the universal moral ideals, such as helping the needy. Beauchamp and Childress's failure to acknowledge that there are universal moral ideals may explain why they do not recognize that our theory, unlike theirs or those of Ross and Frankena, does, in fact, explain the moral decisions and judgments of all morally serious persons. Our account of common morality makes clear that all morally serious persons recognize that common morality consists of more than universally accepted rules; it also includes universally accepted moral ideals. Even many moral codes of particular groups and societies consist of more than binding duties and extraordinary virtues; they also include aspirations that all members of the group are encouraged but not required to follow.

It is universally recognized that when one is not breaking any moral rule, taking a serious risk in order to save the lives of innocent children is morally commendable but not morally required. Nonetheless, when breaking a promise would not involve serious harm, taking a serious risk to save innocent children justifies breaking that promise, even though keeping promises is a "norm that binds." Common morality not only includes universally accepted moral ideals but also includes a procedure for determining whether a violation of a moral rule is strongly justified, weakly justified, or unjustified. Not only do Beauchamp and Childress falsely limit common morality to "norms that bind" but also they ignore all those formal features of common morality that we put forward in our discussion of morality. Furthermore, they do not explicitly acknowledge that common morality allows for some unresolvable moral conflicts.

It is clear that although Beauchamp and Childress use the phrase "moral ideals," they do not mean by it what we mean. They explicitly deny that moral ideals in our sense are part of common morality. They say, "There are two levels of moral standards: ordinary moral standards and extraordinary moral standards. The first level is limited to standards in common morality that pertain to everyone. These standards form the moral minimum" (39). Thus, according to Beauchamp and Childress, common morality is the moral minimum. But, contrary to Beauchamp and Childress's account, all morally serious persons agree that common morality includes more than the moral minimum. All agree that it is morally good to act on the moral ideals whenever one can do so without violating a moral rule. Everyone also agrees that even when acting on an ideal requires breaking a moral rule, it is sometimes justified to break the moral rule. Beauchamp and Childress apparently do not realize that common morality consists of more than moral rules. They fail to include in common morality the moral ideals and the two-step procedure for determining how to act when moral rules conflict or a moral rule conflicts with a moral ideal. Among the consequences of these failures is their holding the mistaken view that common morality, being a system, requires that there be a unique best solution to every moral problem.

Beauchamp and Childress say, "A virtue of our theory is that it requires specification . . . and a problem in Clouser and Gert's account is that it supposes that its 'more concrete' rules escape the need for specification. Only a theory that could put enough content into its norms to escape conflicts and dilemmas in all contexts could live up to the Clouser-Gert demand, but no theory approximates this ideal" (389).[4] This quote demonstrates the fundamental flaw of all forms of principlism, namely that the various principles are not embedded in a system, so everything has to be packed into the principles. But as Beauchamp and Childress admit, there is no way to "put enough content into" any principles in order for them to deal adequately with the complex moral problems that any account of morality must face. We do not claim that our rules escape the need for specification because they are more concrete, but because the rules of common morality are embedded in a comprehensive moral system with a two-step procedure that includes the morally relevant features needed to describe any proposed violation of a rule, and a formula that uses this description when deciding on which way to act. Further, not only do we not claim to "escape conflicts and dilemmas in all contexts," we explicitly claim that some disagreements are unresolvable. But, unlike Beauchamp and Childress, we try to explain why this is so.

Beauchamp and Childress seem to have adopted the concept of "specification" from Henry Richardson. We have already replied to Richardson, but it may be worthwhile to make clear again the advantages of recognizing that the moral rules are embedded in a system, rather than regarding each of the principles as a freestanding principle.[5] When, in our reply, we praised Beauchamp and Childress's "adoption of specification . . . as a way station on the journey to truth—that is to [our] own alternative view of the moral rules governing bioethics," we did not realize that their adoption of Richardson's proposal to improve principlism by means of specification was a last-ditch effort to maintain the view that morality operates with a set of freestanding principles. It is interesting and instructive that Beauchamp and Childress never discuss the possibility that in some circumstances there is no uniquely correct way to specify the principles. They seem to hope that specification will enable them to provide uniquely correct solutions to every moral problem. Thus, they seem to be abandoning the one truly valuable aspect of principlism, namely, that it did not provide uniquely correct solutions to every moral problem. But they are still ambivalent about this, maintaining their original view while at the same time putting forward specification as if it will resolve all disagreements.

The contrast between our theory and that of principlism is stark. Beauchamp and Childress start with freestanding moral or bioethical principles and then modify or specify these principles in order to apply them to particular cases. On the other hand, we start with common morality, a moral system that we neither change nor modify. This system enables us to provide morally relevant descriptions of all the particular cases in a way that makes clear how the moral rules apply to them. Rather than continually reformulating the rules for each particular case, we keep the rules unchanged and instead provide a procedure for determining whether it is morally justified to violate the rule in these circumstances. We even distinguish between strong and weak justification, that is, between the clear cases and the controversial ones. Keeping the moral system unchanged keeps the focus on the facts (where it should be) and avoids the continuing reformulation of the moral rules or principles in order to apply them to each particular case.

And Beauchamp and Childress do adjust, interpret, and specify principles in order to apply them to particular cases. This means that the principles become more complex and are constantly changing, and thus are not known with any precision to anyone. We, on the other hand, keep the moral system constant (morality does not change), and thus it is known to all. However, we provide ways of describing a particular case by means of the morally relevant features, so that it becomes clear how the moral system applies to that case. For us, the work is done in preparing the particular case (e.g., finding out all the facts, categorizing how the morally relevant features fit, etc.) so that the moral system can be applied to it. If the goal is to connect common morality to a particular case, there are two opposing ways to do this. One way is to work on describing the case so that it becomes clear how the moral system applies to it, which is what we do. The other way is to continually specify some principles so that these principles can be applied to the particular case. Since Beauchamp and

Childress have no system, they cannot work on describing the case in the appropriate way and so must adopt the second method.

In deciding between two accounts of morality—one that involves a continual revision of moral principles, such that these principles are unlikely to be known by most of the people to whom they apply, and an account of morality that is known to everyone to whom it applies—the choice seems clear. Further, if the second moral theory focuses on the facts in a way that requires people to describe the moral situation in a way that rules out their personal or cultural biases, whereas the first provides no limits on the way in which the moral principles can be specified, again the choice is clear. Finally, if the second moral theory requires one to view every violation of a moral rule in the way that an impartial rational person would, whereas the first allows one to avoid violations simply by specifying the bioethical principles without involving impartiality at all, again it is obvious which should be chosen.

Specification brings out the ambivalence that Beauchamp and Childress seem to have with regard to the view that a moral theory must provide a unique correct answer to every moral question. On the one hand, they want to hold onto the attractive feature of early principlism, namely, that it did not even pretend to provide a method for arriving at a unique correct answer; on the other, they now want a method for doing just that. They admit that, "in any given problematic or dilemmatic case, several competing specifications may constitute possible resolutions, which returns us to conflicts of the sort that drove us to specification in the first place" (17). Instead of recognizing that not all problematic or dilemmatic cases can be resolved, they say, "We therefore must connect specification as a method with a larger model of justification that will support some specifications over others" (18).

We recognize that not all moral problems have unique best resolutions and do not propose any method whereby they can all be resolved. Beauchamp and Childress seem to accept the standard view of moral theories that common morality always provides a unique correct answer to every moral question about how one morally ought to act. Thus, they are inclined to hold that all moral disagreements must be explained away. Those who disagree must be not equally informed, not impartial, or not rational. If two people who hold this standard view are discussing a controversial moral issue and disagree with each other, each must regard the other as not fully informed, not impartial, or not rational. These are not the attitudes that make for a respectful and fruitful discussion of a controversial moral issue. However, if both hold the view that morality does not provide unique correct answers to all moral questions, then they may conclude, usually correctly, that this is one of these issues. Thus, they need not regard the other person's view as morally unacceptable, and can cooperate in trying to discover a compromise that comes closest to satisfying both of their positions.

It is usually clear if the disagreement is based on a difference about the scope of morality. Most disagreements about abortion and the treatment of animals have their source in that kind of difference, and almost no other moral disagreements have that as their source (see chapter 3). Most other moral disagreements have as their ultimate source a difference in the rankings of the goods and evils or a difference in the estimates of the harmful and beneficial consequences of everyone knowing that a certain kind of violation is allowed. Although differing interpretations of the moral rules are usually based on differences in the rankings or in the estimates, sometimes custom or tradition will determine the interpretation. When there is a conflict among interpretations, an impartial rational person will interpret a moral rule in a way that she regards as resulting in the least amount of overall harm. There is an almost complete parallel in the procedures to be used when deciding what violation of a moral rule is justified and when deciding which of two competing interpretations of a moral rule to adopt.

People who have served on hospital ethics committees or on similar ethical decision-making bodies know how liberating it is to realize that on the most controversial questions no one need be putting forward a wrong answer. This realization allows people to compromise without losing their moral integrity. It allows people to work together to find a solution that, while it may not completely satisfy anyone, satisfies everyone to some degree. It allows those in a subordinate decision-making capacity to accept the decision of the person who has the final authority for making a decision, while at the same time allowing that person to acknowledge the acceptability of alternative views. It allows people to try to persuade one another, without implying that the other person is wrong or lacking in intellect or character.

These features are also of great importance in political theory. To hold the standard view that there is a unique correct answer to every moral question does not naturally incline one to support a democratic form of government. Unless a person holds that there are insuperable epistemological obstacles to finding out the correct answer, the natural result of holding the standard view is to favor a government of those who are most likely to know the correct answers to moral questions. However, if, on the issues about which there are likely to be disagreements, there are often no unique correct answers, then it is most natural for a person to endorse reaching a decision that is favored by the most people. Only a theory that holds that, especially on controversial matters, there is often no unique correct answer provides a moral argument for democracy. Of course, any decision must be one that an impartial rational person could accept, but within these limits, there is often no best moral decision. A theory that does not provide a decision procedure that settles every moral problem allows for unresolvable moral disagreement. Such a theory might seem to be inferior to one that does provide such a decision procedure. However, more careful examination of both kinds of theories shows that the opposite is in fact true.

A complete moral theory should not be taken to be a theory that provides a unique correct answer to every moral question. Rather, a complete moral theory should explain and justify the overwhelming agreement on most moral matters, while at the same time explaining and justifying the limited disagreement on some of the most important moral matters. Moral theories that provide no explanation or justification for unresolvable moral disagreement are incomplete; those that claim there are no unresolvable moral disagreements are false. Beauchamp and Childress do say, "Neither morality nor ethical theory has the resources to provide a single solution to every moral problem" (24). However, they do not seem to realize that a complete moral theory must explain this fact, and must be helpful in pointing out the source of the disagreement. It is interesting that our theory fulfills the "eight conditions for an ethical theory" (338–340) that Beauchamp and Childress propose, far better than any other theory that they discuss, including their own.

A complete moral theory must not only provide analyses of the three concepts that are central to any account of morality, that of morality itself, and of impartiality and rationality, it must also show how these concepts are related to one another. A complete theory must also relate morality to human nature, making it clear why any beings having the essential features of human nature such as fallibility, rationality, and vulnerability would develop a public guide to conduct with all of the features of our common morality. Although common morality is a system, it does not remove the need for human judgment. It is true that common morality is systematic enough that a computer could be programmed so that, provided with the facts of the case, it always comes up with acceptable moral answers. However, another computer could be programmed differently and still always come up with acceptable but different answers. There is no computer program that can tell you which of the competing computer programs you should adopt.

The Principles in Historical Context

To understand the historical background of principlism's pervasive influence, it is helpful to review the "Belmont Report," which is the progenitor of the principles. The principles emerged from the work of the National Commission for the Protection of Human Subjects of Biomedical and Behavioral Research, which was created by Congress in 1974. One of the charges to the Commission was to identify the basic ethical principles that should underlie the conduct of biomedical and behavioral research involving human subjects, and to develop guidelines that should be followed to assure that such research is conducted in accordance with those principles.[6]

At that time there was frustration over the many and various rules for research that were spelled out in the extant codes covering research using human subjects. These codes included the Nuremberg Code of 1947, the Helsinki Declaration of 1964 (revised in 1975), and the 1971 Guidelines issued by the (then) U.S. Department of Health, Education, and Welfare. (The "Guidelines" were codified into U.S. Federal Regulations in 1974.) The assortment of rules seemed at times inadequate, conflicting, and difficult to apply. It therefore became part of the Commission's charge to formulate "broader ethical principles [to] provide a basis on which specific rules may be formulated, criticized and interpreted."[7]

The higher level of generality was achieved by the Commission and articulated as three ethical principles: the principle of respect for persons, the principle of beneficence, and the principle of justice. These principles comprised the "Belmont Report," so named because their articulation was the culmination of intense discussions that took place at the Smithsonian Institution's Belmont Conference Center. In effect, these principles sought to frame in a more general and useful way the moral concerns that underlay the diverse, ambiguous, and (sometimes) conflicting rules comprising the various ethical codes related to research on human subjects.

The work of the Commission was significant. It was insightful and helpful; it elegantly captured in a more general way the basic moral concerns haltingly expressed in the miscellaneous codes. The Commission also went on to delineate some of the more practical consequences of the principles. From the principle of respect for persons came attention to autonomy (which from the Commission's discussion seems more like what is now regarded as "competence") and to informed consent. From the principle of beneficence came the obligation to maximize benefits over risks and the obligation not to harm. From the principle of justice came attention to fairness in the distribution of the benefits and burdens of research.

These principles were clearly intended to be generalized guides for protecting humans as subjects in biomedical and behavioral research. Also, they seem less to have been derived from a theory of any sort and more to be abstractions from ethical rules expressing particular moral concerns. In a summary fashion, the principles generalize and encapsulate a variety of moral considerations especially applicable to research using human subjects. Very likely these formulations additionally accomplished a crucial maneuver for the Commission. They made possible a consensus in a setting where a more detailed account of morality probably never would have been agreed upon.

From these beginnings the application of the principles has grown and now encompasses biomedical ethics in general. Each principle has changed somewhat as its meaning is elaborated, as subdivision takes place, and as another principle or two is added (varying with each author). For example, for Beauchamp and Childress, the principle of beneficence spawns the principle of nonmaleficence. But, in one form or another, these principles have come to dominate the field of bioethics, which is why we are investigating several principles in detail.

Our overall impression of the principles is that they express something very important, something very basic to common moral intuitions. However, they are inadequate and misleading when presented as a general account of common morality, a moral theory, or even an account of morality in medicine or a bio-ethical theory. Our plan is to show how our more systematic account of common morality can encompass and preserve what is good about the principles, while eliminating their unfortunate features. We see them as historically providing a conceptual crutch that allowed the field to achieve certain insights and goals. But having enabled that achievement, the crutch is best set aside because it has prevented further progress and has even become cumbersome.

Critique of Principlism: Our General Approach

Although we have been referring to principlism as a theory, it is not in fact a theory, but rather a collection of "principles" that together are popularly but mistakenly thought to function as a theory in guiding action. Principlism puts forward certain principles that it considers to be the high-level "action guides" most relevant for dealing with issues of biomedical ethics. A variety of principles are claimed by different authors to be "the principles of biomedical ethics," but the best known and most frequently cited principles are those labeled "the principle of autonomy," "the principle of nonmaleficence," "the principle of beneficence," and "the principle of justice." Because these four occur, by far, most frequently together (and thus are more apt to pose as a theory of biomedical ethics) and because these are the ones espoused by Beauchamp and Childress, they are the ones we analyze in order to contrast and compare them with our own account of common morality.

In this chapter we argue that principlism is mistaken about the nature of morality and is misleading about the foundations of ethics. We argue that its "principles" are really misnomers since, when examined carefully, they are not useful action guides at all. They provide a guide only when no guide is needed; when guidance is needed, they are of no use. Traditionally, principles are action guides that summarize and encapsulate a whole theory, as the principle of utility does for utilitarianism. Thus, in a shorthand manner, the principle of utility provides a moral agent with guidance—in this case unfortunately mistaken—in making a moral decision. Those kinds of principles are to be clearly distinguished from those of principlism. We believe that the principles of principlism primarily function to focus attention on issues worth remembering when one is considering a biomedical moral issue. "Consider this . . . consider that . . . remember to look for . . ." is what they tell the agent; they do not provide an articulated, established, and unified moral system capable of providing useful guidance.

These principles presumably follow from several different moral theories, though that connection is not clearly stated by the proponents of principlism.

This is a matter of significant concern, since there seem to be no underlying connections among the principles. They do not grow out of a common foundation and there is no systematic relationship among them. Although each may be an expression of one or another important and traditional concern of morality, their relationship with one another is never discussed. Specification is presented as general procedure for resolving the conflicts that inevitably arise between principles, but there is no guide for how one is supposed to specify a principle. This serves to perpetuate what we have called the "anthology syndrome." This, as described in chapter 1, is a kind of relativism espoused (perhaps unwittingly) by many books (usually anthologies) of bioethics. They parade before the reader a variety of "theories" of ethics (Kantian deontology, utilitarianism, other forms of consequentialism, virtue theory, etc.), and say, in effect, "Choose the theory, maxim, principle, or rule that best suits you." Similarly, although each of the principles of principlism embodies a key concern from one or another theory of morality, no account is given of whether (or how) they are related to one another. We conclude that principlism obscures and confuses moral reasoning by its failure to provide useful action guides and by its eclectic and unsystematic account of morality.

We begin our analysis with a brief discussion of the principles of nonmaleficence and justice in order to set the context for our argument. Then we discuss in more detail the principles of autonomy and beneficence in order to demonstrate the force of our arguments against principlism. These latter two were chosen not only because they are the principles most often employed in discussion of biomedical ethics but also because they best illustrate the more problematic aspects of principlism. In particular, we show that principlism embodies the inadequacies of most previous accounts of morality by failing to appreciate the significance of the distinction between moral rules and moral ideals, by misrepresenting the ordinary concept of duty, and by failing to realize that morality is a public system that applies to all moral agents.

The Principle of Nonmaleficence

This is the one principle for which we have a strong affinity because, as chapter 2 makes clear, the key insight expressed by the principle of nonmaleficence is also a major orientation of our account of morality. This is the only one of the four principles that does not blur the distinction between moral rules and moral ideals. Indeed, this principle is most reasonably interpreted as merely summarizing some of the moral rules. The moral rules "Don't kill," "Don't cause pain," and "Don't disable" are clearly included in this principle, and probably the rule "Don't deprive of pleasure" is as well. Even the rule "Don't deprive of freedom" should be included in the principle of nonmaleficence, but those who follow principlism seem to prefer to give freedom a principle of its own, which they call the principle of autonomy. However, we see no reason for distin-guishing the rule, "Do not deprive of freedom," from the other four rules, for all five of these rules proscribe causing what are universally recognized as evils (or harms), that is, death, pain, disability, loss of freedom, and loss of pleasure.

The principle of nonmaleficence does no more than simply collapse four or five moral rules into one more general rule, "Do not cause harm." That general rule, "*Primum non nocere*," is often taken as the first principle of medicine. It is primarily a matter of purpose and style whether one prefers to list five distinct moral rules or to have one general principle that includes them all. We prefer the former because it makes more salient the fact that there are different kinds of harms (or evils) and that rational persons can and do rank them differently. Not only is neglecting the fact that there are different rational rankings one of the primary causes of unjustified paternalism, it is also one explanation for the popularity of the mistaken view that all moral questions have a unique correct answer. Thus, insofar as recognizing that there are different kinds of harms that morality prohibits causing that must be explicitly and carefully stated sooner or later, the gain in simplicity of having just one general principle is minimal and transitory at best. Nonetheless, this principle, even as it stands, has no major problems. That fact is not surprising since it is the only one of the principles that is not an invention of philosophers, but is a long-standing principle of medicine.

The Principle of Justice

Our discussion of justice is equally brief, but not for the same reasons. Not only is this principle not similar to any specific moral rule, it does not even pretend to provide a guide to action. It is doubtful that even the proponents of principlism put much stock in it as an action guide. The "principle of justice" is the prime example of a principle functioning simply as a checklist of moral concerns. It amounts to no more than saying that one should be concerned with matters of distribution; it recommends just or fair distribution without endorsing any par-ticular account of justice or fairness. Thus, as used by principlism, the principle of justice, in effect, is merely a chapter heading under which one might find sophisticated discussions of various theories of justice. After reading such a chapter one might be better informed and more sensitive to the differing theories of justice, but when dealing with an actual problem of distribution, one would be baffled by the injunction to "apply the principle of justice."

The principle of justice shares an additional problem with the two remaining principles: it blurs the distinction between what is morally required (obeying moral rules) and what is morally encouraged (following moral ideals). Since the principle of justice cannot be taken seriously as an action guide, this blurring is not as obvious as in the two remaining principles. In this, as in other matters, principlism simply takes over errors of those theories that suggested the four principles in the first place. For example, the most prominent contemporary discussion of justice is by John Rawls (1971). In *A Theory of Justice*, Rawls describes what he calls the duty of justice as follows:

This duty requires us to support and to comply with just institutions that exist and apply to us. It also constrains us to further just arrangements not yet established, at least when this can be done without too much cost to ourselves.[8]

Rawls includes in what he regards as a single duty (1) the moral rule requiring one to obey (just) laws, and (2) the moral ideal encouraging one to help make just laws, without even realizing the significant difference between these two guides to action.[9] As we show later, this failure to distinguish between what is morally required (obeying moral rules) and what is morally encouraged (following moral ideals) creates significant problems for codes of ethics and also creates significant confusion in both the principle of autonomy and the principle of beneficence.

The Principle of Autonomy

This principle seems to be the centerpiece of principlism. It is cited more frequently than any of the others and has taken on a life of its own. The concept of autonomy has come to dominate discussions of medical ethics to the point that there is a growing and focused opposition to its supposed predominance. Attention is being drawn to concerns that outweigh autonomy; its primacy over all of the other principles is being questioned. It is to the credit of Beauchamp and Childress that they make it clear that other considerations sometimes outweigh autonomy.[10] But these developments are only symptomatic of deeper theoretical problems with autonomy as a principle. Beauchamp and Childress state the principle of respect for autonomy in two ways:

This principle can be stated as negative obligation and as a positive obligation. As a *negative obligation: Autonomous actions should not be subjected to controlling constraints by others.* The principle asserts a broad, abstract obligation that is free of exceptive clauses, such as "We must respect individuals' views and rights so long as their thoughts and actions do not seriously harm other persons." This principle of respect for autonomy needs specification in particular cases to become a practical action guide." (64)

As stated here it is surprisingly akin to the principle of nonmaleficence and, as such, we, of course, have little disagreement with it. In fact, it seems to pick out just one evil, the loss of freedom, and gives it a principle all to itself. Interpreted simply as an alternative formulation of the moral rule "Do not deprive of freedom," we have no objection to this principle, for it is a genuine action guide in that it prohibits constraining others' actions.[11] However, the principle does not say simply that one should not constrain another's actions and choices, but rather it says that one should not constrain another's *autonomous* actions and choices. The principle does not prohibit constraining non-autonomous choices and actions. Consequently, the distinction between autonomous and non-autonomous actions takes on great moral significance. What counts as an autonomous choice or action becomes a matter of fundamental moral concern; thus, the addition of the word "autonomous" causes many problems in applying the principle of autonomy. These problems manifest themselves in the account of paternalism that Beauchamp and Childress provide.

As a positive obligation, the principle requires respectful treatment in disclosing information and fostering autonomous decision-making. In some cases we are obligated to increase the options available to persons. . . . As some contemporary Kantians declare, the demand that we treat others as ends, requires that we assist persons in achieving their ends and foster their capacities as agents, not merely that we avoid treating them solely as means to our ends.

Here we see the same mistake that Rawls made in describing the duty of justice: including in one so-called duty both a moral rule and a moral ideal. Unless Beauchamp and Childress are describing the professional duties of health care workers, no principle requires us to assist persons in achieving their ends. Beauchamp and Childress do sometimes present their four principles as a way of grouping the special duties of health care workers, but they do this most often when talking about the principles of autonomy and beneficence. It is quite clear that the principle of nonmaleficence is a principle of general morality and is not restricted to health care workers at all. It is difficult to know what to say about the principle of justice, as it does not offer any specific action guide at all. It may be that Beauchamp and Childress's uncertainty about whether to regard the principles of autonomy and beneficence as general moral principles or as ways of grouping the duties of health care workers is what leads them to overlook the important distinction between moral rules and moral ideals.

Autonomous Actions and Choices

In practice, the basic difficulty with autonomy, dogging it throughout all its uses, is knowing whether or not the actions and choices one is concerned with are autonomous. Is one's choice to give up drinking the autonomous choice or is the autonomous choice to continue drinking? Is the choice to withdraw from expensive life-prolonging treatment to save his family money and anguish the autonomous choice, or is the autonomous choice the decision to go on living a while longer? Which choice is it that one is being admonished not to constrain? If there is a conflict between people who differ on which choice of the patient is the autonomous one, each side will appeal to the principle of autonomy for support. One side may favor overruling a patient's refusal using the fact that the refusal is irrational as showing that the choice is not autonomous; whereas the other side may favor going along with the patient's explicitly stated refusal on the grounds that although the refusal is irrational, the patient is competent and therefore the refusal is an autonomous choice. Both sides can sincerely claim that they are acting on the principle of autonomy by respecting the autonomous choice. Autonomy is such a fundamentally ambiguous and disputed concept that "the principle of respect for autonomy" can be used to support two completely opposing ways of acting, even when there is no disagreement on the observable facts of the case and there are no cultural differences. Such a principle is obviously not a useful guide to action.

There are times when it is appropriate to question whether a patient has made an "autonomous" choice, for example, when he is delirious, intoxicated, or under the influence of drugs, and the views he expresses significantly differ from those he expresses when he is in a normal state. But why appeal to autonomy? It is sufficient to appeal to the delirium and the sudden change of views. Those, after all, are the only evidences for a "non-autonomous" choice.

More important, when the significant departure from previously expressed views is not temporary and not explained by medical reasons, then it is misleading and unhelpful to focus on the question of whether a patient's choices are autonomous. The correct application of the metaphysical label of "autonomous" to a patient's choices is a matter of long-standing philosophical dispute. That there is no clear ordinary use of the term that is helpful in resolving any of the difficult cases may explain why Beauchamp and Childress provide no examples of the use of their account of autonomy to solve any such cases. Following the principle of autonomy may even encourage one to act with unjustified paternalism, that is, to overrule the patient's explicit refusal, simply because one views that choice as not being autonomous. Thus, the principle of autonomy may lead one to deprive a person of freedom without an adequate justification for doing so.

A more adequate method for dealing with such problems is by using the concepts of "rational" and "irrational" as presented in chapter 2. Only if a person's decision concerning his own health care is seriously irrational is overruling it justified (see chapter 10). If a person's decision concerning his own health care is rational, overruling that decision is not justified. Suppose, for example, that a patient has thoughtfully and persistently throughout his life insisted that if he contracts terminal cancer he wants no treatment at all. But now that he has cancer that is regarded as terminal (and the patient is anxious, stressed, and drugged), he says he wants life-prolonging treatment. Health care professionals would be hard pressed to decide what to do on the basis of whether or not this was an autonomous decision (after all, it was a sudden change of mind, under the influence of drugs and stress, etc.). However, the patient's current decision in favor of treatment is clearly not irrational, and hence, on our account, should not be overridden. (We discuss this matter in considerable detail in chapters 10 and 12.) It is interesting that Beauchamp and Childress do not even attempt to provide an answer to any controversial case in bioethics.

Moral Rules and Moral Ideals: A Fundamental Distinction

At the core of many problems with the principle of autonomy, as with the principle of beneficence, is its general failure to recognize the significance of the distinction between what is morally encouraged (following the moral ideals) and what is morally required (obeying the moral rules). Many philosophers, including Kant and Mill, have made this distinction, or, rather, one that seems closely related to it, by distinguishing between duties of perfect obligation and duties of imperfect obligation ("perfect" and "imperfect" duties). However, this indiscriminate use of the term "duty" (a matter we discuss later in connection with beneficence) has resulted in this crucial distinction not being made in the correct way. On a correct understanding, the first five moral rules, discussed above in chapter 2, are examples of perfect duties. So also are the second five moral rules requiring one not to deceive, not to cheat, not to break promises, not to disobey the law, and not to neglect one's duty (in the normal sense of that term). A person has no choice in deciding when to follow "perfect duties" or with regard to whom they must be followed; she is allowed to violate a perfect duty only when she has an adequate justification for doing so.

On the other hand, the moral ideals are "imperfect duties," that is, duties in which a person has a choice in deciding when to follow them and with regard to whom. This is because imperfect duties are impossible to follow either impartially or all of the time. Working to help the downtrodden is an example. A person must pick and choose not only which of the downtrodden to help but also when and where she will provide this help. Furthermore, she may even choose not to act on that imperfect duty at all, but rather to act on some other imperfect duty such as preventing the deprivation of freedom of someone, somewhere. It seems as if an imperfect duty is a duty that a person is not required to act on at all; morality certainly does not require people to work for either Oxfam or for Amnesty International, let alone both. It is not morally required to give to or work for any charity, although morality certainly encourages such behavior. Giving to charity is an imperfect duty (moral ideal); it is not a perfect duty (moral rule).

Because this traditional distinction between perfect and imperfect duties embodies a confusion about the notion of duty, we make the distinction in a different and less misleading fashion. Moral rules prohibit acting in ways that cause, or increase the risk of, others suffering some harm or evil. That is precisely what morality requires. Moral ideals, on the other hand, encourage the prevention and relief of harm, but, unless one has a duty to do so, morality does not require following those ideals. A person may have a duty that requires such prevention or relief, but then the circumstances that give rise to the duty are specified and limited (e.g., a nurse has a duty to relieve the pain of her patients). The moral rules must be followed all the time, toward everyone, impartially, but that is impossible in the case of the moral ideals. Doing what morality requires, that is, obeying the moral rules, is usually not praiseworthy; rather, it is expected, and failing to do so makes a person liable to punishment. Doing what morality encourages, that is, following the moral ideals, is usually praiseworthy and failing to do so is not punishable. The distinction between moral rules and moral ideals is crucial for a proper understanding of common morality or the moral system.

The phrases "perfect duties" and "imperfect duties" obscure this crucial distinction between moral rules and moral ideals. The ordinary use of "duty" suggests that a person is required to do what he has a duty to do, and punishment is deserved when he fails to do his duty. After all, it is morally required to obey the moral rules impartially all of the time. For example, depriving persons of their freedom (principlism might call this violating their autonomy) always requires an adequate justification. But, unless a person has a professional duty to do so, she does not need a justification for failing to help persons to achieve their ends (principlism might call this promoting their autonomy). In the absence of such a duty, helping people to achieve their ends is following a moral ideal. Common morality certainly encourages helping people but, except in special circumstances, it does not require doing so.

Autonomy as Rule and Ideal

The principle of autonomy requires respect for autonomy, but it fails to distinguish clearly between "respecting (not violating) autonomy" and "promoting autonomy." Not distinguishing clearly between "respecting autonomy" and "promoting autonomy" inevitably leads to confusion. Compounded by the search for the "genuinely" autonomous actions and choices, the principle of autonomy invites a kind of activism where an agent promotes those choices and actions of another that the agent regards as the other's autonomous choices and actions, even though that involves depriving that person of freedom. For example, suppose a woman is pregnant with a fetus that tests have shown to be severely defective. The woman, who wants to have an abortion, consults a counselor. The counselor, knowing that the woman has always been "a good Catholic" sees her own duty to be that of dissuading the woman from having an abortion. The counselor's reason is that the decision to have an abortion is not an autonomous choice.[12] Such manipulation conflicts with morality itself insofar as it leads one to deprive people of freedom simply in order to promote what one decides is (or should be) their autonomous choice. Thus, principlism's centerpiece "principle of autonomy" embodies a dangerous level of confusion. That confusion is created by unclarity as to what counts as autonomous actions and choices and the additional blurring of a basic moral distinction between moral rules and moral ideals. This unnecessary introduction of the confused and disputed concept of autonomy inevitably results in making it more difficult to think clearly about moral problems. The goal of moral philosophy is to clarify moral thinking, not to introduce new and unnecessary complications.

As an aside, it is worth observing that the principle of autonomy probably caught on so tenaciously in the last three decades for many reasons. One is that Kantian ethics was experiencing a renaissance and that his notion of autonomy was central to his account of morality. A second is that the society became increasingly aware that the medical profession was so markedly paternalistic that patient self-determination was almost nonexistent. A third was that the increase in medical technology resulted in several rational alternative treatments. A fourth was the aging of the population and the resulting increase in chronic diseases that could not be cured, only managed. Many elderly patients often know nearly as much about managing their chronic diseases as their physicians. A fifth, the combination of the increase in medical technology that could keep extremely sick people alive for a long time, together with an aging population that often had a rational desire not to be kept alive, even made it rational to refuse life-prolonging treatment. So the emphasis on autonomy became the banner under which patients rallied to gain more control over their own health care. Allowing the patient to decide what, if any, treatment he would receive became the main issue, and thus momentum and conviction, rather than conceptual clarity or theoretical sound-ness, perpetuated the emphasis on autonomy. Even the fact that the principle of autonomy did not really embody Kant's notion of autonomy did not detract from the overwhelming political appeal of invoking the principle.

An example of how confused the general understanding of autonomy is can be seen by examining Kant's view of autonomy. On Kant's view, a person is not acting autonomously if he kills himself or allows himself to die because of intractable pain. To do so is to allow pleasure and pain (which, according to Kant, are not part of the rational self) to determine one's actions. Thus, such suicide or allowing oneself to die is not an autonomous action of the rational self. To act autonomously one must always act in accord with the Categorical Imperative. In *The Grounding of the Metaphysics of Morals*, Kant explicitly states that the Categorical Imperative requires one not to commit suicide be-cause of pain. By way of contrast, one of the major arguments in favor of allowing people to die when they are suffering from intractable pain is the principle of autonomy. The seeds of confusion were present in the initial planting of the concept of autonomy. This explains, in part, why we prefer the simple rule "Don't deprive of freedom" to the principle of autonomy for pro-tecting the patient from paternalistic intervention.

The Principle of Beneficence

As used by principlism (165), the principle of beneficence suffers shortcom-ings similar to those of autonomy. As popularly used in the biomedical ethics literature, this principle is cited simply to give "validation" both to preventing or relieving harm and to doing good or conferring benefits. Beauchamp and Childress claim, "Positive beneficence requires agents to provide benefits." They now make a distinction between obligatory and ideal beneficence, and realize that "we are not morally required to perform all possible acts of generosity or charity that would benefit others."[13] Nonetheless they claim:

"the principle of positive beneficence does support an array of more specific rules of obligation . . . Examples of these rules of beneficence, in their most general forms, are:

1. Protect and defend the rights of others.
2. Prevent harm from occurring to others.
3. Remove conditions that will cause harm to others.
4. Help persons with disabilities.
5. Rescue persons in danger"[14]

Thus, according to Beauchamp and Childress, we are morally required to follow these rules. But responding to criticism that this mistakenly treats the principle of beneficence as if it were the principle of nonmaleficence, they provide several distinctions between the rules that follow from this principle and the rules that follow from the principle of nonmaleficence. The former rules require positive action and need not be obeyed impartially; failure to follow them normally does not make one liable to punishment. These are just the features that distinguish moral rules from moral ideals, that is, that distinguish what is morally required from what is morally encouraged. Why then do Beauchamp and Childress continue to regard these rules of beneficence as morally required? There are at least two reasons. The first is that sometimes there is a genuine duty to rescue, namely, when the person would suffer great harm if you did not help, it is relatively cost free to help, and you are in physical proximity to the person and in a unique or close to unique position to help. But that you have a duty in these special circumstances does not warrant the general moral requirements that Beauchamp and Childress derive from the principle of benevolence.

The second reason is the result of a common confusion, namely, that only obligations or requirements can override obligations. Beauchamp and Childress say, "Not only do various norms of beneficence establish obligations, but the obligations are sufficiently strong that they sometimes override *obligations of nonmaleficence.* . . . If there were no obligations of beneficence—only moral ideals of beneficence—such actions would be unjustified."[15] Unfortunately, they support this claim by citing actions of governments, without realizing that governments can sometimes be justified in acting on moral and utilitarian ideals when individuals would not be justified to act in this fashion. But their more serious mistake is holding that moral ideals cannot justify violating a moral rule. We have already shown this to be false, but we can do so again, using Beauchamp and Childress's own limited notion of what counts as acting on a moral ideal. I have made a promise to meet someone for dinner, and on my way to dinner, I see a burning building with some children trapped inside. There are many other people watching and I have no special skills or training, but since no one else is making an effort to rescue the children, despite the great risk to myself, I decide to do so. Does my clearly ideal action justify my breaking my promise to meet someone for dinner? If Beauchamp and Childress had a systematic account of morality, they would see immediately that in these circumstances, following a moral ideal strongly justifies the violation of a moral rule.

As is evident from the examples that Beauchamp and Childress offer, the principle of beneficence is now conceived almost entirely as preventing or relieving harms, not with promoting benefits for those who are not deprived. Thus, although they criticize us for making the avoiding and preventing of evil central to morality, as opposed to promoting goods, they have moved almost completely in that former direction. However, since the principle is called the principle of beneficence, they still fail to distinguish between the preventing or relieving of harms and the conferring of benefits (promoting goods). This distinction is especially important in medicine, inasmuch as preventing or relieving harms often justifies violating a moral rule without consent, whereas conferring benefits (or promoting goods) rarely, if ever, does.

Beneficence and the Concept of Duty

Although Beauchamp and Childress have taken our criticisms about their misuse of the term "duty" seriously, and have eliminated the frequent references to "the duty of beneficence," they still say, "Deontological restraints are essentially negative duties—that is, they specify what we cannot justifiably do to others, even in the pursuit of worthy goals."[16] These deontological restraints are what both we and Beauchamp and Childress regard as the rules of common morality. Thus, they still seem to hold that we have a duty not to violate any of the moral rules. But since one of the moral rules is "Do your duty," this would result in people having a duty to do their duty. Such usage distorts and obscures the primary meaning of "duty," which specifically refers to the particular duties that come with one's role, occupation, profession, or special circumstances. Though it is correct to say "One ought not to kill" or "One ought to help the downtrodden," it creates significant confusion to regard these "oughts" as "duties." For some philosophers, "Do your duty" has come to mean no more than "Do what you morally ought to do." But using the term "duty" in this way makes it very difficult to talk about real duties, for example, those associated with people's occupations and whose content is determined by the members of those occupations or professions and the society in which they live. For reasons of conceptual soundness and clarity, we use the term "duty" only in its ordinary sense, that is, to refer to what is required by one's role in society, particularly by one's occupation, profession, relationship as family member, or one's special circumstances. It is not only misleading to talk of the moral ideals as *imperfect* duties, it is also misleading to talk of the moral rules as *perfect* duties.

"Do your duty" is a distinct moral rule on a par with the other moral rules; it is not a meta-rule telling one to obey the other moral rules. However, morality does put a limit on what counts as a duty: there can be no duty to violate unjustifiably any of the other moral rules. "Do your duty" is justified as a moral rule because of the harm, and significantly increased risk of harm that is caused by a person's failure to do that which others are justifiably counting on being done. People are morally required to do their duty, but it generates confusion to say that people have a duty to do their duty.

In medicine it is especially misleading to use the principle of beneficence as if it creates a general duty for all health care workers. Again, this obscures the role of real duties, that is, the special duties that come with one's role or profession. Beauchamp and Childress recognize the significant difference between what they call the general duty of beneficence and the specific duties of beneficence. They state, "Obligations of specific beneficence usually rest on special moral relations (for example, in families and friendships) or on special commitments, such as explicit promises and roles with attendant responsibilities."[17] They are clear that doctors, nurses, and others in the health care field have specific duties to their patients that are determined by their profession and by the practices of their specific institution. To lump these varied and detailed professional duties together with the misconceived "general duty of beneficence" and place them all under one principle of beneficence is to substitute a slogan for substance.

Principlism Versus Common Morality as a Public System

Principlism fails to appreciate that common morality is a public system that applies to all moral agents, thus, it must be known to and understood by all moral agents and it cannot be irrational for any of them to follow it. This failure to recognize that all justified violations of a moral rule must be part of a public system that applies to everyone, that is, that it must be rational to favor everyone knowing that this kind of violation is allowed, is a serious flaw. This failure to appreciate that morality is a public system is most clearly seen in act utilitarianism, a theory that requires everyone always to act so as to produce the best overall consequences in the particular situation, regardless of the consequences of everyone knowing that they are allowed to act in that kind of way.

Rule utilitarianism is, properly speaking, not a consequentialist moral system, for rules as well as consequences are involved in making a moral judgment about a particular act. Nonetheless, even rule utilitarianism does not appreciate the fact that morality is a public system. It claims that those rules that would have the best consequences if generally obeyed are moral rules. It does not require that those rules be known by all those who are subject to them. More important, a rule utilitarian has significant problems in dealing with exceptions to the rules. If a rule utilitarian tries to avoid the problem of justified exceptions by incorporating the exceptions into the rule itself, the rule becomes indefinitely long and, as such, it cannot be part of a public system known by all rational persons. This is similar to what happens in principlism because the principles must be continually modified by being specified. Common morality has rules that are simple, general, that do not change, and are known by all.

If a rule utilitarian adopts simple and general rules, she must determine how particular violations of a rule are justified. She must decide whether to (1) consider only the consequences of her doing this particular act at this particular time, or (2) consider the consequences of everyone knowing that they are allowed to do that kind of act in the same morally relevant circumstances. If a rule utilitarian is contemplating cheating on an exam or deceiving someone and chooses the first option, then her decision is often at odds with what morality requires. If she chooses the second option, she is no longer even a rule utilitarian. Rule utilitarianism must determine justified exceptions by appealing to actual or foreseeable consequences of the particular act. Common morality determines justified exceptions by appealing to the purely hypothetical consequences of *everyone knowing* that they are allowed to break the rule in the same morally relevant circumstances. If those exceptions are better than the consequences of *everyone knowing* that they are not allowed to break the rule, the violation is justified. Common morality requires consideration of these hypothetical consequences because such consideration is essential for obeying the moral rules impartially.

Neither act nor rule utilitarianism appreciates that for an act to be morally acceptable it must be one that can be publicly allowed. Thus, no principle derived from utilitarianism, such as the principle of beneficence, can be relied on to produce valid moral conclusions. Not surprisingly, the principle of beneficence, more than the other principles, is most affected by this failure to appreciate that morality is a public system. When the consequences of a particular violation of a rule (e.g., cheating) are good but the consequences of that kind of violation being publicly allowed are bad, principlism has serious problems. Since the principle of beneficence considers only the consequences, direct and indirect, of a particular violation of a moral rule, it often encourages acting in a kind of way that, if publicly allowed, would lead to bad consequences. Indeed, we suspect that it is because of this tendency of the principle of beneficence to lead to what everyone regards as morally unacceptable conclusions that the principle of autonomy has attained such prominence in principlism. That is, the principle of autonomy is meant to overrule beneficence in all those cases where no rational person would publicly allow the kind of behavior that the principle of beneficence seems to require.

Consider a case in which a physician's breach of confidentiality will result in some very good consequences for her patient. Yet, if intuitively it seems clearly wrong to commit the breach, the principle of autonomy can then be brought in as the reason for not following the principle of beneficence. The problem, of course, is that sometimes beneficence should outweigh autonomy, but principlism provides neither a systematic way of determining which should prevail in any particular conflict nor an explanation of why, in some situations, impartial rational persons will disagree about which should prevail. Proponents of principlism now say that the principles must be specified, but they provide no instructions about how to specify. Nor do they realize that the specified principle is not known to all the people to whom it applies. Thus, principlism simply says to specify the principles involved without providing any instructions on how to do that specification. Common morality has a clear procedure for handing such conflicts: after using the morally relevant features to determine the kind of violation; it compares the consequences of that kind of violation being publicly allowed with the consequences of its not being publicly allowed. Since the only cases in which an account of morality needs to be invoked explicitly are those in which the principles or rules, or rules and ideals conflict, it seems pointless to have an account of morality that provides no guidance on how to deal with or explain such conflicts.

Summary of Objections to the Principles

The traditional concept of an ethical principle has been one that embodies the moral theory that spawns it. As shorthand for the theory, it is used by itself to enunciate a meaningful directive for action because it has an established, unified theory standing behind it: "Do that act which creates the greatest good for the greatest number," "Maximize the amount of liberty compatible with a like liberty for all." The thrust of the directive is clear; its goal and intent are unambiguous. Of course, there are often ambiguities and differing interpretations with respect to how the principle applies to a particular situation, but the principle itself is never used with other principles that are in conflict with it. Furthermore, if a genuine theory has more than one general principle, the relationship between them is clearly stated, as in the case of Rawls's two principles of justice. Principlism, however, invokes four independent and often conflicting principles, and not only is there no ranking of these principles (which is good), there is no guide on how to resolve or explain the conflicts between them (which is bad).

The principles of principlism seem to function more as reminders of topics or concerns that the moral decision maker should review prior to decision. Except for the principle of nonmaleficence, they are not true action guides. The principle of justice is the clearest example of this. The principle of nonmaleficence is acceptable since it simply prohibits the causing of harm, and as such merely summarizes the first four or five moral rules. But since it does not specify what counts as the prohibited harms, it is less useful than it might be. Furthermore, since it does not make clear that there are different harms that different people rank differently, it is more misleading than it might be. Nonetheless, insofar as the principle of nonmaleficence is interpreted as "Don't cause harm," it at least meets the criterion of being morally required.

The principles of autonomy and of beneficence are more complicated. They actually sound like action guides; they seem to tell one how to act. But closer inspection shows that they generate confusion. If the principle of autonomy were an action guide, like nonmaleficence, simply telling one not to deprive of freedom, then of course we would have no objection to it because it is now synonymous with that moral rule. But, unhappily, the principle of autonomy goes beyond that clear and defensible rule. It injects confusion because there is confusion and disagreement over the proper meaning of "autonomous action." Another troubling feature, as shown earlier, is that the principle also requires that moral agents promote one another's autonomy. That move, which fails to recognize the crucial moral distinction between moral rules and moral ideals means that the principle cannot be taken seriously as a moral requirement. If the principle is interpreted loosely to mean simply "Respect persons" (the original principle from which the principle of autonomy seems to have been derived), it is still not clear what that entails. At best it might mean, "Morality forbids you from treating others simply as you please. Some ways are acceptable and some are not. Think about it." So then one is back to interpreting the principles as a list of concerns.

The principle of beneficence also has an action guide appearance. It seems to be saying one has a duty to prevent harm as well as to help others. But Beauchamp and Childress now recognize that this principle is significantly different from the principle of nonmaleficence, for a person cannot possibly follow this principle impartially, all the time. Although Beauchamp and Childress now interpret this principle as being primarily concerned with moral ideals (the prevention of harms), they still do not explicitly distinguish these moral ideals from utilitarian ideals (the promotion of goods) that, except when special circumstances apply, cannot be used to justify the violation of a moral rule. Like utilitarianism, from which this principle is derived, having one follow it might lead to unjustified transgressions of moral rules toward the few in order to confer benefits on the many, thus triggering the use of the principle of autonomy.

Finally, we highlighted the more general difficulties with principlism. We noted that even if the individual principles are interpreted as action guides, they often conflict with one another. Since individual principles are not part of a public system, there is no agreed upon method for resolving these conflicts or understanding why a particular conflict cannot be resolved. Since they do not share a common ground, there is no underlying theory to appeal to for help in understanding or resolving conflicts. Indeed, each of the principles, in effect, seems to be a surrogate for the theory from which it is derived. The use of the principles seems to be an unwitting effort to allow the use of whatever ethical theory seems best suited to the particular problem one is considering. It is simply a sophisticated technique for dealing with problems ad hoc.

The appeal of principlism is that it makes use of some features of standard ethical theories that have popular support. But there is no attempt to see how these different features can be blended together as integrated parts of a single adequate theory, rather than disparate features derived from several competing theories. So, in effect, principlism tells agents to pick and choose as they see fit, as if one can sometimes be a Kantian and sometimes a utilitarian and sometimes something else, without worrying about consistency or whether the theory one is using is adequate or not. Principlism does not recognize that in order for a moral decision to be correct, it must be one that can be publicly allowed. It not only does not recognize the unified and systematic nature of morality, it does not recognize that the common moral system, or common morality, must be public.

The upshot of having principles with an unclear content, which are not part of any unified public system, is that an agent is not aware of the real grounds for his moral decision. Because the principles are not clear and direct imperatives at all, but simply a collection of suggestions and observations, occasionally conflicting, the agent cannot know what is really guiding his action. Nor do these principles tell him what facts are morally relevant, such that a change in them could change what he should do; thus, he is not able to propose better alternatives. Although the language of principlism suggests that the agent should apply principles that are morally well established, a closer look shows that he has looked at and weighed many diverse moral considerations, which are only superficially interrelated, having no unified, systematic, underlying foundation. Principles seem to be involved in complex decisions only in a purely verbal way; the real guiding influences on the moral decision are not the ones the agent believes them to be. Rather, the agent is, in fact, guided by his basic understanding of common morality, and only later cites principles when stating his conclusions, giving the illusion of theoretical support.

Concerning Specification

Our critiques of principlism have led those espousing it to search for a method of transforming the principles into actual action guides instead of a checklist of concerns.[18] The most prominent of these methods is known as "specification." Several articles put this method forth as the solution to some problems of principlism that we have pointed out.[19] Beauchamp and Childress completely embrace the notion in their most recent revision of *Principles of Biomedical Ethics*.[20] The embracing of specification by principlism shows that those supporting principlism recognize the need for a theory to explain and support it.

However, as far as we know, there is no explanation of where the appropriate specifications come from or how the narrowing of the application of the norms takes place. The moral system that we describe in chapter 2 makes it unnecessary to specify the rules, because common morality includes a two-step procedure for determining when it is justified to violate a moral rule. We do not, however, attempt to eliminate all disagreement. We not only acknowledge, we emphasize that equally informed, impartial, rational persons can differ, not only in how they rank the harms and benefits but also in their estimates of the consequences of everyone knowing that they are allowed to break the rule in the same morally relevant circumstances. Furthermore, as we made clear in chapter 3, we also allow impartial rational persons to differ about who is included in the group that is impartially protected, or protected at all, by morality. It is clear that in applying a principle or rule to a particular situation, one must identify the morally relevant features of the situation. However, without a detailed description of common morality, principlism provides no clue about how one determines what those morally relevant features are.

We conclude that the embrace of specification shows that principlism knows that it has serious problems. However, because specification accepts the view of principlism, it cannot move principlism very far. Specification does nothing about the crucial flaw of principlism, that it conceives of morality as consisting of several freestanding principles rather than recognizing that these principles must be embedded in a system. This system does not consist solely of the moral rules and ideals, it also includes the two-step procedure for deciding if a kind of violation of a moral rule is strongly justified, weakly justified, or unjustified. This procedure includes the morally relevant features of the situation that determine what counts as the same kind of violation. After providing a sufficiently detailed account of the common morality that thoughtful people use, usually implicitly, when making moral decisions and judgment, a moral theory must justify this system.

In most cases, our account of morality shows that the immorality of an action can be deduced from its description. For example, a clear-cut case of deception that results in significant harm to others in order to gain some benefits for the deceiver is immediately seen to be immoral by "deduction" from the moral rule prohibiting deception. However, although that is the most common and frequent kind of application of a moral rule to a situation, it is almost never discussed because there is no practical or theoretical reason to discuss it. No one doubts that the action is immoral, and because of this there is no point in discussing it. But an adequate moral theory must account for the common and uninteresting cases as well as the uncommon and interesting ones.

For these uncommon and interesting cases, the ones that are described in the medical ethics case books and discussed in all of the medical ethics anthologies and textbooks, our account of morality not only does not yield easy answers but also recognizes that there are unresolvable disagreements about what is the best solution to some of these problems. What our critics do not appreciate is that we recognize that morality is an *informal* public system. Like sandlot baseball, there is unspoken agreement on the point of the game and all of the fundamental rules. What causes problems is how one interprets the rules in the non-obvious cases. But without overwhelming agreement on most matters, the game would never even get started. Similarly, there is overwhelming agreement on the point of morality, the lessening of the suffering of evil or harm, and on all of the fundamental rules. But equally informed, rational, impartial persons can disagree on almost all interesting, non-obvious cases.

Our account of the moral system gives an account of how this can happen, for example, people can disagree on the ranking of harms to be avoided, they can disagree on the consequences of publicly allowing a kind of violation, they can disagree on the interpretation of the particular moral rule, or they can disagree on the scope of morality. We do not believe, and common morality does not require, that one and only one solution exists for each moral problem. We do not criticize principlism because it does not provide a unique answer to every moral problem, but rather because it does not explain in any useful way what is responsible for the disagreement and, hence, provides no help in resolving the disagreement.

Like principlism, our theory includes features from all of the classical theories. Unlike principlism, we do not merely formulate principles that call attention to the insights from these theories. Our theory incorporates the best features of each of these theories and eliminates those features of the previous theories that result in so many devastating counterexamples. Our theory, unlike all of the standard theories, not only explains and justifies the overwhelming agreement on most moral matters but also, as shown in chapter 3, explains the unresolvable disagreement on important controversial issues such as abortion. We look forward to continuing the dialogue we have had with Tom Beauchamp and James Childress. We have learned much from their criticisms and our theory is improved because of it. We find their discussions of particular issues to be among the best that we have read. Our criticisms of them are only on the level of theory, a level that was initially not an important concern of theirs. We think that they should continue to concentrate on the particular issues that are of concern to those in the health care fields. We believe that their discussion of these issues might even be improved if they come to appreciate that the systematic character of common morality does not conflict with unresolvable disagreement on some important controversial issues.

Notes

1. Perhaps in response to our previous criticisms, Beauchamp and Childress now claim that common morality is the basis of principlism. However, their account of common morality makes it sound remarkably like principlism. It consists solely of prohibitions and requirements, and there is no systematic procedure for resolving conflicts or showing that

they cannot be resolved. It is somewhat ironic that they claim that common morality is the basis of principlism, for we have continually used common morality as the basis of our criticism of principlism. See Clouser and Gert (1990 and 1994), Clouser (1995), Gert, Culver, and Clouser (2000), and Clouser and Gert (2004). It might be worth noting that the title of a recent version of Gert's moral theory is *Common Morality: Deciding What to Do* (2004).

2. Beauchamp and Childress (1979, 1983, 1989, 1994, and 2001).

3. See Emanuel (1995).

4. In a note (409n9) they acknowledge that we do provide a method for dealing with conflicts between rules, but not surprisingly, they criticize this method because it does not yield a unique answer to every conflict.

5. See Gert, Culver, and Clouser (2000).

6. This section is based on the Federal Register 44, no. 76 (1979): 23192–23197 (1974).

7. Ibid., 23193.

8. See Rawls (1971, 115); see also 334.

9. For further discussion of Rawls on this point, see Gert (1988), chapter 13.

10. Beauchamp and Childress (2001, 57): "A misguided criticism of our account is that the principle of respect for autonomy overrides all other principles. This we firmly deny."

11. Our earlier account of this rule was too narrow, corresponding closely with the statement of negative obligation of the principle of autonomy. We have benefited from criticism by James Childress and now include in the actions prohibited by this rule, touching without consent, and also some cases of unconsented to listening to and looking at.

12. For a more detailed account of the problems caused by autonomy in genetic counseling, and of the way in which using the common moral system can help deal with these problems, see chapter 6 of Gert, et al. (1996).

13. Beauchamp and Childress (2001, 167).

14. Ibid.

15. Ibid., 168.

16. Ibid., 353.

17. Ibid., 173.

18. See Clouser and Gert (1990, 219–236), and Clouser and Gert (1994, 251–266).

19. For example, DeGrazia (1992).

20. See Beauchamp and Childress (2001).

6

Malady

Introduction

The proper definition of "disease" (we subsume "disease" under our concept of "malady") is an issue that has been weaving in and out of bioethics for a long time.[1] There are some bioethical matters for which the concept of disease has seemed pivotal, while there are others in which it has seemed to play little or no role at all. Furthermore, not everyone agrees about when the concept applies and when it does not. Especially now, with the mapping of the human genome, the concept of (disease) malady deserves an in-depth explication, for example, there is no way to make the distinction between genetic therapy and genetic enhancement without a clear concept of genetic (disease) malady.

The concept of disease is interesting in and of itself, apart from any moral implications. It is the central concept of medicine and yet, at its core, it involves values, though what values and to what extent they play a role in defining the concept constitutes much of the debate in the literature. Compare medicine's basic concept of disease with the basic concepts of other sciences—cell, molecule, gene, neuron, electron, proton, positron—all of which are empirically, operationally, or contextually defined, without any element of values. Admittedly, medicine may not be a science, but it is certainly very closely related to science and is considered by many to be a science, so the possibility of a value element at its core is noteworthy.

Our plan is to explicate the concept of (disease) malady because it is so basic and because we believe it does enter into important bioethical issues, especially in genetics and psychiatry. It also has important implications for the kinds of conditions that should be covered by various health plans. A direct and significant consequence of our analysis is the clear conclusion that abnormality alone does not constitute a malady, and thus deviancy (e.g., having a genetic mutation or engaging in unusual sexual behavior) is not in and of itself sufficient for a condition to be a malady. This link between psychiatry and genetics is not accidental. The definition of mental disorder in the three most recent volumes of the *Diagnostic and Statistical Manual of Mental Disorders* (*DSM*) of the American Psychiatric Association have removed deviancy as a sufficient condition for a person being labeled as having a mental disorder. Some deviant behavior, for example, homosexual behavior, is no longer even included in the list of paraphilias. But when homosexuality was claimed to be linked to a deviant allele, some people said that this showed that homosexuality actually was a malady.

An Overview of Malady

Such terms as "disease," "illness," "sickness," "lesion," and "disorder" are often used interchangeably, but each has a unique connotation. Although "disease" is sometimes used to include all of these terms (e.g., medical textbooks sometimes call an injury a traumatic disease), such all-inclusiveness can be awkward in certain contexts. It is often misleading to use "disease" to refer to an injury, wound, defect, syndrome, trauma, or disfigurement. All these terms have specific connotations so that in certain situations one term is the most accurate label; for example, "wound" is more accurate if one has been stabbed with a knife. It is odd to refer to a knife wound or a leg broken in an accident as a "disease"; it is even more odd to refer to chickenpox as an injury. Nausea or a headache is probably better called an illness than a disease, since "illness" connotes the presence of symptoms, that is, that the afflicted individual is aware of pain or discomfort. On the other hand, "disease" suggests an identifiable underlying physiological process with an etiology and with distinct stages of development, all the signs of which may be present without the victim being aware of them, that is, without experiencing any symptoms. In fact, many people have diseases but do not feel ill at all, and may even feel better than normal, for example, those suffering from high blood pressure or from mania or hypomania.

Additional confusion exists because the conditions to which these terms refer overlap to some extent and the terms do not have consistent connotations. Ordinarily, syndromes advance to being diseases as the causes and stages become more clearly understood, yet often the syndrome label persists simply because of tradition, for example, Down syndrome. Another example of the somewhat arbitrary nature of disease-concept labeling is the condition experienced by deep-sea divers who return from the depths too quickly. It is called either "caisson disease" or "decompression illness," yet essentially all the ill effects are due to the cellular injury caused by nitrogen bubbles forming in various bodily tissues. Other conditions do not fit comfortably into any of the standard disease terms, for example, hernias and allergies.

Because of the plethora of terms with overlapping meanings and special connotations, we propose to give a new sense to the infrequently used general term "malady" so that it includes the referents of all of the other terms. As we use the term, "malady" refers to that which all the following words have in common: injury, illness, sickness, disease, trauma, wound, disorder, lesion, allergy, headache, and syndrome. We call all of them "maladies." What do they all have in common? Answering that question constitutes much of the work of this chapter. Our analysis of malady can be taken as an analysis of the expanded sense of "disease" as it is often used in medical textbooks (where, e.g., an injury is sometimes called a traumatic disease), namely to include the referents of all the terms listed above. We choose to use the term "malady" because such an expanded sense for the word "disease" is a significant distortion of the ordinary use of that term among both health professionals and lay individuals.

We approach the analysis of malady much as we approached the analysis of common morality in chapter 2. We want to capture what is common in the meaning of all the terms listed in the previous paragraph. We are not inventing a new concept, but we are making explicit and thereby calling attention to what is common in the meaning of all these terms. We are giving that commonality the name "malady," which is an old but very useful term that carries its meaning on its sleeve. There is no word in the English language that serves this overarching purpose, that is, one that is a genus term, of which "disease," "injury," and so on, are species terms.[2] However, there is a need for such a word in order to refer to all of these conditions without being locked in to one or another of their special connotations. The all-encompassing word "malady" also helps to maintain focus on the search for what the referents of all of the individual terms have in common.

During the last thirty years, analyses of the concept of disease have dwelled on the term's purported subjectivity and value-ladenness as if those two terms necessarily went together. But as we showed in the chapter on morality, some values, that is, goods and evils or harms and benefits, are universal and their presence or absence can be objectively determined. We argue strongly for malady being value laden but nevertheless objective. Our goal is to put the concept on a more stable footing, less subject to whimsy and manipulation. In the past, a malady label, especially "mental disorder," has been used to try to accomplish a variety of personal and political agendas, in particular to enforce conformity. This is one of the reasons to deny that abnormality is sufficient for a condition to be considered a malady. Malady labels such as "mental disorder" have been manipulated to force "treatment," to block entry into a country, to deny reimbursement, to forbid marriage, to restrict freedom, to enforce morals, and to "medicalize" a variety of human conditions.

An ordinary example of a malady term being manipulated is "alcoholism." When it is important to impress upon the alcoholic that he must share some of the responsibility for his condition, and that he must exercise some control over his behavior, he may be told that alcoholism is not a disease, but more of a bad habit. But when it is important for the alcoholic to be freed from a burden of guilt and blame, it may be emphasized that alcoholism is a disease, the connotation of which is that it is an unfortunate condition that has befallen the alcoholic, victimizing him, and requiring expert medical treatment. Our concept of malady makes it clear that although alcoholism is a malady, the alcoholic must bear some responsibility for controlling the symptoms of that malady and, perhaps, even for coming to have that malady. This is not simply due to alcoholism being a mental malady; the same is true for a physical malady such as diabetes. The diabetic must bear some responsibility for controlling the symptoms of that malady and, perhaps in some cases, even for coming to have that malady.

On our account, mental maladies do not differ from physical maladies in any significant way. The fourth edition of the *DSM* (*DSM-IV*) almost apologizes for having "mental disorders" in its title: "Although this volume is titled the *Diagnostic and Statistical Manual of Mental Disorders*, the term *mental disorder* unfortunately implies a distinction between 'mental' disorders and 'physical' disorders that is a reductionistic anachronism of mind/body dualism. A compelling literature documents that there is much 'physical' in 'mental disorders' and much 'mental' in 'physical disorders.'"[3]

Mental maladies are usually distinguished from physical maladies largely by their primary symptoms. This is made clear by the definition of mental disorder that is provided in *DSM-IV* and its text revision, *DSM-IV-TR*. "In *DSM-IV* each of the mental disorders is conceptualized as a clinically significant behavioral or psychological syndrome or pattern that occurs in a person and that is associated with present distress (a painful symptom) or disability (impairment in one or more important areas of functioning) or with a significantly increased risk of suffering death, pain, disability, or an important loss of freedom."[4] Sometimes it seems simply a historical accident whether some malady is considered a physical malady or a mental malady. However, because mental disorders or maladies present some philosophical problems not presented by physical maladies, we will devote the next chapter to examining the concept of mental disorder in more detail.

Physical maladies usually affect particular parts of the body. This is obviously true of injuries such as a broken leg, but it also is true of diseases such as eczema, cancer, and the flu. Mental maladies usually involve behavioral or psychological symptoms with no particular bodily location. Both physical and mental maladies may have genetic causes, and some physical maladies have mental causes while some mental maladies have physical causes. Stress causes both physical and mental maladies. Drugs not only cause both kinds of maladies, they can also be used to treat both physical and mental maladies. Mental maladies are not distinguished from physical maladies by their causes or cures but by their dominant symptoms. Both physical maladies and mental maladies can involve pain or disability, but the kind of pain and disability will usually be different. Physical maladies necessarily involve something being wrong with a particular part of the body, and what is wrong with this part of the body involves either physical pain or a physical disability. Mental maladies involve something being wrong with the person's way of feeling or thinking, and this often involves mental pain or a volitional disability. Moreover, both physical and mental maladies often involve an increased risk of death, pain, disability, loss of freedom, or loss of pleasure. Unless we specifically say otherwise, everything we say about maladies applies equally to both physical and mental maladies.

Our account eliminates as much subjectivity as possible, allowing far less room for arbitrariness and manipulation. We provide a precise and systematic account of maladies, thus enabling a more fruitful discussion of controversial cases. Nevertheless, there are places where some vagueness remains. We give an account of these vague cases, showing what causes the vagueness and why some vagueness may be unavoidable. Our explication also shows what aspects of some conditions make them borderline cases and what about these conditions would have to change for them to be clear cases of maladies or clearly not maladies.

Surprisingly, at least when first presented, the values that are an essential part of the concept of punishment are also an essential part of the concept of malady. Maladies have some important conceptual connections to morality. This is one of the unexpected benefits of having a systematic account. The harms that rational individuals want to avoid when they are inflicted as punishment are the very harms or risks of harms that, when caused in a certain way, constitute maladies. So, like morality, the concept of malady is grounded in universal and universally agreed-upon features of human nature. This means that although values remain at the core of the concept of malady, the specific values are objective and universal. Our account of malady includes mental as well as physical maladies. The harms that are included in our definition of malady encompass all the harms that are referred to by any of the particular malady terms, such as "disease," "illness," and "injury." All of the other essential features that these terms share are also included in our definition.

To summarize: (1) We believe that all the particular terms such as "disease," "illness," and "injury" have something in common; (2) We use the term "malady" to capture that commonality; and (3) Our account of the concept of malady is grounded in the same universal values that ground our account of the concept of morality and punishment.

We provide an objective analysis of the concept of malady. The objective criteria we specify describe the necessary and sufficient conditions under which terms such as "disease," "illness," and "injury" are actually used in ordinary language. We are not introducing a new concept, only a new word, in order to make the concept more salient and objective. However, although analyses of concepts should not be used to change the concept, they can be used to sharpen it. A good analysis can make people more aware of the essential features of a concept than they were previously and they may then be less apt to use the concept in a loose or misleading way. Good analyses of concepts also can help in classifying some previously borderline conditions, and sometimes settle long-standing disputes about whether the concept applies. Even if the application of a concept to a particular condition does remain borderline, the analysis usually makes it clear why the condition is in fact borderline. We consider several borderline conditions later in the chapter.

Some Background

There have been many attempts to set out a formal definition of "disease," but among medical professionals "disease" has been used in a technical sense, not in its ordinary language sense in which there is a distinction between a disease, an illness, and an injury. Consequently, "disease" is often used interchangeably with "illness," and injuries are regarded merely as a subclass of diseases. What most formal definitions of disease have been intending to define is what we call a malady, that is, they have taken "disease" to refer to injuries, illnesses, headaches, lesions, disorders, and so on.

A characteristic definition is the following one from a pathology textbook:

Disease is any disturbance of the structure or function of the body or any of its parts; an imbalance between the individual and his environment; a lack of perfect health.[5]

This offers three separate but presumably equivalent definitions. According to the first definition, recently clipped toenails and puberty are diseases, as is asymptomatic *situs inversus* (right-left reversal of the position of some internal bodily organs). The second definition is too vague to be of any use, and the third is circular. Although the "disturbance of the structure or function of the body" is inadequate when considered as a complete definition, it can be incorporated as a feature of a more complex and adequate definition.

Another medical textbook definition states that:

disease may be defined as deprivation or lack of ease, a discomfort or an annoyance, or a morbid condition of the body or of some organ or part thereof.[6]

Here two separate definitions are offered. The second one is obviously circular and hence of no help. The first may characterize many illnesses but certainly includes far too much. It rightly includes heartburn, an earache, and an infected toe, but it also includes an overheated room, tight-fitting shoes, and irritating neighbors. Our definition of malady avoids this problem by requiring as a necessary condition that the malady be a "condition of the individual."

An early definition of disease expresses what many subsequent definitions have emphasized, portraying the disease as a result of an unfortunate interaction between the individual and his environment:

Disease can only be that state of the organism that for the time being, at least, is fighting a losing game whether the battle be with temperature, water, microorganisms, disappointment or what not. In any instance, it may be visualized as the reaction of the organism to some sort of energy impact, addition or deprivation.[7]

On this definition, one wrestler held down by another or an individual getting increasingly annoyed by loud music is suffering from a disease. We avoid the flaw in such definitions by requiring that the harm being suffered have no "distinct sustaining cause."

Several authors have correctly identified various aspects of the concept of disease. Robert Spitzer and Jean Endicott include in their definition of "a medical disorder" that it is intrinsically associated with distress, disability, or certain types of disadvantage.[8] We think this definition is on the right track. It begins to sort out the specific harms that are at the core of disease, but it fails to capture all of them, and does not include the condition of an increased risk of suffering these harms.

Donald Goodwin and Samuel Guze significantly improve on Spitzer and Endicott's list of harms in their 1979 definition and add the condition mentioned above that most others fail to consider. Goodwin and Guze define disease as:

any condition associated with discomfort, pain, disability, death, or an increased liability to these states.[9]

We discuss and clarify in our definition of malady this important added feature: "increased liability." It is a necessary amendment if asymptomatic conditions such as high blood pressure are to count as maladies.

The foregoing examples of definitions are typical of those found in medical and pathology textbooks. Our primary interest is not in criticizing them, but in using them to introduce our concept of malady. They show there is a need for a more adequate definition, and they suggest and exemplify some of the flaws that need to be avoided.

One kind of definition in particular directly raises moral issues: that kind of definition that makes abnormality a central feature of disease. We have not yet cited an example of this kind of definition, but many formal definitions in the literature make this feature central. For example, in the 1992 (third) edition of *Medicine for the Practicing Physician*, editor-in-chief J. Willis Hurst, in his own chapter "Practicing Medicine," says, "A disease is defined as an abnormal process." And he defines abnormality as "a deviation from the normal range."[10] The concept of disease that one adopts has wide-ranging repercussions for everything from establishing the goals of medicine to the distribution of health care in society, but for us the "abnormality" definition of disease has the most immediate moral implications. As we show in our explication of malady, abnormality, although it is a necessary feature of a malady, is clearly not a sufficient feature. Abnormality also plays an important though limited role in defining some of the terms that we use in our definition of malady. Thus, it does play a significant role in the determination of some maladies, a role that needs careful discussion and specification.

Constructing a Definition of Malady

Our plan for this section is to lead the reader through a series of steps in order to produce a definition of malady. This is in contrast to simply stating the definition and defending it against possible objections. We believe this "method of discovery" process helps with comprehension of the problem, its subproblems, and the subproblems' solutions. A step-by-step process should make the nuances and maneuvers more accessible to the reader.

Something Is Wrong

In the very broadest sense, when one of the malady terms correctly applies to an individual or, as we say from now on, when an individual has a malady, there is something wrong with that individual. As we showed in our earlier discussion of textbook definitions, however, to note only that "something is wrong" is much too inclusive. Many things can be wrong in an individual's life without her having a malady, for example, living in poverty, being neglected, or being in a runaway truck. But before we specify when having "something wrong" with oneself does constitute having a malady, we must make clear what it is to have "something wrong" with oneself. What is wrong with someone who has a malady?

A typical and frequent answer is "He is in pain," "He is disabled," "He is dying." But do these states or conditions have anything in common? What is the genus of which pain, disability, and death are species? The answer is: they are all harms (or evils).[11] Harm (or evil) is the genus of which pain, disability, and death are species. What characterizes these harms is the fact that no one wants them. In fact, everyone wants to avoid them. At least all individuals acting rationally want to avoid them unless they have an adequate reason not to, as elaborated in chapter 2. The very definition of an irrational action is that it is an action of an individual who does not avoid harm for himself even though he has no adequate reason for not avoiding that harm. However, people who choose to die rather than suffer unrelenting pain, or who choose to endure great pain to avoid a certain disability are not acting irrationally because they have adequate reasons for choosing the particular harm in question.

"Pain," as we use the term, includes unpleasant feelings of anxiety, disgust, displeasure, and sadness, and all the other kinds of mental suffering. Similarly, disabilities are not limited to physical disabilities, but include cognitive disabilities and volitional disabilities as well. Examples of cognitive disabilities are receptive aphasia and dementia; volitional disabilities include addictions, compulsions, and phobias.

Furthermore, death, pain, and disability are not the only basic harms. Two other significant harms are loss of freedom and loss of pleasure. So we anticipate that these also play a role in maladies, even though they do not immediately suggest themselves when one considers maladies. However, there are instances where one or the other of these latter two harms underlies conditions that are intuitively considered maladies. For example, if an individual has an allergy, he may be able to avoid the circumstances or the places that trigger the allergic reaction, so that, in effect, he appears not to be suffering any harm. However, his freedom, with respect to those circumstances and places, has been limited, so he is, in fact, suffering a harm, namely, the loss of freedom. The loss of pleasure, independent of the other harms, is fairly limited in scope, but one example is anhedonia, which is the failure to feel pleasure. It is sometimes associated with schizophrenia, although its presence is neither necessary nor sufficient to establish that diagnosis. However, any condition of an individual that was characterized solely by a significant loss of pleasure, even without such negative feelings as sadness or anxiety, would qualify as a malady. Possible examples are a condition that leads to failure to experience sexual pleasure or a stroke that affects the limbic system, blocking out the experience of pleasure. Some forms of mutilative operations on a young woman's genitalia result in her later failure to experience sexual pleasure, so that condition counts as a malady as well.

Maladies vary in the intensity of the harms being suffered from relatively minor to very great. However a threshold exists in applying the concept such that trivial harms are not usually regarded as maladies. The day following a mild degree of exercise, an individual might experience a slight twinge of muscle stiffness in one of his legs. This twinge qualifies as a physical pain, but it is quite trivial, and without the addition of the phrase "nontrivial" the condition would satisfy all the criteria for applying the concept of malady (see below), even though the condition is not ordinarily regarded as a malady. We use the phrase "nontrivial" to modify "harms" because it both makes clear that trivial harms are not sufficient to make a condition a malady and it explains one source of some disagreement in labeling a condition a malady. We prefer to make the locus of those disagreements as obvious as possible, so it is helpful to realize that people may not always agree on when a harm is "trivial."

Thus far, then, we can say that a malady is a condition that involves the suffering of nontrivial harms. All the harms involved are instances of the basic harms: death, pain, disability, loss of freedom, and loss of pleasure. These are harms that every individual acting rationally wants to avoid. This explains why and in what way "malady" (or "disease") is a normative term. The concept involves values, but they are objective and universal values. Like colors, these values are universal and objective because there is almost complete agreement about what conditions are harms. Most people distinguish between different colors, for example, between red and green; those who cannot are regarded as color-blind. There is a similar, almost universal agreement among people about what the basic harms are and, unless one has an adequate reason for desiring these harms, about the undesirability of experiencing any of them. For a term to involve values in no way entails that the application of that term is subjective, whimsical, or "culturally relative."

Significantly Increased Risk of Suffering Nontrivial Harms

The notion of malady (or disease) involves more than an individual currently experiencing a nontrivial harm, for example, pain or disability. Many maladies do not initially involve suffering a harm; they can be at first asymptomatic. Such a condition may be regarded as a malady, even though it is not yet causing any suffering of harms, if it is a condition that will either definitely lead to the eventual suffering of nontrivial harms (e.g., a positive HIV antibody status), or if it has a significantly increased risk of leading to the suffering of nontrivial harms (e.g., highly elevated blood pressure).

We use the adverb "significantly" to modify "increased risk" because it highlights not only that insignificantly increased risks are not sufficient to make a condition a malady but also because it explains another source of some disagreement in labeling a condition a malady. The locus of those disagreements should be as obvious as possible, so it is helpful to realize that people do not always agree on when an increased risk is "significant." Other variables enter into determining whether or not to call something a malady on the basis of increased risk. A small increase in the risk of suffering a serious harm is likely to lead to labeling that condition of an individual as a malady, whereas a greater increase of a mild harm might not. For example, a condition of a twenty-year-old associated with a 10% greater risk of dying before the age of fifty would probably be regarded as a malady, while a 3 to 5% greater risk of experiencing mild joint pain before the age of 50 probably would not. Still another variable may be whether or not there is a cure. If a cure is available, there is some advantage to labeling a condition as a malady, even if the increase in risk that justifies the labeling is for a relatively mild harm in the relatively distant future. Our point in stressing the role of "significantly" in the important component of our definition "significantly increased risk of harms," is to make explicit a source of reasonable variation in how and what conditions are labeled maladies.

Whether an increased risk is significant enough to warrant regarding the person with that condition as having a malady may become a more frequently asked question as more is learned about the morbidity and mortality associated with various ascertainable genetic mutations. For example, a twenty-five-year-old person with the Huntington's disease mutation is 100% certain to experience intense suffering and disability in the future and so, on our account, would certainly have a malady. Similarly a woman with a BRAC1/BRAC2 mutation, whose probability of having breast cancer in the future is 60 to 70%, compared with a base rate of, say, 8 to 10% for women in her cohort, would also, on our account, have a malady. However, our account does not settle the question of whether a thirty-year-old person with a genetic mutation that raises his chances of having a heart attack before age sixty-five by 2 to 3% has a malady. It is not clear whether that increase is significant enough to warrant labeling the condition a malady.

A Condition of the Individual

That an individual is at a significantly increased risk of suffering nontrivial harms is not sufficient for regarding him as having a malady. There must be an identifiable condition of the individual that is associated with the predicted harm. It is not sufficient that the individual be at risk of harm simply by being in a statistical cohort of some sort. For example, if all families living within a ten-mile radius of an atomic power plant have a 2% greater risk of developing thyroid problems than a matched cohort living elsewhere, it does not follow that all of these individuals have a malady. Similarly, women whose mothers or sisters have or have had breast cancer may be at increased risk of getting breast cancer themselves, but they do not all, therefore, have maladies. Also, having a certain history, for example, having been abused as a child, may make a person more likely to develop a mental malady, but being in a statistical cohort is not a condition of the individual. Unless the condition that leads to the increased risk is identified as a condition of the individual, we do not say that she has a malady.

Thus, we need to add to our nascent definition of malady that it is a condition of the individual that involves suffering a harm or the significantly increased risk of suffering a nontrivial harm. The condition must pertain only to what is within the integument of an individual's body; it is limited to what is contained within that zone marked by the outer surface of the skin and inward. This distinguishes the condition from the situation or circumstances the individual is in. For example, an individual could be in an elevator with a broken cable, hurling downward. That individual is at significantly increased risk of harm, yet it is incorrect to describe him as having a malady, at least at the moment. Likewise, an individual who is in jail is suffering a harm, namely, a loss of freedom. Yet this surely is not a malady. It is a situation the individual is in, rather than a condition of the individual himself.

The condition that significantly increases the risk of suffering harm must have a locus within an individual. This requirement distinguishes it from a mere statistical probability associated with membership in a group, in which case there is no identifiable condition having a locus within the individual person that causes the increased risk of suffering a harm. There is also no identifiable condition having a locus within the individual person that is correlated with that person's age. How old a woman is, that is, the date on which she was born, is a historic fact about her, but it is not a condition of the person in the sense that we are using that phrase. That an individual is at increased risk of harm simply by being in a statistical cohort of people of the same age is not sufficient for her to have a malady.

In order to make sure that the malady is within the individual and not identified with some circumstance of the individual, this aspect of malady must be more carefully described. We started our construction of the malady definition by talking about an individual with whom something was wrong. Occasionally we have used the phrase "condition of an individual." It is tempting to speak of a "bodily condition" in order to emphasize that the malady must be in the body and not a situation the body is in. That phrase, however, makes it impossible to include mental disorders within the malady label because, though at least some mental maladies are very likely to be conditions of the body, they need not be in order to qualify as maladies (see the next chapter). Referring to "a condition of an individual" leaves the condition's ontological status an open question but still guarantees that our definition will not include any condition as a malady that is not normally classified as such.

"Malady" not only has the same meaning in "mental maladies" as in "physical maladies" but it also has the same meaning when applied throughout the plant and animal world, at least insofar as particular plants and animals are capable of suffering any of the basic harms. Therefore, we properly should refer to the locus of maladies as "a condition of an individual organism." That phrase, however, seems somewhat stilted, and given that our primary concern is with human maladies, we shall continue to use the simpler phrase "a condition of an individual" or occasionally "a condition of the person."

Exception for Rational Beliefs and Desires

So far, our developing but still incomplete definition of malady is "a condition of an individual such that he is suffering or is at significantly increased risk of suffering some nontrivial harm (death, pain, disability, or loss of freedom or pleasure)." But "condition of an individual" includes more than is appropriate, so a certain narrowing and certain exclusions are necessary. Beliefs and desires are conditions of an individual and certain beliefs and desires can have the effect of causing harm or increasing his risk of suffering harm. When a rational belief that one has lost all his money in the stock market, or when a rational belief that one's child is very sick causes suffering, a person is not regarded as having a malady. Similarly, desires to climb mountains, ride motorcycles, and fly hang gliders are conditions of individuals that result in an increased risk of suffering harms, yet no one regards having those desires as constituting maladies.

On the other hand, there are beliefs and desires that not only cause harms to be suffered, but are themselves symptoms of maladies, usually mental maladies, for example, irrational beliefs and desires. A person might have a belief that he is being tortured by demons and thus be currently suffering. Or he might believe that he could fly if he leaped from a high window, and thus be at increased risk of suffering harms. A desire to commit suicide to see what it would be like to be dead puts one at significantly increased risk of harm. These cases do seem like maladies, and they do involve beliefs and desires.

The way we sort this out is to make "rational beliefs and desires" an exception to the conditions of individuals that can be maladies. Our expanded definition of malady thus reads, "A condition of an individual, other than his rational beliefs and desires, such that he is suffering or is at significantly increased risk of suffering some nontrivial harm (death, pain, disability, or loss of freedom or pleasure)." As shown in the previous paragraph, irrational beliefs and desires must not be ruled out as being involved in maladies since they may, in fact, constitute maladies. A belief is irrational only if its falsity is obvious to almost everyone with similar knowledge and intelligence.[12] A desire is irrational when it is a desire for any of the harms or a desire for something that one knows (or should know, i.e., almost everyone with similar knowledge and intelligence does know) will result in her suffering a harm, and she does not have an adequate reason for that desire.

Distinct Sustaining Cause

We have focused on the condition constituting the malady within the individual organism; now it must be noted that although that condition is necessary for having a malady, it is not a sufficient condition. There are many instances of conditions within individuals that cause their suffering harms not because of a rational belief or desire, and yet no one regards that particular condition as a malady. A wrestler could be experiencing the pain induced by an opponent's hammerlock; a gardener could be experiencing the discomfort of the relentless sun beating down on her; an individual might be trapped in a tightly closed space and therefore be experiencing aching muscles and anxiety, yet none of these people necessarily has a malady. We need to make some kind of conceptual move in order to distinguish these cases from those conditions that are regarded as maladies. We need to distinguish between those harms being suffered by the individual due to factors within the individual and those caused from without.

Many harms are, of course, caused by agents from outside the individual (e.g., allergens, bacteria, car accidents, and bright sunrays). Nevertheless, as long as the external circumstances are actively responsible for perpetuating the harm (e.g., the anxiety is being suffered because one is in a runaway car), then we do not regard that anxiety as constituting a malady. If someone suffers a loss of freedom due to something internal to the individual, for example, because of allergies or a fear of heights or open spaces, then we say he has a malady. But if his freedom is restricted by being in jail, we do not. When a change in the external circumstances immediately, or almost immediately, removes the harm being suffered, we do not call the condition a malady. We believe that all of this is in accord with the ordinary use of malady terms, such as "disease" and "injury."

To accomplish this conceptual move with a bit more finesse, we introduce the notion of a sustaining cause. As long as the harms are sustained by a cause distinct from the individual, the harms do not constitute a malady even though they do involve a condition of that individual. Thus, we include as a necessary condition for a malady that the condition of the individual giving rise to his suffering harms has no sustaining cause that is distinct from the individual. The distinct sustaining cause, in addition to its being distinct from the individual, must be one whose effects come and go simultaneously, or nearly so, with the cause's respective presence or absence. A wrestler's hammerlock may be painful, but it is not a malady because when the hammerlock ceases, so does that individual's pain. Of course, if the pain persists for a considerable length of time after the hammerlock ceases, then a malady is present because the pain, initially caused by an external source, is now being generated by the condition of the individual himself. A malady is a condition of an individual such that, whatever its original cause, it is now part of the individual and cannot be removed simply by changing his physical or social environment.

Our definition of malady now looks like this: An individual has a malady if and only if she (he) has a condition, other than her (his) rational beliefs or desires, such that she (he) is suffering, or is at significantly increased risk of suffering, a nontrivial harm or evil (death, pain, disability, loss of freedom, or loss of pleasure) in the absence of a distinct sustaining cause.

The Role of Abnormality: Disabilities, Significantly Increased Risk, and Distinct Sustaining Cause

Thus far we have developed our definition of maladies without including any reference to abnormality. However, we noted in our discussion of something being wrong that we would not say something was wrong with an individual if he was normal in all respects. Nonetheless, we regarded an individual having something wrong with himself to mean primarily, with respect to maladies, for him to be suffering a harm or to be at significantly increased risk of suffering a harm. And we have explained under what circumstances suffering a harm counts as a malady. We neglected to include abnormality in our developing definition and now realize that our definition of malady should include the term "abnormal." It should read: An individual has a malady if and only if she (he) has an *abnormal* condition, other than her (his) rational beliefs or desires, such that she (he) is suffering, or is at significantly increased risk of suffering, a nontrivial harm or evil (death, pain, disability, loss of freedom, or loss of pleasure) in the absence of a distinct sustaining cause.

But there are other features of the definition of malady in which further reference to the notion of abnormality is necessary. One reason for devoting a separate section to abnormality is to make clear that, contrary to most definitions of disease, abnormality, although necessary, is not sufficient for applying the disease or malady label. Earlier, we provided a recent example where abnormality was cited as the essence of disease in a book on medicine for the practicing physician. As we show in the next chapter, some editors of earlier editions of the American Psychiatric Association's *DSM* made this same error. We believe that this was both wrong and potentially dangerous. Making abnormality the essence of disease has serious harmful consequences, and that is why we need a clear account of abnormality's proper role. Labeling sheer deviancy as a disease mislabels, misdirects, and eventually may even lead to mistreatment. However, abnormality, besides being a necessary condition for something being wrong with an individual, is also a necessary feature in determining what counts as a disability, what counts as a significantly increased risk, and what counts as a distinct sustaining cause.

Disabilities and Inabilities

One of the basic harms whose presence can, in part, define a malady is a disability. However, determining what counts as a disability requires using the concept of normality.

How do we determine when someone has a disability? Most cases are clear: if a person cannot see, she has a disability; if an adult cannot walk, or has a limited range of motion in his joints, then he has a disability. But problems of labeling come in the borderline cases. Does an individual have a disability if he can walk but cannot run, if he does not have full and complete range of motion in all his joints, or if he has less than perfect vision? What if someone who is only four months old cannot walk? Or what if an individual cannot jump to the top of a two-story building at any age? What if an individual cannot walk more than a quarter mile without tiring? These are the kinds of labeling problems that need to be worked through in order to have a grasp of the variables at work in the use of malady labels.

It is obvious that the lack of some abilities is properly called an inability rather than a disability. That humans cannot fly is a clear example of an inability. No human can fly. Further, there are some extraordinary abilities that a very few humans have, but that does not mean that everyone else is disabled. It is at this point that the concept of the norm for the species becomes relevant. The lack of an ability to run a mile in four minutes is an inability rather than a disability. Even though there are a handful of humans who can actually run that fast, it is so far from the norm that there is no question that an individual is not disabled because he cannot do it. Labeling is more difficult as less rare abilities are considered. Just how far should one be able to walk or run, and how quickly, in order not to be considered disabled? Invariably, the norm for the species must be consulted, and that which takes special training, for example, pole vaulting, jumping hurdles, or playing chess, must be taken into account. Many athletes can do extraordinary things, but again that does not mean that everyone else is disabled. For one thing, the athlete's feats are outside the normal range of what people can do, and for another, they require special training that others may not have an opportunity to acquire. If an ability is present in only a small subset of the human species, the lack of that ability is not regarded as a disability; and if an ability requires special training, the lack of that ability is also not regarded as a disability. In both cases, the lack of ability is more accurately described as an inability.

A baby is unable to walk when she is only four months old. Is she disabled? Many very elderly persons cannot walk even a hundred feet. Do they have a disability? The baby does not have a disability but the very elderly individual does. We believe that a clarifying conceptual move in this regard, and one that parallels the intuitive understanding of the matter, is to conceive of a stage in normal human development when abilities are at their peak. Until an individual reaches that point, she may lack the ability but is not properly said to have a disability. It would simply be said that she is unable to do such and such or that she cannot yet do such and such; for example, the baby cannot yet walk. If she still does not have the ability in question after the time when it usually appears in the human species, or if she once had it but no longer does, then the lack of the ability is regarded as a disability, and hence a malady. For common abilities, after particular points in human development, when almost all persons in their prime have that ability, the ability in question is simply regarded as the norm. By "in their prime" we mean the time of life in which it is normal for people to have children. After that maturation point, whoever does not have the ability has a disability no matter how many of the population at that stage of life, for example, 95%, also do not have the ability. It is not inconsistent to say, "It is normal for the very elderly to have a significant loss of flexibility." Just because it is normal in one sense (that is, statistically common) does not mean that it is not a disability, at least not after one has reached that stage of life when having the ability is the norm.

In summary, both inabilities and disabilities involve the lack of abilities. An inability is not a malady. A lack of ability is an inability if either (1) the lack is characteristic of the species or of members of the species prior to a certain level of maturation, or (2) the lack is due to the lack of some specialized training not naturally provided to all or almost all members of the species. A lack of ability is a disability if one has reached a stage of life at which that ability is the norm for the species. Furthermore, having reached that point of maturation, one has a disability even if most others in his age group also lack that same ability. Abilities that only one gender has are not abilities that are the norm for the species, thus, lacking that ability is not a disability in those of a different gender (woman do, but men do not, have a disability if they cannot bear children). However, if a male or a female lacks an ability that is the norm for males or females, that is, almost all adult males or females in their prime have that ability, then that person does have a disability.

Low ability. That disabilities exist along a continuum leads to some vagueness in using the malady label. When should a low level of an ability be called a disability? The gradations are often so gradual that there is no definitive way to draw lines. Obviously one must rely considerably on the norms for the species, the norms apart from any special training to enhance abilities. For example, an individual who cannot walk even after the maturation point at which almost all members of the human species acquire that ability obviously has a malady. But how far must he be able to walk so as not to be considered as having a malady? If he is limited to a few steps, or even to fifty yards, he is considered disabled. But a mile? Two miles? One must rely on a comparison with the ability of the vast majority of humans at their prime for that ability. If that ability is distributed along a normal curve, as abilities commonly are, then almost all of those falling within that range are considered normal, that is, without a disability. However, those few at the very low-ability end of the curve are usually regarded as disabled, though, of course, those few at the high end of the curve are not. They have super abilities.

Something of this sort is already done in general intelligence testing. Intellectual ability is normally distributed and an IQ of 100 denotes average intelligence. Those having somewhat lesser IQ scores, for example, between seventy and eighty, are not regarded as mentally disabled but merely as having lesser ability. But those scoring sixty-nine and under are regarded as being mentally disabled to varying degrees. Although this is two standard deviations below the mean of 100, there is no bright line distinguishing those who have a lesser normal intelligence (e.g., an IQ of seventy-one) and those who are mentally retarded (e.g., an IQ of sixty-nine), so that using this cutoff is somewhat arbitrary.

An individual who develops an extraordinary ability (e.g., the ability to run a marathon in less than three hours), and then subsequently loses that ability, does not thereby have a disability, even if she loses it because of disease or injury. As long as she still falls within the normal range of ability, she is not disabled even though her own ability is significantly less than it was. Only if she reaches a point where she falls below the normal range of ability (e.g., can barely walk) is she said to have a disability. And that is true no matter how many individuals her age have the same problem. The comparison group for making these determinations is always the human species at its prime for that particular ability.

Significantly Increased Risk

We want to forestall some conceptual confusions that can arise from the notion of "being at significantly increased risk." As has been shown, this is an important phrase in our definition. These possible confusions relate to the matter of normality in the species.

We noted earlier that it was necessary to use the phrase "being at significantly increased risk." This is because some conditions of the individual that need to be labeled maladies are not yet causing perceptible harm, but they nevertheless put one at significantly increased risk for eventually suffering harm. High blood pressure is a good example, as is presymptomatic arteriosclerosis or having the Huntington's disease gene at age ten. In these examples, it is clear that the significantly increased risk is based on empirical studies showing that having the condition often or always leads to suffering some harm in the future. In most of these cases even the causal mechanism is well understood. So the clearest instances of "significantly increased risk" are empirically based.

One of the possible interpretations of "increased risk" that we want to avoid is the one that applies to an individual who had been in extraordinarily good health and has now slipped from that peak condition. Perhaps she had been a highly trained athlete who ate carefully and exercised vigorously. But now she has ceased training and has relaxed her nutritional regimen. She is now more at risk for a malady (e.g., arthritis, high blood pressure, obesity) than she had been before. We do not label this kind of increased risk as a malady. The increased risk criterion is not a matter of having a greater risk than you had before, but a matter of having a condition that puts you at significantly increased risk compared with most human beings in their prime.

The key to understanding the meaning of "increased risk" is seeing it as a comparison with what is normal for the human species. Given that the human condition itself puts one at risk for all kinds of harms, the only conditions that count as maladies are those that significantly increase the risk of such harms. Maladies designate those conditions of individuals that put them at a significant risk of harm over and above what is normal for members of the species in their prime, or in the case of death, a significant risk of suffering that harm much earlier than what is normal for members of the species in their prime.

Allergy, Abnormality, and Distinct Sustaining Cause

Many maladies become apparent only in certain settings. When an individual is suffering discomfort and pain, or intense itching during an allergy episode, there is no doubt about his having a malady. At first impression it might seem as though this is a case of a distinct sustaining cause, since removing the allergen would cause the bad effects of the malady to disappear. But usually that does not happen quickly, and the individual continues to suffer for a period of time even in a changed environment.

But what about such an individual who is in an environment free of allergens. Does he still have a malady? Certainly he has a condition that puts him at risk of a malady. If he is living in a place where there are no allergens, then he is not at significantly increased risk, although he still has the malady because, as explained earlier, he is suffering a harm, namely, the loss of freedom. His choices of environment are limited because of his condition. Hence, he definitely has a malady, though it may not be a very disturbing one for him.

It is in this context that another need for the concept of normality becomes evident. It is necessary for determining which reactions to one's environment are normal and which ones are indicative of a malady. If all humans gasp for air in a room densely filled with smoke, then the act of gasping for air in a room densely filled with smoke does not indicate that one has a malady. The harm is regarded as being caused by the environment, not by something within the individual. If only a small number of individuals develop shortness of breath in the presence of a cat, then the problem is regarded as being within those individuals. They have a malady and the harm is regarded as being caused by their condition, not by a distinct sustaining cause. Similarly, if an individual becomes anxious in the presence of almost everyone she meets, then she has a malady. In certain circumstances almost everyone becomes anxious, but if someone becomes anxious in circumstances where most others do not, she has a condition that is causing the problem. The cause is not in the environment, but in her. Thus, "abnormality" is important here too in deciding whether someone has a malady, for it determines whether an experienced harm does or does not have a distinct sustaining cause.

Society's Reaction

The question about what counts as a distinct sustaining cause is a particularly difficult problem when it is society's reaction to a person that is related to the harm a person is suffering. Consider the following question: If a malady is a condition of the individual such that he suffers harms, then might not race be a malady? Race, after all, can lead to individuals suffering death, pain, disability, loss of freedom, and loss of pleasure. But it is certainly wrong and counterintuitive to think of race, ethnic origin, or gender as a malady. On the other hand, how should a grotesque deformity, a significant disfiguration caused by accidents or surgery, or an extreme abnormality of someone's body be regarded? A significant part of the suffering associated with these latter conditions may be based on people's reaction to the condition, and here the malady label seems more appropriate. If the latter set of conditions are maladies, how can they be distinguished from the first set that are not regarded as maladies?

It may seem that in the case of race, society's reaction could be regarded as a sustaining cause that is clearly distinct from the individual, and therefore that race (or gender, or ethnic origin) is not a malady. But what of the deformities, disfigurations, and extreme abnormalities? Do these not also depend upon society's reaction? Since extreme deformities usually involve some pain and disability, that alone makes them maladies without even considering the reaction of others to the deformity. For example, there is often organ and joint involvement in extreme abnormalities of size; there can be difficulties in using one's hands and legs in deformities; there can be disabilities of seeing, blinking, breathing, and hearing in cranial or facial disfigurations. So, in general, the pain and disabilities connected with abnormalities and deformities are sufficient themselves to classify the conditions as maladies.

Suppose, however, that there were no disability or pain connected with a severe disfigurement. Is the disfigurement or deformity still a malady? If there is a "natural" or "universal" shock to others who first observe such individuals (e.g., a person without a nose), they do have a malady according to our definition. If this is not a learned, acculturated response, but rather is a basic emotional response of almost all humans upon first encountering these abnormal features, then the condition is a malady. In this sense, such conditions are similar to allergies. In allergies, a condition of the individual interacts with certain elements of the environment resulting in harmful effects to the individual. One can avoid that environment, but having to do so constitutes another harm the individual is suffering, namely, loss of freedom. The natural, spontaneous reaction of other humans to these physical abnormalities is like the natural environment. The abnormalities of the individual, not the natural reaction of others, are regarded as the cause of the pain and suffering to the individual. As a general rule, any deformity, abnormality, or disfigurement that is highly unusual and naturally and reflexively provokes an unpleasant response by others should be regarded as a malady. That, of course, leaves a certain amount of vagueness, but at least the features essential for deliberating about each case are now clearer.

Race was dismissed as a malady because society's negative reactions were considered to be a distinct sustaining cause. But this is an inadequate reason. Allergies also have a distinct sustaining cause, but the condition of the individual is regarded as a malady because the overwhelming majority of the species does not suffer harm when they encounter that environment. So are race and similar features such as ethnic origin really maladies? They are not, because the cause of the harm, unlike the example of disfigurement, is not normal for the species. Indeed, in other societies, an individual being of that race or ethnic origin might provoke a positive response. When the reaction is characteristic only of a society, not of the species as a whole, we regard the reaction as a distinct sustaining cause, and do not regard the object of that reaction, for example, the race of the person, as a malady.

This suggests that if animals or insects are significantly more likely to cause harm to individuals who have a certain condition, that condition is a malady since it puts the individuals at significantly increased risk of harm and deprives them of freedom. We accept that implication. Some individuals attract mosquitoes significantly more than others do, and that condition should be regarded as a malady, although usually not a major one. All humans attract mosquitoes to some extent, so do they all have maladies? No, because attracting mosquitoes to some extent is normal and thus they do not have a condition that puts them at significantly increased risk of harm. This is an instance of our meaning of "significantly increased risk" in the sense of one being at risk "significantly more than is normal for individuals in their prime." This is how it is determined if it is the individual who has the malady or if it is simply an abnormal environment. As noted earlier, if submerged in water or closeted in a smoke-filled room, all humans have difficulty breathing; such difficulty is caused not by an abnormal condition of the individuals involved, but by an abnormal environment. That is because the standard is what is normal for the species. It is the norm for the species to be unable to breathe underwater or in dense smoke. So the problem is not in particular individuals. However, if an individual cannot breathe because there is a cat in the room, then the problem is within that particular individual, because it is normal for individuals to be able to breathe in such circumstances.

Thus, establishing the norm for the species is essential for determining whether the lack of an ability counts as a disability or only as an inability. It is also essential for determining what counts as a significantly increased risk of harm. Finally, what is normal for the species sometimes even determines whether the harm has a distinct sustaining cause and, consequently, whether the individual suffering that harm has a malady.

Some Special Concerns

Crosscultural Issues

One sometimes hears accounts of diseases that appear to conflict with the labeling of one's own culture. For example, conditions that American society regards as maladies, other cultures regard as a sign of beauty or a gift of the gods. The condition known as St. Vitus's dance, a neurological disorder associated with uncontrolled movements, is claimed by some to be a visitation from the gods; *dyschromia spiraccotosis*, a bacterial infestation, is regarded by some as a beauty mark. Is the labeling of maladies purely a relative matter?

We believe the relativity of maladies is analogous to the relativity of morality. We regard both maladies and morality as basically universal, because both involve those harms that all rational persons everywhere avoid unless they have an adequate reason not to.

However, a different culture could have a rational belief that leads it to interpret a particular pain, disability, or loss of freedom differently from other cultures. In our definition of malady, we have excluded rational beliefs and desires as conditions of the individual that can count as maladies. Thus, we do not deny that another culture may welcome a condition that most cultures regard as a malady, but this does not show that the concept of malady is society-relative. In all cultures, a malady is occasionally welcomed: for example, to avoid work, to avoid being drafted, to avoid being chosen for a dangerous mission, or to receive compensation. But the condition involved is still a malady if, intrinsically, it causes death, pain, disability, the loss of freedom or pleasure, or a significant risk of suffering these harms. For example, St. Vitus's dance is a disability in any culture, yet it may still, on balance, be desired if it is thought to be a favor of the gods. In short, though maladies are intrinsically bad, they can be instrumentally good.

The matter is sometimes even more complex. What are regarded as good or bad ends are sometimes a function of the beliefs of that culture. For example, some cultures have ceremoniously inflicted severe wounds on members of their group because of beliefs that regard these wounds as being associated with significant goods such as purification, the passage to manhood, or some other personal benefit. Although these wounds may not be thought of as maladies by those cultures, one suspects that a closer look at behavior would reveal that those wounds were attended to in the same manner that similar wounds incurred under different circumstances are managed. It also seems likely that a similar wound on some other part of the body—not involved in the belief system—would be regarded and treated as a malady.

There is another reason that the very same condition of an individual might not be labeled as a malady by all societies. Some societies may not know that a certain condition is a malady because it is so endemic in their culture (e.g., schistosomiasis, a parasitic infestation) that they believe its signs and symptoms are a normal feature of the species. However, they can be mistaken about this, just as they can be mistaken about any matter of fact.

Distinct Sustaining Cause within an Individual

Another point of possible ambiguity concerns distinct sustaining causes. The issue at hand is whether the harmful effects experienced by the individual stop when the external cause ceases. The clear case is the wrestler's hammerlock, or being in jail, where the pain or the loss of freedom may stop immediately and simultaneously with the cause being withdrawn. But sometimes there are lingering pains or disabilities. Here, as in many of these issues, practical considerations guide the labeling process. Someone who coughs for only one or two minutes after leaving a smoke-filled room is not said to have a malady. There is little point in so labeling her momentary condition. If the coughing continues for a significant amount of time, such as several hours, depending on its severity, it might be regarded as a malady. That is because what had been a distinct sustaining cause is now seen to have caused a condition within the individual that continues independently of the original cause. At that point the cause of the pain and suffering is not distinct from the individual. Similar reasoning applies to the wrestler's hammerlock if the pain continues for a significant time after the hold is released. At some point, what is producing the pain is not distinct from that individual. To state it somewhat more precisely, we say that the individual has a malady if and only if the harm she is suffering does not have a sustaining cause that is distinct from the individual. That keeps us from having to locate the harm precisely within the individual; rather, it requires only that it be shown that the harm is not in continuing dependence on the distinct sustaining cause.

Our account of a distinct sustaining cause may suggest that these causes are always externally located, that is, outside the individual's body. Most are, but an increased risk of harm may have a sustaining cause that, though "clearly distinct" from the individual, is nevertheless within that individual, for example, a cyanide capsule held in the mouth. What if the poison capsule is swallowed but is still undissolved? At what point does a "clearly distinct" sustaining cause become one not so clearly distinct from the individual? A quantity of heavily encapsulated cyanide inside an individual's mouth is a "clearly distinct" sustaining cause because it has not yet been biologically integrated into the individual's body and it can be easily and quickly removed. If it were removed, the individual would instantaneously be rid of the risk of harm. If it is swallowed and in the body of the individual, so that it cannot be easily and quickly removed, it is no longer a distinct sustaining cause; if it causes a significant increase in the risk of harm, its presence constitutes a malady.

An example of a foreign substance in the body that is not a distinct sustaining cause is the defoliative poison dioxin. It may become absorbed in the body's fat tissue and not have a harmful effect until the individual loses weight and the dioxin is released into the body, becoming metabolized within the body's circulation. Thus, the individual whose body is storing dioxin certainly has a malady because he has a condition that increases the risk of his suffering an evil. This case is even clearer than the encapsulated cyanide that has been swallowed, for the dioxin has been biologically integrated within his body, even though it has not yet caused any harm.

When we speak of biological integration of a substance we mean that the substance has become a part of the individual, unlike, say, a marble that a child has swallowed. Biological integration means that body cells are invaded and interacted with, biochemical exchanges take place, or bodily defenses react, or all of these. But biological integration is not necessary for something in the body to cease to be a distinct sustaining cause. We do not consider a clamp or sponge in the stomach (left after surgery) or food in the windpipe to be distinct sustaining causes. They may appear to be instances of internal distinct sustaining causes because they are not biologically integrated but, for us, anything in the body that is difficult to remove without special training, skill, technology, or all of these, does not count as a distinct sustaining cause.

It is universally recognized that if the cause of harm or increased risk of harm is inside the body and has become biologically integrated or physiologically obstructive, then the cause is not a distinct sustaining cause and the individual has a malady. It has not been universally recognized that if the cause of harm or increased risk of harm is inside the body and cannot be quickly and easily removed without special training or skill or equipment, then the cause is not a distinct sustaining cause and the individual has a malady. Conditions involving these items significantly increase the risk of suffering harm and so, when discovered, require swift medical intervention. Such conditions have all the features of a malady even though there is no ordinary malady term that refers to them. In persisting to the fine points of using the malady label, we are making distinctions at a level not ordinarily recognized or considered. We regard the ability of our analysis of the concept of malady to provide guidance, not provided by ordinary disease terminology, as an indication of its utility and precision.

Borderline and Difficult Cases

In this section we explicitly address some conditions that may be difficult to classify. This discussion, while making additional clarifications, also functions as a working review, showing how the concept of malady works in some problematic cases. The first two cases concern women; the next three apply equally to men and women.

Menopause

Menopause meets the criteria of a malady, even though it might be welcomed by the individual. It is a condition of the woman that necessarily involves a disability, though the lack of the ability to become pregnant is often not unwanted. The fact that menopause is entirely normal at a certain age does not keep it from being a malady. Similarly, a vasectomy in a man should be regarded as causing a malady, an iatrogenic malady, even if the resulting disability is exactly what is desired. Though the procedure was elected by a male patient and performed by a physician, the result is still a malady since it is a condition of the individual such that not only is he no longer able to do something that he had the ability to do before, but that ability that he once had is an ability characteristic of the human species in its prime. That menopause is universal in women after a certain age does not exclude it from being a malady any more than an enlarged prostate being universal among men after a certain age excludes it from being a malady. Almost all persons over a certain age suffer a significant loss of hearing and of short-term memory, but that does not exclude the resulting conditions as maladies. Natural selection plays a significant role in shaping the characteristics that human beings have in their prime; it does not play this same role in shaping the characteristics that human beings have after they have passed their prime.

Pregnancy

Pregnancy is perhaps the condition that we have had the most difficulty in classifying. It is a condition of the individual, other than her rational beliefs or desires, such that she is suffering, especially in the final trimester, some pain, much discomfort, and significant disability, all in the absence of a distinct sustaining cause. Labor and delivery, the inevitable culmination of pregnancies that come to term, are often uncomfortable and confining, and of course can be extremely painful, although this may be in significant part the result of changes in lifestyle due to civilization. Also, throughout pregnancy the woman is at a significantly increased risk of suffering a variety of harms. Thus, at the present time, pregnancy seems to have all the objective features of a malady.

However, it is counterintuitive to regard pregnancy as a malady. It is not generally regarded as a disease or, for that matter, as a disorder, a trauma, or an injury. None of those terms seem quite right. Nor do we think that a woman who is pregnant has something wrong with her. On the other hand, women who are pregnant often suffer nausea, feel terrible, and, especially in the last month or so, suffer significant loss of their ability to move around. Perhaps, most striking, if pregnancy is not a malady, it is the only nonmalady whose treatment is routinely paid for by medical insurance.

Despite the objective features that pregnancy shares with other conditions readily labeled as maladies, it is easy to see why the malady label does not seem to apply to pregnancy. Malady, and other disease terms, refer to conditions that people avoid unless there is an adequate reason for having them, but many or most women want to become pregnant. Moreover, the adequate reason for becoming pregnant, having a baby, is an intrinsic feature of the condition. There are no other maladies that have such an intrinsic feature. Pregnancy is unique. Pregnant women tolerate pregnancy in order to achieve the desired end. If there were no child at the end of the process, no one would voluntarily become pregnant.

Our emphasis in discussing malady has been on the harms suffered as a result of the condition of the individual, and pregnancy seems clearly to be a condition of the individual that causes harm. Some might be tempted to regard the fetus as an internal distinct sustaining cause, in which case pregnancy, carrying the fetus to term, is not a malady. Although eventually the fetus becomes distinct, during most of the pregnancy it is not only biologically integrated in the body of the pregnant woman it is also not easily and quickly removable without special skill, technology, and training. Therefore, according to our criteria, the fetus cannot be an internal distinct sustaining cause.

We had previously claimed that not labeling pregnancy a "malady" because pregnancy is normal was a bad reason. We acknowledged that pregnancy was normal, but since we regarded it as a mistake to take abnormality to be the essence of a disease or disorder, we concluded that it was irrelevant that pregnancy was normal. We still think it is a mistake to take abnormality to be the essence of a disease or disorder, but we now recognize that abnormality is relevant to the malady status of a condition. We now think that the fact that a condition is normal, that is, in accord with what Christopher Boorse calls "species design," for people in their prime is a sufficient condition for it not being a malady.[13] We would not say of someone that she had something wrong with her if there was nothing abnormal about her condition. Thus, it is not a bad reason for saying pregnancy cannot be a disease or malady because there is nothing abnormal about pregnancy. Given that there is an adequate reason, intrinsic to this condition, for undergoing the harms involved in pregnancy, and that pregnancy is a normal condition for women in their prime, we have modified our definition of malady so that pregnancy no longer counts as a malady. This was accomplished simply by adding the word "abnormal" to our definition in the section on abnormality at the beginning of this chapter. Our complete definition of malady now looks like this: An individual has a malady if and only if she (he) has an abnormal condition, other than her (his) rational beliefs or desires, such that she (he) is suffering, or is at significantly increased risk of suffering, a nontrivial harm or evil (death, pain, disability, loss of freedom, or loss of pleasure) in the absence of a distinct sustaining cause.

Shortness of Stature

Shortness of stature is similar to many contenders for the malady label in that it seems that the physical (or mental) characteristic in question is a disadvantage only in particular social milieus. In a society that values height, shortness is seen as a disadvantage. The disadvantage is most likely to be stated in terms of loss of freedom (opportunity) (e.g., freedom to play sports, to become a model, or whatever). But, of course, being short may be an advantage for becoming a jockey. Certainly there need not be any pain, disability, or increased risk of death. The only problem seems to be falling short of societal expectations or value by virtue of the condition of the individual. We see no grounds for classifying such conditions as maladies. Of course if the shortness of height is associated, as it often is in severe cases, with disabilities and painful conditions, then the condition would satisfy the definition of a malady.

Earlier we discussed the role of society's reaction to an individual's condition. In the case of shortness, any loss of freedom that is experienced is a direct result of a particular society's reaction. There is no natural, universal human reaction of shock or revulsion to shortness of stature, so there is no malady. There is nothing in the condition of the individual that itself causes harm to the individual; the problem comes about only as that condition interacts with the values and beliefs of particular societies. That may be a social problem, but it is not a malady. Furthermore, whether shortness of stature, which does not involve disabilities, is caused by a deficiency of human growth hormone or simply by genetic inheritance makes no difference as to whether or not it is a malady.

Therapies are interventions whose intention is to reduce or eliminate the harms that are due to maladies. The most popular definition of enhancements is as interventions directed toward increasing the personal goods of the person (e.g., abilities [including knowledge], freedom, and pleasure). On this definition, interventions not directed toward increasing another's personal goods are not enhancements. Although this definition seems to correctly classify all cases of enhancements, it creates borderline cases.[14] How is one to classify an intervention whose intention is to reduce or eliminate harms, when these harms are caused by a particular society's reaction? For example, how should one classify the administration of growth hormone to a child destined to be very short, but who suffers from no pain or disabilities? As we stated above, whether shortness of stature, which does not involve disabilities, is caused by a deficiency of human growth hormone or simply by genetic inheritance makes no difference as to whether or not it is a malady.

However, because the administration of growth hormone to a child destined to be very short is intended to eliminate harms rather than to increase goods, it is often regarded as therapy rather than enhancement. Especially when the shortness is caused by a deficiency of human growth hormone, it is very tempting to regard the intervention as a therapy and hence to regard the condition as a malady. This disagreement is due to defining enhancement as limited to increasing the personal goods. If it were defined as including decreasing harms that are the result of society's reactions, then it would be clear that treating shortness of stature is an enhancement rather than a therapy.

The practical question is whether this intervention should be paid for by medical insurance. When the shortness of stature is caused by a deficiency of human growth hormone, the only difference between this condition and maladies as we define them is that the harms have a distinct sustaining cause, that is, they are caused by a particular society's reaction.[15] Thus, it is not surprising that shortness of stature is regarded as a malady. We are not opposed to having this condition paid for by medical insurance, and as a practical matter, it may be necessary to limit payments to those whose condition is caused by a deficiency of human growth hormone. But theoretically, we see no reason to make any such distinction, or to treat shortness of stature without pain or disability, no matter what it is caused by, as a malady.

Old Age

On the surface it seems that old age is the epitome of a malady, for people who are very old almost always suffer pain, disability, loss of freedom or pleasure, or are at significantly increased risk of all those harms. However, there are several reasons for not calling old age a malady, even though it is usually accompanied by diverse maladies, but the most important is that age is not a condition of the individual. Cirrhosis of the liver, a broken leg, a colon polyp, and a missing clotting factor are all conditions of the individual. That a person was born at a certain time is a historic fact about him; it shows only that he belongs to a certain cohort. Therefore, age alone, the mere passage of time, is not a condition of a person but a historic fact about him, a fact like "the individual swam in the river yesterday," or "he has lived through two world wars." Cells of the body do change with age and different organs of the body change in a variety of ways, but the degree of change depends on the environment that the cells and organs have individually lived through. Thus, it is not helpful to characterize an individual's malady status with respect to age alone. Individual systems—cardiovascular, renal, endocrine, and so forth—are likely to have deteriorated with age, but they need not have done so. In any case, insofar as they have, these conditions of the organism are what are responsible for the suffering of harms or significantly increased risk of harm, and so they are the maladies, not the age of the person.

Artificial and Transplanted Body Parts

Does the individual who has an artificial or transplanted body part still have a malady? This is not a contentious issue, but it is interesting to test the logic of our account of malady. It is fairly straightforward to apply the malady label. If an individual who had suffered from a chronic malady and, because of available therapy, is now no longer suffering or at increased risk of suffering any harm, then we say that he no longer has a malady. He is suffering nothing. Of course, realistically, if the individual has received a transplanted organ, very likely he is at increased risk of harm, and hence still has a malady. Normally, he is at less risk of harm than he was before the transplantation, but the comparison for determining the relative risk, as we have pointed out, is not with his previous condition but with the norm for the species. After the transplantation, this individual's malady is normally less serious than his previous malady, but compared with individuals in their prime, he is still suffering from a significantly increased risk of harm.

Suppose a woman had hypothyroidism, and physicians were able to implant in her a lifetime supply of completely safe and effective replacement hormone, so that none of the harms of the hypothyroidism were present and there was no increased risk of harm. We would say that she has no malady. The same is true of a formerly diabetic patient who now has an indwelling insulin pump, providing that the harms of diabetes were gone and the risks of harm were no greater than normal for the species. An artificial hip and an artificial lens implant in the eye are other examples. However, if these artificial or transplanted parts developed problems, the individual would have a malady. Now the individual is suffering a harm or would be at significantly increased risk of suffering a harm due to a condition of that individual and there is no distinct sustaining cause involved.

Genetic Maladies

We explore in this section several interesting issues concerning the application of the term "malady" to an individual's genetic status. It is likely that soon it will be possible to map an individual's entire genome and sequence her individual genes. When that happens it is also likely that a great deal will be learned about the correlation between individual genes and the occurrence of particular physical and psychological conditions, some of them maladies, some of them not. In some cases, the discovered correlation will be between a single gene (either a dominant gene as in Huntington's disease or a recessive gene as in Tay-Sachs disease) that is only slightly modulated by other genes, and its physical or behavioral mani-festations. In other cases, the manifestations will be under polygenic control. Sometimes this correlation may be exact, with the environment controlling only the timing and the severity of the malady. Thus, the discovery of particular genetic sequences early in life may predict unerringly the appearance of a par-ticular malady in the future. In other cases, the correlation between the genes and the malady will be lower, for example, some specific environmental circum-stances may be necessary for the malady's appearance, but knowledge of the individual's genome will still allow better predictions than are now possible.

What conditions qualify as genetic maladies? When, according to our definition, is it true that conditions that are correlated with particular DNA sequences constitute genetic maladies?

An individual clearly has a genetic malady if he is directly suffering harms because of his genetic condition (e.g., he has Tay-Sachs disease) or his chro-mosomal structure (e.g., he has Down's syndrome). Such conditions qualify ac-cording to the definition because harms are being suffered (e.g., mental and physical disabilities) and these harms are caused by the individual's genetic makeup or his chromosomal structure.

By contrast, there are a great many conditions that are genetically determined, fully or partially, but that are not maladies because they do not involve the suffering of harms. Eye color and fingerprint patterns are two clear examples.

Having hazel eyes is not a malady. Neither is having all ten fingers each with a fingerprint pattern of an arch (or having ten loop patterns, or ten whorls), though this is statistically extremely rare. Although eye color and fingerprint pattern are genetically determined, neither condition involves suffering or an increased risk of suffering harms. Therefore, neither can be considered a malady; hence, they cannot be genetic maladies, either intuitively or according to our definition.

It also follows from the definition that an individual has a genetic malady if her genetic structure is primarily responsible for her having a significantly increased risk of suffering harms in the future. Huntington's disease is a clear example; if a young woman in her twenties is discovered to have the Huntington's disease gene, she is usually regarded as having a genetic malady even though she is not yet suffering any symptoms. The definition thus accords with ordinary intuitions. The situation is similar to someone having a significantly elevated blood pressure but not yet having any target organ symptoms, or someone being HIV positive but not yet symptomatic with AIDS. The Huntington's positive and the HIV positive individual will certainly or nearly certainly suffer harms in the not too distant future. The individual with the Huntington's disease gene is even more likely than the hypertensive individual to suffer harms in the future, and nonsymptomatic hypertension is widely regarded as a malady.

Genetic testing may soon reveal many conditions that, if suitable prophylactic measures are taken, will not develop symptoms. Phenylketonuria (PKU) is a present example of this kind of condition: if the condition is diagnosed suffi- ciently early and appropriate dietary precautions are followed, serious symptoms may be prevented. Other conditions may be discovered in the future in which a suitable diet or the chronic administration of a drug may prevent symptoms from occurring. However, even in the fortunate cases where prophylaxis results in the genetic malady's symptoms being completely avoided, people would still be regarded as having a genetic malady. This is because they suffer the loss of freedom to eat certain foods that other people without this disease can eat, at least for some period of time. As long as one cannot eat certain foods, or must take some drugs chronically, then one continues to have the genetic malady. This situation is closely analogous to the condition of having an allergy. An allergy is a malady even if the individual can eliminate symptoms totally by taking a drug or moving to another part of the country; her freedom has been curtailed by having always to take the drug, or by having to live in one place and not another. Indeed, it is quite likely that allergies are genetic maladies.

Genetic maladies (e.g., Huntington's disease and PKU) are far more likely than nongenetic maladies to include conditions in which harms are not currently being suffered, but rather conditions in which there is a significantly increased risk, compared with most people, that they will be suffered in the future. Indi- viduals with conditions like Huntington's disease may suffer no harms for a long period of time, but the harms, when they do appear, may be quite severe.

Sometimes, as in Huntington's disease, the harms are certain to appear and there is no preventive treatment. Sometimes, as in PKU, the price of forestalling those harms is to employ treatment regimes that themselves involve the suffering of other nontrivial harms. It is for these reasons that it is in accord with common intuitions to consider individuals with nonsymptomatic Huntington's disease or those still being treated for PKU to be suffering from genetic maladies.

New genetic discoveries also may make available knowledge about genetic conditions that involves being at increased risk of suffering relatively mild future harms. Suppose that a four-year-old boy, because of his particular genetic condition, has a 50% probability of experiencing some mild skin condition— annoying but not disfiguring, like eczema of the scalp—in his thirties. He satisfies the definition of a genetic malady, that is, he is at significantly increased risk, compared with the general population, of suffering harms in the future because of a particular genetic condition. If there were no way to prevent those symptoms, it might seem questionable to regard him as currently having a malady at age four. Some may claim that since the harms, even when they occur, are mild, and there is only a 50% probability of those harms occurring, and even then not for thirty years, the condition is too trivial to be classified as a malady when he is four years old. However, if a low-cost and low-risk intervention were discovered that would prevent the eczema-like condition, we believe people would be much more likely to regard the four-year-old boy as having a genetic malady, albeit a very mild one.

Genetic maladies and risk of occurrence. Whether genetic conditions that, if not treated, involve possible or certain future harms are regarded as genetic maladies seems to be a joint function of several variables. Two seem particularly important: (1) the magnitude of the probability that the malady will occur, and (2) the likely age of the individual when it might occur.

(1) The higher the probability of future occurrence, compared with the population as a whole, the more likely the individual will be regarded, in advance of the harms occurring, as having a malady. Thus, a twenty-five-year-old man with a genome indicating he had a 50% chance of developing leukemia before age sixty would probably be regarded as having a malady. But if he were only 2% more likely to develop leukemia than others of his age, he probably would not be regarded as having a malady. This is consistent with our definition of malady. As discussed earlier, "being at significantly increased risk" in the definition refers to being at increased risk over and above what is normal for the species.

(2) The age of occurrence seems a separate important factor. If, on the basis of his genome, it could be predicted that a twenty-five-year-old man had a 50% chance of developing a serious malady (e.g., leukemia) if he survived until his nineties, he would not be regarded at age twenty-five as having a malady. In fact, even if the likelihood of his developing leukemia approached 100% if he survived to his nineties, he still would not be regarded at twenty-five as having

a genetic malady. Of course, this is based on the assumption that one's average life span is in the mid-eighties or lower.

Someone with the Huntington's disease gene is regarded by everyone as having a genetic malady because of the seriousness of the symptoms, the certainty they will occur, and the fact that death will occur prematurely. Although Huntington's disease can be accurately diagnosed decades before any symptoms occur, and the individual may feel entirely well during this presymptomatic period, the affected individual is still regarded as having a malady. Even though there is presently no treatment that may postpone or ameliorate its symptoms, if an expensive genetic treatment became available that would prevent the malady from developing symptoms at least 50% of the time, impartial rational persons would favor including it in health insurance coverage.

In the future, many significant linkages between genes and maladies may be found. Thus, the number of individuals who know or could discover at a relatively young age that they have a condition, without a distinct sustaining cause that is associated with a significantly increased risk of suffering serious harms in the future—including a significantly increased risk of premature death—could increase significantly. For example, the age of occurrence of heart disease and cancer, the two diseases associated with the highest death rates in the United States, has been proved to have significant genetic correlates that can be measured at an early age. This could result in one frequently noted ethical problem: the extent to which genetic information about individuals could and should be kept confidential and unavailable to employers and life insurance companies. But it could also result in a large number of young individuals considering themselves and being considered by others as suffering from maladies because of the significantly increased probability they will become seriously symptomatic during middle age.

Being at higher risk: group membership versus a condition of an individual. Some individuals are known to be at increased risk of prematurely developing diseases such as heart disease and cancer because of their family histories. However, as we noted earlier, there is a difference between (1) knowing that an individual is at increased risk because he has a particular individual genetic structure associated with a high risk of prematurely suffering a fatal malady, and (2) knowing that he is at increased risk because of being a member of a group, some of whose members will prematurely suffer that malady, while others will not. Both of these points must be distinguished, for it is known that the former individual has a malady, whereas it is not known that the latter has a malady. This is true even when the objective level of risk is the same.

Consider this example: Jane is born into a family in which 25% of female members develop breast cancer before the age of forty. It is ordinarily said of

Jane, at age twenty, that she is at increased risk, compared with other women, of developing a malady, but not that she currently has a malady. Now suppose that Jill is born into a family, in which no female member has ever, so far as is known, developed breast cancer before the age of forty. However, in mapping Jill's genome it is discovered that she has a 25% chance of developing breast cancer before the age of forty. Jill is much more likely to be regarded as having a malady than Jane. Since Jill has a demonstrated aberrant genetic sequence, it is clear she has something wrong with her. It is not yet known whether Jane has something wrong with her, for example, with one of her genetic sequences, even though her risk is objectively the same. Although Jill now has a genetic malady, it is not yet known whether Jane has.

Our definition of genetic malady does distinguish between Jane and Jill. "Condition," in the definition, means condition of the individual. Jill is at increased risk because of an aberrant genetic sequence, and this genetic sequence is clearly a condition of the individual. Jane, by contrast, is at the same increased risk, but it is not known if this is because of some condition of her person; being a member of a group (her family) is not what is meant by a condition of the individual. If Jane does develop breast cancer this will almost certainly be because of an aberrant genetic sequence, as is true with Jill, but it is not yet known whether Jane has an aberrant genetic sequence.

We think it is more likely to be said of two individuals at equal objective risk of suffering genetically caused harms in the future that the one with a demonstrable genetic aberrancy has a malady, compared with the other who only may have a genetic aberrancy. If true, this shows the power that the new knowledge of linkages between a person's genome and maladies could have in altering perceptions of individuals' malady status. Thus, discovering genetic conditions of individuals that significantly increase their risk of suffering future maladies will result in many more people knowing they have maladies at much younger ages. By increasing the importance of having a significantly increased risk of suffering harms, it will decrease the close connection between presently suffering symptoms and having a malady. Many more people who have no present symptoms may nevertheless be regarded as having maladies.

Advantages of the Concept of Malady

A subtle benefit of using "malady" in this new technical sense described here is that it is apparently the first explicit term in any language with the appropriately high level of generality. No language that we have investigated (English, French, German, Russian, Chinese, or Hebrew) contains a clearly recognized genus term of which "disease" and "injury" are species terms. Each term in the usual cluster of disease terms has specific connotations that guide and significantly narrow its use. That is as it should be if specificity is desired and justified. "Disease," "injury," "illness," "dysfunction," and other such terms overlap somewhat, yet each has its own distinct connotations.

The advantage of "malady" comes by way of the term's generality, by way of its referring to all those conditions that are referred to by terms that have their own individual though overlapping referents and connotations. This by no means makes the old terms irrelevant; rather, "malady" is useful precisely in those contexts where generality is important. One such situation is when nothing is known about a patient's condition that justifies the connotations of any of the other terms (injury, disease, sickness, etc.). All these words have connotations with respect to what it is and how it was caused. Inappropriate use of these terms can lead to wrong expectations and, hence, lead one temporarily down the wrong path of diagnosis. "Malady" is general and noncommittal with respect to particular connotations. It is useful as a beginning point for labeling a phenomenon. Thus, though it is not as informative as other disease words like "wound," "injury," "disease," "lesion," and "disorder," it is a useful term when none of these circumstances is known.

The search for a general term initiated the question: What do all the human conditions designated by the various disease terms have in common? This is the question that this chapter has tried to answer, and in doing so, has arrived at an analysis of the variables that enter into the labeling of these various human conditions. Our account of malady led to the recognition that all maladies involve either suffering at least one of the harms—namely, death, pain, disability, loss of freedom, or loss of pleasure—or being at significantly increased risk of suffering them. Because these harms are objective, that is, all rational persons agree that the items listed are harms, the influence of ideologies, politics, and self-serving goals in manipulating malady labels is considerably diminished. The possibility for some subjectivity does remain, as we have pointed out, but given the above explication of malady, exactly what elements are open to subjective bias can be determined. In short, our definition clarifies what may be causing the disagreement, and, hence, may facilitate efforts to resolve it.

The concept of malady has values at its core, but the values are universal and objective. Thus, our explication shows the inadequacy of either regarding disease as being totally value free or as being completely determined by subjective, cultural, and ideological factors. We have also tried to show how culture influences malady labeling in those few instances in which it does.

An important feature of our account of malady is that it shows that although abnormality is a necessary condition, it is not a sufficient condition for the application of any disease or related terms. Although we would not say that a person had something wrong with him if everything was normal, abnormality becomes important in certain contexts, which we have specified, namely, in the determination of disabilities, distinct sustaining causes, and increased risks. It does not play the major role that many other definitions have assumed it plays. Labeling a behavior or a condition as a malady simply because it is abnormal sometimes leads to unfortunate consequences, as with some paraphilias that we discuss in the next chapter. All of the various disease terms, such as "disorder" or "dysfunction" require more than abnormality for proper application; all require suffering, or significantly increased risk of suffering, one or more of the harms. Deviancy is not sufficient for using any disease term and the consequences of so regarding it can be significant. One tendency in the medical-scientific world has been to establish a normal range for this or that (some component of the human body), and ipso facto to have "discovered" two new maladies: hyper- and hypo- this or that.[16] Our account makes it clear that this use of abnormality represents a misunderstanding of the concept of malady.

A final advantage of our explication of malady, as we will show in more detail in the following chapter, is that its basic elements, concepts, principles, and arguments are the same when applied to mental maladies. The usual bifurcation between mental and physical maladies disappears. As we have seen in numerous examples throughout this chapter, significantly increased risk of premature death, pain, disability, loss of freedom and pleasure, and the absence of distinct sustaining causes are applicable to the mental domain as well as to the physical.

Notes

1. Our introduction of this technical use of "malady" and our earliest treatment of the concept appeared in Clouser, Culver, and Gert (1981).
2. This seems to be true in all other languages as well; see p. 161.
3. See American Psychiatric Association (1994, xxx).
4. Ibid., xxx. Loss of pleasure should also have been included as a symptom of a mental malady. It probably was not included because of a failure to distinguish between loss of pleasure and pain, or perhaps it might have been thought that any condition of a person that results in his suffering a loss of pleasure involves a disability.
5. See Peery and Miller (1971).
6. See Talso and Remenchik (1968).
7. See White (1926).
8. See Spitzer and Endicott (1978).
9. See Goodwin and Guze (1979).
10. Butterworth-Heinemann (1992, 14).
11. A connotation of "having something wrong with oneself" is that something is not the way it should be, that something is not normal. We now realize that it is true that if everything is normal, we would not say that the person has something wrong with himself.
12. What we call irrational beliefs, psychiatrists refer to as delusions. For a further discussion of the relationship between irrational beliefs, irrational desires, and mental disorders, see Gert (1990b).
13. See Boorse (2004). Although we still hold that the suffering of harm, not abnormality, is the essential feature of a malady, we agree with Boorse's criticism of our previous view that if something is in accord with species design, it cannot be a malady. However, what is in accord with species design is only determined by the features of

human beings in their prime. This is why we talked about disabilities being determined by whether the overwhelming majority of people had that ability in their prime. It is not part of what we regard as species design that people deteriorate as they get older. Evolution may not select for features that have no effect upon people until after their reproductive years.

14. An extensive project ("The Enhancement Project") sponsored by the Hasting Center concluded that the two terms—enhancement and intervention—could not be defined clearly and could serve only as "conversation starters." They say, "Like many distinctions, the treatment/enhancement distinction is permeable, unstable, and can be used for pernicious purposes." See Parens (1998, 25). We think the terms can be defined clearly and that one advantage of clear definitions is that they decrease the likelihood of any pernicious applications of the terms defined.

15. Juengst (1998, 29–47) and Daniels (1994, 110–132) also use the concept of malady in distinguishing between therapies and enhancements although Daniels's definition of malady differs from ours.

16. See Bailey, Robinson, and Dawson (1977).

7

Mental Maladies

In our analysis of maladies thus far, we have used as examples primarily physical conditions of the individual. A person is diagnosed as having a physical malady like cancer on the basis of accompanying bodily alterations. Even a person who has a significantly increased risk of a physical malady like cancer, because of a cohort to which he belongs or because of the circumstances he is in, counts as having a malady only when he has some bodily alteration, for example an aberrant genetic mutation. Yet our definition of malady contains no reference to bodily organs or genetic sequences, or to biochemical or physiological processes. The presence or absence of these physical conditions or processes does not determine, on our account, whether a condition is considered to be a malady.

Many conditions manifested primarily by psychological symptoms qualify as maladies on our definition. Someone with a severe endogenous depression, for example, is suffering a serious harm (mental pain) that is unrelated to any rational belief or desire, and that exists in the absence of a distinct sustaining cause. Our definition makes no distinction between physical and mental harms because we believe that, in defining maladies, both should be included. Both kinds of harms exist on a continuum of severity. In both physical and mental maladies there can be an increased risk of death as well as other harms suffered. To require of someone suffering psychological harms that an alteration of physical functioning be present before labeling her condition as a malady is to accept a reductionistic materialist view that is not, in fact, used by physicians and for which there is no justification.

To illustrate that altered bodily processes are not necessary to establish the existence of a malady, consider the case of schizophrenia. This psychosis is a condition manifested symptomatically primarily by a collection of psychological dysphorias and disabilities. Its etiology is not well understood. Some believe that schizophrenia is caused primarily by certain inherited neurochemical and neuropathological abnormalities; others believe that particular kinds of early psychological experiences play the predominant etiological role; and still others hypothesize that both these factors are conjointly necessary to produce the condition.

Suppose there are three different etiological paths to schizophrenia. (1) Some people inherit certain nervous system abnormalities so that schizophrenia develops no matter what the quality of their early psychological experiences; (2) other people have such psychologically traumatic early childhoods that schizophrenia develops even if they initially inherited a normal nervous system; and (3) still other individuals develop schizophrenia only because they have both an inherited central nervous system abnormality and a traumatic childhood.

Suppose further that these groups are phenotypically indistinguishable in terms of the psychological symptoms they manifest, the course of their condition, and the most effective treatment for them. Imagine, however, that with sophisticated neurochemical assays one can detect enzymatic abnormalities in the first and third groups that are not present in the second group. (We assume that cerebral processes are a necessary substrate for the symptoms of the second group but that this group does not show the enzymatic abnormalities.)

If the pathogenesis of schizophrenia turns out to resemble the above model, which it very well could, then those who believe that bodily abnormalities are a necessary condition for malady status would presumably believe that only the first and third groups qualify. We maintain that if the second group manifested the same symptoms, course, response to treatment, and so on, it would be pointless to deny that it shared the same malady status. The patients would suffer the same harms, would be treated by the same physicians in the same way, and should be covered by the same kind of health insurance coverage. Schizophrenia is a malady regardless of whether some, all, or no schizophrenics are eventually proved to have inherited central nervous system abnormalities. Physical maladies are distinguished from mental maladies primarily in terms of their most salient symptoms, but there is no fundamental difference in cause or severity between physical and mental maladies.

We discuss in this chapter three important issues concerning mental maladies: (1) the relationship between classifying behavior as deviant and classifying behavior as constituting a mental malady; (2) the pervasive role of the volitional disabilities in defining many kinds of mental disorders; and (3) the extent to which definitions of mental disorders rely upon value judgments that can easily vary from culture to culture. In discussing these issues we refer frequently to statements found in the most recent edition (2000) of the American Psychiatric Association's *Diagnostic and Statistical Manual of Mental Disorders, DSM-IV-TR*.

Mental Maladies and Deviancy

Perhaps the most serious cause of mistaken definitions of mental maladies is the pervasive temptation to equate behavior that is deviant with behavior that is a symptom of a mental illness. While it is true that the symptoms of mental maladies are deviant, in the sense that they are statistically uncommon (relatively few people mutilate themselves or speak with someone whom no one else can see or hear), it is not true that behavior and traits that are statistically uncommon are necessarily symptomatic of a mental illness. Being left-handed, having a passion for skydiving, or being able to wiggle one's ears are not symptoms of maladies.

Nowhere has the error of equating deviancy with illness been more frequent than in the area of human sexuality. There has frequently been the inclination, on theoretical or other grounds, to believe that normal heterosexual functioning is ideal and healthy, and that engaging in statistically less common kinds of sexual activities is undesirable and sick, independent of whether the individuals involved suffer in any way because of their unusual sexual preferences.

There exists in the field of psychiatry a set of conditions, once called *perversions* but more recently labeled by the American Psychiatric Association (APA) as *paraphilias*, whose malady-status and defining criteria have changed over recent decades.[1] This kind of diagnostic uncertainty is not unknown in psychiatry—witness the current discussion about whether premenstrual dysphoria should be counted as a psychiatric disorder—but probably with respect to no other condition(s) has it been more pronounced.[2]

Are the paraphilias listed by the APA in its series of volumes of the *Diagnostic and Statistical Manual*[3] actually mental disorders? At first blush there seems a straightforward way to answer this question. The *DSM* volumes supply a general definition of mental disorder. How adequate is that definition, and how well do the paraphilias described in the volume satisfy the definition?

We believe that the *DSM-IV-TR* definition of a mental disorder is a good definition.[4] It states:

In *DSM-IV*, each of the mental disorders is conceptualized as a clinically significant behavioral or psychological syndrome or pattern that occurs in an individual and that is associated with present distress (e.g., a painful symptom) or disability (i.e., impairment in one or more important areas of functioning) or with a significantly increased risk of suffering death, pain, disability, or an important loss of freedom.[5] In addition, this syndrome or pattern must not be merely an expectable and culturally sanctioned response to a particular event, for example, the loss of a loved one. Whatever its original cause, it must currently be considered a manifestation of a behavioral, psychological, or biological dysfunction in the individual. Neither deviant behavior (e.g., political, religious, or sexual) nor conflicts that are primarily between the individual and society are mental disorders unless the deviance or conflict is a symptom of a dysfunction in the individual, as described above.[6]

The first sentence in the definition provides the essential features of mental disorders and distinguishes them from physical disorders. The definition makes clear that mental disorders involve behavioral or psychological features rather than the physical features of the person. Normally, what makes a disorder a mental disorder is its symptoms, not its cause or etiology.

For both mental and physical disorders, the symptoms must be associated with present distress or disability (functional impairment) or with an increased risk of death, pain, and so forth. For example, arthritis is a physical disorder that involves both present distress and disability. High blood pressure is a physical disorder that may not involve present distress or disability, but does involve an increased risk of death or disability in the future. Phobias are mental disorders that are associated with both present distress and disability. That no condition is a disorder, either mental or physical, unless it is associated with present distress and disability (or a significantly increased risk of these and other harms) is important, for it helps to establish the objectivity of the concept of a disorder. The presence or absence of these symptoms can, in general, be objectively verified. Mental disorders, properly understood, like physical disorders, are not merely labels for conditions that some culture or society has arbitrarily picked out for special calumny or treatment.

Mental disorders, since they involve distress, disability, or significant risks of these and other harms, are conditions that no one wants for himself or herself (or for a beloved person), at least not without an adequate reason. Sometimes, as explained in the previous chapter, one might choose or want to suffer a minor disorder in order to gain an advantage; for example, mild asthma may result in a deferment from a wartime draft. But, as this example shows, although social circumstances may make it advantageous to have a disorder, having a disorder nevertheless involves at least an increased risk of suffering some harm or evil that, without an adequate reason, everyone would prefer to do without.

According to this notion of a disorder, suffering, distress, disability, or significant risks of these and other harms, though necessary features of a mental or physical disorder, are not sufficient; more things cause suffering than mental or physical disorders. We often suffer because something has gone wrong—not with us, but with the world outside us. A loved one dies; someone threatens us with serious physical harm; poverty prevents us from providing adequate food or clothing for our children. All these circumstances cause one to experience distress, although this distress is not a symptom of mental disorder if it is merely an expectable and culturally sanctioned response to a particular event.

However, these conditions, especially if prolonged, can bring about changes in a person. The point is that even were the original cause of the symptoms to cease, the individual may still feel distress. The distress brought about by the strains or tensions of real-world events can cause a dysfunction in the individual that persists even after these strains or tensions have been removed. One example is post-traumatic stress disorder (PTSD). The parallel here with physical disorders is exact. For example, prolonged exposure to extreme heat or cold may not only make a person experience distress but may also cause a change in the person so that he or she now has a dysfunction that involves being afflicted with symptoms even after the external temperature has returned to normal (see Culver and Gert [1982, 72–74]).

Sometimes external conditions may not cause present distress or disability, but may affect the individual in such a way that he or she suffers significantly increased risk of death, pain, and so forth. Continuing strain and tension may cause high blood pressure. Continuing to smoke, to drink alcohol, or to take various drugs recreationally may result in a person acquiring a substance abuse disorder that significantly increases his or her risk of death, pain, and so forth. Substance abuse, like the physical disorder of high blood pressure, undoubtedly is sometimes made more likely by a person's genetic predisposition. This fact reinforces the view that what distinguishes mental from physical disorders is their symptoms, not their etiology.

The *DSM*'s definition of mental disorder concludes by asserting that merely deviant behavior (political, religious, even sexual), or conflicts between an individual and his or her society, is not a mental disorder—unless the deviance or conflict is a symptom of a dysfunction in the person. Simply holding, even promulgating, unpopular or strange political or religious ideas is not a mental disorder. But most important and, because of its importance, what should be made explicit by the definition, is that nothing is a *dysfunction* unless it is associated with present distress, disability, or increased risk of death, pain, and so forth. It is not as if some dysfunctions are associated with these harms and risks, while others are benign dysfunctions that have no harms or risks at all. A mild dysfunction is associated with mild symptoms or lower risks, but there can be no dysfunction that has no symptoms or no increased risks. Rigorous adherence to this definition of mental disorder frees psychiatry from any temptation to enforce social conformity in the name of mental health and contributes to psychiatry's simply being one more medical specialty. But rigorous adherence requires that deviant behavior (in the absence of a painful symptom, impairment in functioning, or increased risk of death, pain, and so forth) is no more regarded as a mental disorder than asymptomatic *situs inversus* or being able to wiggle one's ears are regarded as physical disorders. However, when discussing the paraphilias, the various editions of *DSM* over the years have not always abided by their own definition of mental disorder.

The definition of mental disorder has remained essentially the same from *DSM-III-R to DSM-IV-TR*, but the volumes' discussion of the various paraphilias and the defining characteristics necessary to diagnose them have significantly changed. In particular, the diagnostic roles of *behavioral deviance* and of *the suffering of harms* have varied. Sometimes, especially in *DSM-III-R*, the existence of behavioral deviancy alone is sufficient to diagnose a paraphilia (and thus a mental disorder). By contrast, in *DSM-IV*, distress plays a major and necessary role in defining all the paraphilias. But *DSM-IV-TR* offers a more complex picture: it continues to stipulate (in the fashion of *DSM-IV*) that the suffering of harms is necessary—but only for *some* paraphilias; thus, *DSM-IV-TR* asserts that the suffering of harms is *not* necessary for others (in the fashion of *DSM-III-R*).

Examine, for example, the defining criteria of the paraphilia transvestic fetishism, the *DSM* term for men who experience sexual excitement by dressing in women's clothing. Compare two sets of defining criteria:

DSM-III-R (1987, 288–289):
A. Over a period of at least six months, in a heterosexual male, recurrent intense sexual urges and sexually arousing fantasies involving cross-dressing.
B. The person has acted on these urges, or is markedly distressed by them.

DSM-IV (1994, 530–531); *DSM-IV-TR* (2000, 574–575):
A. Over a period of at least six months, in a heterosexual male, recurrent, intense sexually arousing fantasies, sexual urges, or behaviors involving cross-dressing.
B. The fantasies, sexual urges, or behaviors cause clinically significant distress or impairment in social, occupational, or other important areas of functioning.

Now consider Mr. X, a forty-year-old man who for years has found it sexually arousing to put on women's underwear. Once or twice a month, in the privacy of his bedroom, he dresses in lingerie, becomes sexually excited, and masturbates to orgasm. He considers himself heterosexual and has had reasonably satisfying sexual relations during his two marriages and more recently with several women he has dated. He finds cross-dressing exciting and has no desire to change. He has never engaged in any homosexual behavior and has never desired to be in public fully dressed as a woman. His social demeanor is (to use *DSM-IV-TR*'s term) unremarkably masculine. No acquaintance, male or female, knows about his cross-dressing, except one girlfriend. He once vaguely described his activities to her, but she seemed mostly amused and the subject never came up again. Mr. X is usually able to cross-dress when he has the urge.

How would Mr. X be diagnosed? According to *DSM-III-R*, Mr. X has a mental disorder: he has cross-dressed persistently over the years (criterion A) in order to become sexually excited (criterion B). In fact, essentially all cross-dressers would have a disorder because they would satisfy not only criterion A but also the first part of B: it would be highly unusual to find a man with recurrent intense sexual urges and sexually arousing fantasies involving cross-dressing who never acted on them. Thus, criterion B would be satisfied even if its second half—being markedly distressed—were not satisfied. Deviance without distress would constitute a mental disorder. However, according to *DSM-IV* and *DSM-IV-TR*, Mr. X does not have a mental disorder. He satisfies criterion A: he has become sexually aroused through cross-dressing for a period of at least six months. He does not, however, satisfy criterion B: his cross-dressing fantasies, urges, and behaviors have not, over the years, caused him clinically significant distress or functional impairment. Indeed, they have caused him little if any distress or impairment of any kind and he would not want to eliminate his urge to cross-dress, even if doing so were possible.

An important difference between the two sets of *DSM* criteria (between *DSM-III-R*, on the one hand, and *DSM-IV* and *DSM-IV-TR*, on the other) is that behavioral deviance or abnormality alone is sufficient to warrant a diagnosis of mental disorder in the first set. This is true despite the fact that the *DSM-III-R* definition of mental disorder (see above) clearly states that deviance alone is *not* sufficient for mental disorder. The authors of the *DSM-III-R* criteria of transvestism seemingly ignored *DSM-III-R*'s own definition of mental disorder (see Gert [1992], on this problem). In *DSM-IV* and *DSM-IV-TR*, by contrast, deviance is not sufficient for the diagnosis; the behavior must be accompanied by significant distress or dysfunction. Even so, it would have been useful for the authors of *DSM-IV* and *DSM-IV-TR* to have been more precise. Suppose Mr. X feels comfortable with his transvestite experiences, but his cross-dressing is accidentally discovered by a friend who tells other people about it, and Mr. X suffers significant social rejection as a result. On one interpretation of criterion B, it could be said that Mr. X's behavior *has* led to (i.e., caused) his experiencing significant social distress. This interpretation is almost certainly not what the *DSM-IV* and *DSM-IV-TR* authors would endorse—otherwise a gay person who was distressed by encountering hostile homophobic behaviors would have to be said to have a mental disorder. Both the *DSM-IV* and *DSM-IV-TR* should have stated that the transvestite fantasies, sexual urges, or behaviors that cause clinically significant distress or impairment in social, occupational, or other important areas of functioning are not the result of conflicts that are primarily between the individual and society. The situation seems entirely analogous to that of ego-syntonic homosexuality, which the APA removed from the list of *DSM* mental disorders in the 1970s (see Conrad and Schneider [1980]). Why this was done for distress-free homosexuality but not for any other conditions involving statistically uncommon sexual behaviors is a mystery that *DSM* never addresses (for a discussion of this issue, see Soble, [2004]).

Although the defining criteria for transvestism in *DSM-IV* and *DSM-IV-TR* are compatible with the *DSM* definition of mental disorder, the same cannot be said for *DSM-IV-TR*'s defining criteria for some of the other paraphilias. Although *DSM-IV*'s account of all of the paraphilias included distress as a necessary component, *DSM-IV-TR* has regressed. In *DSM-IV-TR*, the diagnosis of five of the eight paraphilias does not require distress: exhibitionism, frotteurism, pedophilia, sadism, and voyeurism. For each of these five paraphilias, criterion B states: The person has acted on these sexual urges, or the sexual urges or fantasies cause marked distress or interpersonal difficulty. The first "or" makes it clear that simply acting on these sexual urges or fantasies, without any distress or impairment, constitutes a disorder.

Why did *DSM-IV-TR* go back to the *DSM-III-R* form of criterion B for five paraphilias? *DSM-IV-TR* does not say. Consider a voyeur who is not distressed by his voyeurism. In 1987 he had a disorder (he acted on his urges, *DSM-III-R*); in 1994 he did not have a disorder (he did not suffer clinically significant distress, *DSM-IV*); but in 2000 he once again had a disorder (he acted on his urges, *DSM-IV-TR*). If the psychiatric profession's authoritative diagnostic manual changes a condition's disorder-status every time a revised edition is issued, one would think that significant theoretical or empirical reasons for doing so existed and they would be fully discussed. Not so. Appendix D in *DSM-IV-TR* ("Highlights of Changes in *DSM-IV* Text Revision") notes this change in diagnosing some of the paraphilias (840), but no attempt is made to explain or justify it.

This regression to the *DSM-III-R* criterion for these five paraphilias is a mistake because it confuses criminal or immoral behavior with having a mental disorder. For a person to have a mental disorder, the individual suffering harm must be the person with the disorder, not someone else (the victim in the criminal or moral sense). This is abundantly clear from *DSM*'s definition of mental disorder. Once again it appears that the crafters of *DSM* have ignored their own definition of mental disorder.

Paraphilias Described in Psychiatric Texts

We have seen that the American Psychiatric Association in *DSM-III-R* started with a valid definition of the general term "mental disorder." There was a lack of correspondence in *DSM-III-R* between that definition and the sets of criteria that APA proposed for the various paraphilias, but the correspondence grew closer with the publication of *DSM-IV*, then regressed noticeably with *DSM-IV-TR*. An important question to raise is to what extent does the *DSM* actually influence psychiatric diagnostic behavior? For example, do psychiatrists refrain from diagnosing a paraphilia in a person who satisfies criterion A of the *DSM-IV* definition of a particular paraphilia but does not satisfy criterion B? We know of no data that address this important question.

However, there is a kind of surrogate for the actual behavior of psychiatrists that can be examined. Psychiatrists are active writers of psychiatric textbooks. To what extent do the descriptions and the discussions of the paraphilias in psychiatric texts run true to the definition of psychiatric disorder or to the criteria for these disorders stipulated by the *DSM* volumes? Most psychiatric texts rely heavily on the *DSM* criteria in their discussion of the disorders, so finding a high correspondence between *DSM* criteria and a psychiatric text might reflect little about how psychiatrists actually behave in clinical practice. Finding a low correspondence might be more worrisome.

We examined the discussions of the paraphilias in eight fairly recent psychiatric texts. Half came from one of our bookshelves and the others came from the new textbook department of a local medical bookstore. We make no claims that this is a scientifically based random sample, but we know of no reason to think it is unrepresentative.

We examined in particular whether a text had any discussion of the issue of whether deviancy alone was sufficient for the diagnosis of a paraphilia or whether significant distress on the patient's part was a necessary criterion for the diagnosis. Two or three of the texts (which we quote below) explicitly or fairly explicitly addressed this issue and presented it in a way consistent with the *DSM-IV* and *DSM-IV-TR* definition of mental disorder, and with the *DSM-IV* criteria, but contrary to *DSM-IV-TR* criteria.

However, some of the books made comments inconsistent with the *DSM-IV* and *DSM-IV-TR* definition and the *DSM-IV* criteria. For example, Bruce Cohen[7] states, "In other cases however the individual believes that the cravings are acceptable and even desirable, such that the cravings are considered 'ego syntonic.'" This is also the case with the paraphilias. Howard Goldman[8], in a similar vein, states, "Individuals with paraphilias may not report feeling distress and may justify their sexual interests as variant sexualities." And Robert Hales and Stuart Yudofsky[9] write, "In diagnosing all of the paraphilias, a further criterion is that the person has acted on the urges or is markedly distressed by them. Finally, David Tomb[10] states, "These patients [paraphiliacs] may not be troubled by their desires (ego-syntonic) and thus are difficult to treat, although depression, anxiety, and guilt do occur."

The problem with these authors' comments is not that they (correctly) recognize that some persons with unusual objects of sexual desire are not distressed either by having or acting on these desires. The problem is that the authors fail to see that persons with these characteristics do not satisfy the *DSM-IV* and *DSM-IV-TR* definition of having a mental disorder.

One short text by Michael Murphy, Ronald Cowan, and Lloyd Sederer[11], although containing the most abbreviated discussion of the paraphilias of any of the texts, is trenchant and to the point. Its entire discussion of the paraphilias is limited to three sentences:

Paraphilias include sexual disorders related to culturally unusual sexual activity. A key criterion for the diagnosis of a paraphilia (as in all psychiatric disorders) is that the disorder must cause an individual to experience significant distress or impairment in social or occupational functioning. In other words, an individual with unusual sexual practices who does not suffer significant distress or impairment would not be diagnosed with a psychiatric illness.

Another text by Benjamin Sadock and Virginia Sadock[12] shows a perceptive sensitivity to some of the issues involved. They state, in a discussion of transvestic fetishism:

Socially, dual-role transvestites, transgenderists, and transsexuals come together in organizations that are formed to provide environments that enable these men to appear as women. These cross-dressers network, build relationships, and learn more about their life possibilities at regional and national meetings. Participants have occasionally been the object of questionnaire studies and are the source of information from non-patient transvestites. These samples raise the possibility that there are some transvestites who are not paraphiliac because they sense no occupational, relationship, or other impairment. Such studies point to the fact that the gratifying aspects of networking and displaying the self as a female represents a good adaptation to this proclivity. It contrasts to those socially isolated men who cross-dress in private and who remain mortified at the possibility of anyone knowing about their situation.

The notion of a nonparaphiliac cross-dressing man nicely captures the important distinctions that need to be made. The situation seems entirely analogous to that of ego-syntonic homosexuality, which APA removed from the list of *DSM* disorders many years ago. Why this was done for homosexuality, but not for any of the other conditions involving statistically unusual sexual object choices is a mystery that *DSM* never addresses.[13]

Volitional Disabilities as a Kind of Mental Malady

One of the most significant evils associated with mental maladies is a particular type of disability, namely, a volitional disability. The concept of a volitional disability not only enables one to make explicit what phobias and compulsions have in common but also makes clear that addictions share this common feature. Indeed, a volitional disability is what compulsions, phobias, addictions (including alcoholism), and some kinds of noncompliant patient behaviors all have in common. An analysis of the concept of volitional disability helps to explain why mental maladies sometimes involve irrational behavior. The concept of a volitional disability was developed as part of an effort to provide a clear account of what it is to lack free will, as free will is understood in discussions of the philosophical problem of free will.[14] However, it turns out that it also plays an essential part in providing an adequate explanation of some psychiatric diagnoses (e.g., factitious disorders).

Voluntary Abilities

In order to fully understand the concept of a volitional disability, it is necessary to understand what a volitional ability is and how volitional abilities and disabilities are related to other abilities and disabilities, such as cognitive abilities and disabilities and physical abilities and disabilities.[15] These different kinds of abilities do not manifest themselves independently of one another; rather, volitional abilities, together with cognitive and physical abilities, make up what we call voluntary abilities. Voluntary abilities are abilities to do a kind of voluntary action, for example, to throw a ball, to recite a poem, or to pick up a snake. We do not usually distinguish between the various abilities that are the components of voluntary abilities—cognitive, physical, and volitional abilities—except when someone lacks one of those component abilities, that is, unless someone is disabled in a particular way.

Cognitive and physical abilities have an identical analysis. They differ from each other only in that physical abilities are essentially related to some particular part or parts of the body other than the brain, and cognitive abilities are not. For both kinds of abilities, the following analysis seems to capture what is essential. A has the cognitive (physical) ability to do X (a kind of action) if, and only if, for a reasonable number of times, A were to will to do a particular act of kind X, then, given a reasonable opportunity, A would do that particular act of kind X. Someone has a cognitive (physical) disability if he lacks the cognitive (physical) ability to do a kind of act after having reached a stage of life at which the ability to do that kind of act is the norm for the species. Furthermore, having reached that point of maturation, one has a disability even if most others in his age group also lack that same ability.

The way to test if someone has the cognitive ability to memorize ten lines of poetry or the physical ability to touch his toes is to provide situations in which he wills to demonstrate his ability and has a reasonable opportunity to do so. If he does exercise that ability a reasonable number of times (it is not necessary that he touch his toes every time he tries, or that he never fails to recite the ten lines correctly), then he has the ability in question. What counts as a reasonable number of times depends in part on the probability of doing that kind of action by luck. For example, swimming the English Channel needs to be done only once out of several attempts in order to demonstrate the voluntary ability to do so, whereas flipping a coin and making it land heads only once out of several attempts does not count at all in favor of having that ability.

Sometimes we know that someone has a cognitive (physical) ability even though we have never seen him demonstrate it, because he has demonstrated other more complex cognitive (physical) abilities. And since cognitive (physical) abilities do not depend on context, other than a reasonable opportunity, someone who demonstrates a cognitive (physical) ability in one context but not in another justifies us in concluding that it is not the cognitive (physical) ability that comes and goes, but that in one context he does not will to exercise that ability, but not necessarily that he lacks the relevant ability to will.

Volitional Disability

A volitional disability, like all other disabilities, is always related to a kind of action. When we say that A has a volitional disability with regard to willing to do X, X stands for a kind of action, such as entering elevators. Or the kind of action may be described in more general terms, such as entering small enclosed spaces. Since we are interested in volitional disabilities, we usually describe the kind of action as the most general kind of action with regard to which the person has a volitional disability. This is because it is the most general feature that is psychologically significant and, hence, most accurately describes the volitional disability.

If someone has a severe phobia with regard to being in elevators, he may have a volitional disability with regard to willing himself to enter an elevator or, more generally, with regard to entering small enclosed spaces. (We say "may" rather than "does" because phobias do not always involve a volitional disability; they sometimes involve only the suffering of inappropriate anxiety. We will discuss this later in the chapter.) Someone who has the requisite physical abilities but has a volitional disability with regard to willing to exercise these physical abilities when confronted with entering a small enclosed space has claustrophobia.

Our analysis of a volitional disability is as follows: S has a volitional disability with regard to willing to do X, if and only if one or more of the following statements is false.

(1) If S believes that there are coercive incentives for doing a particular act of kind X, he would almost always will to do it.

(2) If S believes that there are noncoercive incentives for doing a particular act of kind X, he would at least sometimes will to do it.

(3) If S believes that there are coercive incentives for not doing a particular act of kind X, he would almost always will not to do it.

(4) If S believes that there are noncoercive incentives for not doing a particular act of kind X, he would at least sometimes will not to do it.

(5) S has the ability to believe that there are coercive and noncoercive incentives, both for doing and for refraining from doing an act of kind X. That is, if S were presented with what almost everyone with similar knowledge and intelligence would regard as overwhelming evidence that there are coercive or noncoercive incentives for doing an act of kind X, S would believe that there are coercive or noncoercive incentives for doing an act of kind X, and if S were presented with what almost everyone with similar knowledge and intelligence would regard as overwhelming evidence that there are coercive or noncoercive incentives for refraining from doing an act of kind X, S would believe that there are coercive or noncoercive incentives for refraining from doing an act of kind X.

A coercive incentive is one that it would be unreasonable to expect any rational person not to act on, and hence provides an excuse for so acting, while a noncoercive incentive is, as its name implies, an incentive that is not coercive.

There are many different kinds of incentive: moral, prudential, patriotic, and so on. Moreover, while money can serve as an incentive, one sum of money, such as $5,000, is obviously a stronger incentive than a smaller sum of money, such as $100. However, in normal circumstances, no amount of money is a coercive incentive. Coercive incentives must involve suffering or the threat of suffering significant evils, such as death or serious disability, for only these can provide the kind of incentive that it would be unreasonable to expect any rational person not to act on. (To be subject to coercive incentives does not mean one is a victim of coercion. Coercion always involves an intentional threat by another person, but coercive incentives can come from anywhere.) However, even significant evils are not always coercive incentives. Whether an incentive is coercive or noncoercive depends not only on the strength of the incentive but also on the act for which it provides the incentive. That one will die by not undergoing the slight pain of an injection provides a coercive incentive for having the injection. However, the same incentive, dying, is not a coercive incentive for accepting a life-prolonging operation when one is suffering from chronic severe pain and permanent significant physical disabilities.

A compulsive hand washer who believes that there are both coercive and noncoercive incentives for not washing his hands once every waking hour and yet does not act in accordance with these incentives—and indeed laments his failure to act—is a paradigm example of someone who has a volitional disability. Such a person has a volitional disability with regard to washing his hands once every waking hour. Even though he does intentionally wash his hands, he does not do so voluntarily. Compulsive action of this kind provides the clearest example of someone who acts intentionally yet not voluntarily. This category of action requires the concept of a volitional disability, for acting voluntarily requires having the volitional ability to will to do that kind of action. Because having a volitional ability requires refraining from doing particular acts of the relevant kind when there are appropriate incentives for refraining, it is possible to perform an action intentionally, but not voluntarily.

Although we talk of willing and the volitional ability to will, we do not hold that there is some special faculty of the will or some special internal act of willing. For us, a person wills to do X if and only if he intentionally does X or tries to do X. We offer no philosophical analysis of willing, noting only that, as we use the term, there is no temporal gap between willing and doing. But, as we noted above, willing to do X does not imply having the volitional ability to will to do X, just as shaking by a palsy victim does not imply the physical ability to shake. To have the volitional ability to do X one must be able both to will (try to do or intentionally do) X, and refrain from willing (try to do or intentionally refrain from doing) X.

We do not make any claims about what is responsible for a particular volitional disability. What we say is compatible with the claims of those who claim that volitional disabilities are the result of genetic factors; early childhood training;

chemical, neurological, or physical problems with the brain; or a combination of these factors. Concerning the compulsive hand washer, his actions may result from guilt feelings due to real or imagined doing of some forbidden act, such as masturbation, that creates such anxiety that he has a volitional disability with regard to willing to refrain from washing his hands; or it may be that he has a volitional disability because he was conditioned to behave according to a particular schedule of reinforcement; or there may be genetic or chemical factors, or any combination of the above.

The Ability to Believe

We have characterized volitional disability primarily in a hypothetical manner that seems similar to the hypothetical manner in which cognitive and physical abilities were analyzed. However, whereas one need not lack one of these latter abilities even if he never wills to exercise it, one may lack the volitional ability to do X if he never believes in the existence of coercive and noncoercive incentives for doing X. This can happen if he lacks the ability to believe in the existence of incentives for certain kinds of actions. Thus, though he might have the volitional ability if he believed, he lacks the ability to believe. The volitional ability to will to do X (a kind of action) includes the ability to believe that there are incentives for and against doing X. But the ability to believe is not limited to beliefs about incentives for doing and refraining from doing an act of kind X.

We propose the following analysis of the general ability to believe: S has the ability to believe some proposition (P), if and only if, S were presented with what almost everyone with similar knowledge and intelligence would regard as overwhelming evidence that P were true, then S would believe that P was true. And if S were presented with what almost everyone with similar knowledge and intelligence would regard as overwhelming evidence that P were not true, then S would believe that P was not true.

This analysis of the general ability to believe is not limited to beliefs that there are coercive and noncoercive incentives for both doing and not doing X. The ability to believe or the lack of that ability applies to all kinds of beliefs, for example, that one has cancer, that one's wife is faithful, or that one's son has been killed. It is interesting to note the strong connection between holding an irrational belief (see chapter 2) and lacking the ability to believe. Irrational beliefs may be symptoms of mental maladies because they count as evidence that the person lacks the relevant ability to believe. What is wrong with having psychotic delusions, such as paranoid delusions, is not that they are false but rather that they show the person does not have the ability to believe; he does not respond to the overwhelming evidence in a way that is appropriate for someone with his knowledge and intelligence. This explains in a more precise way why holding irrational beliefs is a symptom of a mental malady.

A Classification of Actions

The concept of a volitional disability allows us to provide a general and complete framework for classifying human behavior with regard to excuses. Excuses are usually invoked in order to lessen or eliminate responsibility for doing something wrong or for the bad consequences of something one has done. Generally speaking, in offering excuses, a person is trying to show that his relationship to the bad consequences for which he is being held responsible differs in a significant way from a case in which he must accept full responsibility, that is, one in which (1) he acted intentionally in order to bring about those bad consequences; (2) he did not, at the time, suffer from any relevant volitional disability; and (3) his intentional action was not due to his being subject to coercive incentives.

In other words, the paradigm case of being held fully responsible for bringing about bad consequences is that of a person who acted intentionally, voluntarily, and freely. We call such actions free actions (A). Thus, in offering excuses, one move is to try to show that what was done was not done freely, that is, it was the result of coercive incentives. We call such actions unfree actions (B). A second move is to show that the action was not done voluntarily, that is, it was due to some volitional disability. We call such actions unvoluntary actions (C). A third move is to deny that the person intended to bring about the consequences for which he is being held responsible. We call such actions nonintentional (D). A fourth move is to claim that though the consequence stems from some movement (or lack of movement) of his body, that movement is not properly described as an action of his at all. We call such movements (or lack of movements) nonactions (E). The diagram on the following page shows how these various categories are related to one another.

We do not claim that it is always possible to categorize a given movement clearly. But often no distinction is made between category E and category D; both are simply lumped together as nonintentional actions. However, though there are significant borderline cases, there are also clear examples of each category. If A is pushed by B against C, then when C complains of being pushed, A can truthfully say, "I didn't do anything; I was pushed by B." This kind of case is the clearest example of nonaction. But there are other cases that also seem to be nonactions, such as movements of a person in an epileptic seizure, reflexive behavior such as knee jerks and eye blinks, and all the movements of a newborn infant. Thus, what some call involuntary actions, we regard as nonactions. Less clear cases would be complex movements made during sleep, or movements made by someone experiencing a sleepwalking disorder (*DSM-IV-TR* [2000, 639–644]). We think that providing for a distinct category of nonactions allows us to use the term "action" in a philosophically more fruitful fashion.

The clearest examples of actions fitting into category D are accidents (e.g., in reaching for the salt, I knock over my glass of water) and mistakes (e.g., I put

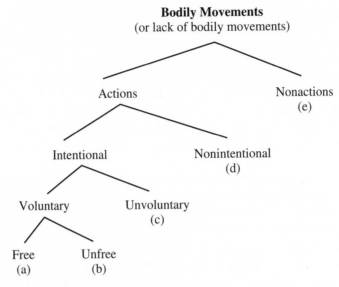

Figure 7.1

a teaspoon of salt instead of sugar into my tea). All of the clear cases of actions that fit into category D involve a person who is intentionally doing something but not intentionally doing the action (bringing about the consequences) at issue: for example, a hunter who, while shooting at a bird, wounds the picnicker behind the bush. Category D, therefore, unlike category E, typically involves some intentional action on the part of the agent.

Before we discuss category C, unvoluntary action, some discussion of the two categories of voluntary action, that is, A, a free action, and B, an unfree action, is in order. All voluntary action is intentional; what makes it voluntary is that it is willed by someone with the volitional ability to will it. An act done freely, or a free action (A), is thus one that is both intentional and voluntary; that is, it is willed by a person who has the volitional ability to do that kind of action, and what makes it free is the fact that no coercive incentives are responsible for the occurrence of the action. Normally, an unfree action is also one that is done by someone with the volitional ability to do that kind of action. It is unfree because there are coercive incentives that are responsible for that particular action's occurrence. A classical example of such an unfree though voluntary act is Aristotle's case of the sea captain who, in order to save his ship and crew, jettisons his cargo in a storm.

Some writers have combined categories B and C and regarded both as examples of actions done because of compulsion. However, in order to avoid confusion, it is important to distinguish between unfree actions (B) and unvoluntary ones (C). Unfree actions are those that are caused by something distinct from the agent, namely, coercive incentives. Were these coercive incentives removed, the person would be free to refrain from doing the contemplated action. However, unvoluntary actions are those caused by something about the agent himself, namely, a specific volitional disability. In no normal situation would such a person act differently than he did in fact act. The typical use of the term "compulsion" to cover both categories B and C is unfortunate, for it leads one to regard inner compulsion as identical to external compulsion, such as coercion, in all respects, except that it comes from within the person rather than from without. But this obscures the fact that external compulsion, such as coercion, typically involves the doing of particular actions—your money (here and now) or your life—whereas inner compulsion, that is, a volitional disability, always involves doing or refraining from doing kinds of actions.

Category C is not only the most important category with regard to the philosophical problem of free will, it is also the most interesting with regard to psychiatric problems. In addition to a tendency to equate categories C and B, there is an even stronger tendency to equate categories C and D. "Voluntary" and "intentional" are sometimes used as synonyms, and thus it is natural to equate unvoluntary with nonintentional action. But the recognition of the concept of a volitional disability shows clearly that there is an important distinction between voluntary and intentional actions. An action can be done intentionally but not voluntarily because the person has a volitional disability with regard to doing that kind of action. The standard confusion has arisen because it was assumed that if one willed (tried to do or intentionally did) X, then one must have had the volitional ability to do X. Consideration of the compulsive hand washer shows the falsity of this assumption. The compulsive hand washer intentionally washes his hands: he deliberately goes to the sink, takes the soap and lathers up. He knows what he is doing and intentionally does it. However, he does not do so voluntarily. He has a volitional disability with regard to washing his hands. This paradoxical situation, of intentionally doing what one does not have the volitional ability to do, arises because having the volitional ability to do X includes as a necessary feature willing not to do (trying not to do or intentionally not doing) X in appropriate circumstances. The volitional ability to do X requires the ability to refrain from doing X. A compulsive hand washer intentionally washes his hands, but since he has a volitional disability with regard to not washing his hands, he does not wash his hands voluntarily. Similarly, the claustrophobic intentionally refrains from entering the elevator but he does not refrain voluntarily if he cannot believe that there are coercive incentives for entering the elevator, or he would not intentionally enter the elevator even if he believed that there were coercive incentives.

It is the concept of a volitional disability that allows us to distinguish category C from both categories B and D and to make an unvoluntary action a category of its own. In applying this classification scheme to psychiatry, category C is especially important, for some significant psychiatric disorders involve this category.

Applications to Psychiatry

It is instructive to apply the above classification of actions to various conditions seen by psychiatrists. The symptoms of a great many mental maladies are characterized, at least in part, by some type of unvoluntary behavior, but other categories of actions are also relevant. We will give examples of conditions in four categories: free, intentional, voluntary actions (category A); intentional, unvoluntary actions (C); nonintentional actions (D), and nonactions (E). Since coercive incentives are seldom, if ever, involved in classifying actions for psychiatric use, we do not discuss Category B, that is, unfree actions, and we postulate that no coercive incentives are involved in the other categories we discuss. Failure to recognize category C leads to special problems in describing certain conditions such as factitious disorders.

Intentional Voluntary Actions (Category A)

Malingering is an example of a voluntary action that sometimes confronts physicians. The person who feigns symptoms does so intentionally and has the relevant volitional ability to feign or not to feign. The malingerer is regarded as acting both intentionally and voluntarily and, therefore, as being fully responsible for his behavior.

Malingerers do not suffer from a mental malady. Malingering is not even a condition of the person; it is the name given to a particular kind of action that is intentionally and voluntarily performed. The action is often quite rational in that the benefits the person may gain are worth the risks of discovery.

Malingering is a voluntary action. The essential feature is the voluntary production and presentation of false or grossly exaggerated physical or psychological symptoms, motivated by external incentives such as avoiding military duty, avoiding work, obtaining financial compensation, evading criminal prosecution, or obtaining drugs (*DSM-IV-TR* [2000, 739]). It might be preferable to say that malingering involves the intentional and voluntary production of symptoms, thereby explicitly noting that the malingerer not only intentionally produces the exaggerated symptoms of a malady but also that he has the volitional ability to produce them. This facilitates a distinction between a malingerer and someone suffering from a factitious disorder (e.g., Munchausen's syndrome, discussed later in this chapter). Both produce their symptoms intentionally, but the malingerer has the volitional ability to produce them and so their production is voluntary, whereas someone suffering from a factitious disorder has a relevant volitional disability and so the symptom production, although intentional, is not voluntary.

Intentional Unvoluntary Actions (Category C)

There are many behaviors of interest to psychiatrists that fall into this category. These actions all involve the patient's having a volitional disability. Compulsions and phobias are obvious examples and have been alluded to above. The patient carries out his compulsion intentionally. For example, he wills to wash his hands repetitively, but he does not do so voluntarily since he cannot refrain from washing his hands frequently over a period of time. It is, in fact, correct to say that he has a volitional disability with regard to washing his hands frequently over a period of time since having that volitional ability requires refraining from washing one's hands in the presence of appropriate coercive and noncoercive incentives, and this he cannot do.

Not all intentional unvoluntary actions are compulsions. Addictions are distinguished from compulsions, and they also involve intentional unvoluntary action. Indeed, the category of intentional, unvoluntary action brings out the obvious similarity between compulsions and addictions. The difference between them is that addictions involve substances that we know cause physiological changes in the body, whereas compulsions do not.

Phobias are also frequently associated with intentional unvoluntary behavior. Phobias are defined chiefly in terms of the patient's excessive or unreasonable fear when in the presence of the phobic stimulus. As a result of this fear, situations containing the phobic stimulus are either avoided or else are endured with intense anxiety or distress (*DSM-IV-TR* [2000, 449–450]). If the phobic person always or nearly always avoids the object of his fears (e.g., he refuses to enter small enclosed spaces like elevators), then he suffers from a volitional disability; if he is able to force himself to enter such spaces, but only with great anxiety, then he does not suffer from a volitional disability but rather from intense, inappropriate anxiety. In either event, he clearly has a mental disorder on our and on *DSM*'s definition.

Another interesting example of intentional, unvoluntary behavior is found in the *factitious disorders*. These are disorders in which the patient produces for the physician various symptoms that are either fabricated or self-induced. Because these disorders are not widely known, we will first quote from the *DSM-IV-TR* description of them (2000, 513).

The essential feature of Factitious Disorders is the intentional production of physical or psychological signs or symptoms. The presentation may include fabrication of subjective complaints (e.g., complaints of acute abdominal pain in the absence of any such pain), falsification of objective signs (e.g., manipulating a thermometer to create the illusion of fever), self-inflicted conditions (e.g., the production of abscesses by injection of saliva into the skin), exaggeration or exacerbation of pre-existing general medical conditions (e.g., feigning of a grand mal seizure by an individual with a previous history of seizure disorder), or any combination or variation of these. The motivation for the behavior is to assume the sick role. External incentives for the behavior (e.g., economic gain, avoiding legal responsibility, or improving physical well-being, as in Malingering) are absent.

This disorder differs from malingering in two important ways. The first is that patients who malinger are usually acting rationally (though immorally, because they unjustifiably intend to deceive), whereas patients with factitious disorder are not. They have no adequate reason for subjecting themselves to the repeated trials of hospitalization, diagnostic tests, and the significant risk of discovery that they generally experience. Indeed, they have both coercive and noncoercive incentives for not subjecting themselves to these risks, and yet they do so. The malingerer will rarely if ever go through with a painful or dangerous operation; indeed, one sometimes discovers malingerers by presenting them with the possibility of such an operation. However, operations usually do not discourage those suffering from factitious disorder.

Nonintentional Actions (Category D)

An example of a psychiatrically interesting condition that involves nonintentional actions is accident-proneness. Accident-prone individuals behave in ways that result in nonintentional self-injury. Essentially everyone manifests such behavior on occasion, but when an individual consistently does so with a frequency that seems too high to be due to chance alone, then he is often said to be accident-prone. It is part of the usual theory of accident-proneness that these accidents are not just bad luck, although it is acknowledged that they are not intentional. Rather, they are usually attributed to unconscious needs or motives, such as guilt. The condition of accident-proneness is not listed in *DSM-IV-TR*, but it does satisfy the definition of a mental disorder in that accident-prone individuals do have an increased risk of suffering evils. We can see no reason why accident-proneness, at least in its more extreme and obvious form, should not be a *DSM-IV-TR* disorder. Of course, there are many borderline cases in which one is not certain whether to attribute a person's frequent accidents to the person himself or to uncommonly bad luck, so malady status should not be conferred except when there is a clear pattern of accident-causing behavior.

A final example of psychiatrically relevant nonintentional action is a slip of the tongue, which is often referred to as a Freudian slip. In these cases, a person intends to say one thing but actually says something else, often in basic conflict with the intended utterance. The person nonintentionally uses a word that is inconsistent with the meaning he intends to express but consistent with some second meaning, often opposed to the first, which seems to express attitudes or feelings that there is good reason to believe the speaker has. Freud provided many examples of such slips, some of them undeniably demonstrating the nonintentional character of these actions.

Nonactions (Category E)

Movements made during major motor epileptic seizures represent a clear case of a nonaction. They are independent of the will of the patient, who is unconscious, and they have physical rather than mental causes. Tourette's syndrome (*DSM-IV-TR* [2000, 111–114]) is a similar condition occurring in patients who are not unconscious. These individuals have a malady in which they experience multiple motor and one or more vocal tics many times a day nearly every day. Many patients with this disorder also manifest a condition called coprolalia, in which they periodically bark out obscenities without intending to do so.

The vocal tics of Tourette's patients are not merely nonintentional; they do not seem to be actions at all. As we use the term "action," the movement (or lack of movement) must include, at least in part, willing to do something. Most nonintentional actions, such as wounding the picnicker, involve an intentional action, such as shooting at the bird. But the symptoms of Tourette's syndrome, such as barking out obscene words, involve no willing at all. Thus, we do not regard these utterances as actions, in our sense of the term. Similarly, we do not count reflex actions such as knee jerks and eye blinks as genuine actions, but only as bodily movements.

Psychiatrically interesting cases of bodily movements that are not actions may include hysterical seizures. These seizures resemble epileptic seizures, do not seem intentional, and do not seem to involve any willing. They come over the patient in a manner closely resembling that of epileptic seizures. However, we know that there is no brain disorder, so that these bodily movements, though not considered actions, are nonetheless psychologically caused. The existence of such bodily movements independent of the will, but clearly having mental rather than physical causes, reinforces Freud's view about unconscious mental processes. These movements are also compatible with mental causation for what seem like normal physical disabilities, such as hysterical blindness and hysterical paralysis. In addition, these movements fit well with mental causation of genuine bodily changes, such as burnlike blisters on the skin from the hypnotic suggestion that a lighted cigarette has been ground into one's palm. The fact that very similar symptoms can have either psychological or physical causes reinforces our view that there is no essential distinction between physical and mental maladies.

Criticisms of the *DSM-III-R*, *DSM-IV*, and *DSM-IV-TR* Definition of Mental Disorder

The definition of mental disorder offered by *DSM-III-R*, *DSM-IV*, and *DSM-IV-TR* is in conflict with two quite distinct and opposing views. The first kind of definition, whose most prominent exponent is Christopher Boorse, provides an objective account of mental disorders solely in value-free scientific terms. The second kind of definition, which is represented by Tristam H. Engelhardt and Peter Sedgwick, defines mental disorder solely in society-based value terms. R. E. Kendell is talking about these two opposing views when he says the following.

"The most fundamental issue, and also the most contentious one, is whether disease and illness are normative concepts based on value judgments, or whether they are value-free scientific terms; in other words, whether they are biomedical terms or sociopolitical ones."[16] Thus, Kendell, in a paradigm of the fallacy of assumed equivalence, accepts the view that biomedical terms are value-free scientific terms and that normative concepts based on value judgments are sociopolitical terms. That some biomedical terms such as "disease" or "mental disorder" are objective value terms is not even considered as a possibility.

Jerome Wakefield, while agreeing with Kendell that value terms are sociopolitical, attempts to provide an account that reconciles the two opposing views of mental disorder that Kendell mentions. Against these two extreme accounts, Wakefield says, "I argue that disorder lies on the boundary between the given natural world and the constructed social world; a disorder exists when the failure of a person's internal mechanisms to perform their functions as designed by nature impinges harmfully on the person's well-being as defined by social values and meaning."[17] Wakefield defines a disorder as "a harmful dysfunction, wherein harmful is a value term based on social norms, and dysfunction is a scientific term referring to the failure of a mental mechanism to perform a natural function for which it was designed by evolution."[18] It is useful to examine Wakefield's attempt at compromise in some detail as it illustrates the problems with both of the views that he is attempting to bring together.

The first problem involves the claim that a dysfunction is "the failure of a person's internal mechanisms to perform their functions as designed by nature."[19] This view is reminiscent of Kant, who says, "In the natural constitution of an organized being, let us take it as a principle that in such a being no organ is to be found for any end unless it be the most fit and the best adapted for that end."[20] Kant simply assumes a teleological account of nature, derived from the view that God designed the best possible world. Wakefield's account of dysfunctions as failures "of a person's internal mechanisms to perform their functions as designed by nature" has the same characteristic. There is no reason to believe that *every* dysfunction is a failure of nature's design. Evolution may not be quite as perfect as Wakefield takes it to be. A person is suffering from a dysfunction when she is suffering one of the harms mentioned in the definition of mental disorder in *DSM-III-R*, *DSM-IV*, and *DSM-IV-TR*, and there is no sustaining cause distinct from the person responsible for her suffering that harm. This is what the definition means by saying that the harm must be due to "a dysfunction in the person." This would have been clearer if the *DSM*'s definition explicitly included the concept of a distinct sustaining cause.

Although Wakefield claims that there is a dysfunction only if there is a "failure of a person's internal mechanisms to perform their functions as designed by nature," he actually relies on there being no distinct sustaining cause indicating a dysfunction. He says, "The fact that in Post-Traumatic Stress Disorder (PTSD) the person's coping mechanisms often fail to bring the person back to functional equilibrium months and even years after the danger is gone, and that PTSD reactions are dramatically out of proportion to the actual posttraumatic danger, suggests that the response is indeed independent of any environmental maintaining cause and therefore is a dysfunction."[21] It is from the fact that there is no "environmental maintaining cause" that he infers that the person's distress is due to a dysfunction. He does not and cannot know directly that there is a "failure of a person's internal mechanisms to perform their functions as designed by nature." The claim that a dysfunction is a failure of nature's design is often unverifiable. Perhaps nature designed people to deteriorate and die in order to allow for the species to develop. Regardless of nature's design, if a person is suffering or is at a significantly increased risk of suffering death, pain, disability, or an important loss of freedom or pleasure, and there is no distinct sustaining cause, he has a dysfunction. It is significant that Wakefield never mentions conditions that significantly increase the risk of suffering harm such as very high blood pressure as a disorder for, on his view, until there is a failure of nature's design, there is no dysfunction.[22]

Societal Values and the Definition of Mental Disorder

Wakefield's second problem is his acceptance of the common view of social scientists that values are constructed by particular societies. By accepting this account, he opens the door to the kind of relativity that the definitions of mental disorder in *DSM-III-R*, *DSM-IV*, and *DSM-IV-TR* were designed to close. He does not seem to realize that if harms are determined primarily by social norms, then this opens the door to the criticism of psychiatry as primarily enforcing social norms. Wakefield claims, "The requirement that there be harm also accounts for why albinism, reversal of heart position, and fused toes are not considered disorders even though each results from a breakdown in the way some mechanism is designed to function."[23] Since Wakefield claims that albinism is a failure of nature's design, a particular society that negatively evaluates albinism means it is a disorder in that society, but not a disorder in a society that does not negatively evaluate it. A person can cease to have a disorder simply by moving from one society to another.

Also, if homosexuality and sexual deviations are taken as involving a breakdown in the way some mechanism is designed to function, homosexuality and other sexual deviations would be mental disorders in those societies where they are negatively evaluated and not in those societies where they are not so evaluated. His suggested definition would reverse the progress that was made in *DSM-III-R*, *DSM-IV*, and *DSM-IV-TR*, when "conflicts that are primarily between the individual and society" were explicitly ruled out as a criterion of mental disorder.

Only traits that would result in conflict with all societies count as a dysfunction in the person. This is the way in which the additional criterion that was added to the list of criteria for the paraphilias in *DSM-IV* should be understood. "The fantasies, sexual urges, or behaviors cause clinically significant distress or impairment in social, occupational, or other important areas of functioning."[24]

Wakefield's acceptance of the common view of social scientists, that values are constructed by particular societies, is what leads him to think that harm cannot be defined in universal terms. However, as we showed in chapter 2, it is universally true that, in the absence of reasons to hold otherwise, rational persons in every society regard death, pain, disability, and loss of freedom or pleasure as harms. No person who is considered rational wants to suffer any of these harms unless he has some belief that he or someone else will avoid what is considered by a significant number of persons as either a greater harm, or a compensating benefit, such as greater consciousness, ability, freedom, or pleasure. The universality of these harms and benefits is shown by the fact that nothing counts as a disorder unless it involves one of these harms or a significantly increased risk of suffering one of these harms, and nothing counts as a punishment unless it involves the infliction of one of these harms.[25]

The agreement of rational persons in all societies about the universality of the basic harms is extremely important, for it establishes the objectivity of the concept of a disorder. Disorders, mental or physical, are conditions that are associated with suffering distress or disability or a significantly increased risk of suffering death, pain, disability, or an important loss of freedom or pleasure. Mental disorders, properly understood, like physical disorders, are not merely labels for conditions that some culture or society has arbitrarily picked out for special treatment.[26] Mental disorders are conditions that no rational person in any society wants himself, or anyone he cares for, to suffer, unless there is some compensating benefit.

It is not a symptom of a mental disorder to be distressed on discovering that one has a physical disorder (e.g., cancer), because the physical disorder counts as an event in the world just as the death of a loved one and one's distress is an expectable and culturally sanctioned response to this situation. However, if the distress goes beyond an expectable and culturally sanctioned response to a particular situation, then one may be suffering a mental disorder that the physical disorder, just like other unfortunate events in the world, may have played a significant role in causing. What counts as an expectable and culturally sanctioned response to a particular event often differs from society to society and from culture to culture within large multicultural societies like the United States. But suffering distress, disability, or a significantly increased risk of suffering death, pain, disability, or an important loss of freedom is a necessary feature of any disorder, mental or physical.

The fact that it is primarily on the basis of their symptoms that mental disorders differ from physical disorders makes it clear that "neither deviant behavior (e.g., political, religious, or sexual) nor conflicts that are primarily between the individual and society are mental disorders unless the deviance or conflict is a symptom of a dysfunction in the person." However, if the conflicts between a person and society are such that they would occur in all societies, this is a symptom of a dysfunction in the person. Although deviance, by itself, is not sufficient to count as a disorder, some deviance seems to be so closely related to distress, disability, or a significantly increased risk of suffering death, pain, disability, or an important loss of freedom or pleasure that it is often classified as a disorder. Thus, having a third eye in one's head might actually give one greater visual ability than those having the normal number of eyes. Nonetheless, normal human responses to this kind of deviance may so regularly involve either pain or an important loss of freedom or pleasure that the deviance itself is regarded as a physical disorder. Similarly, normal human responses to some deviant behavior, for example, sexual intercourse with corpses, may normally call forth such a universal negative human response that the condition is itself regarded as a mental disorder. However, for the reactions of others to any deviance, either physical or mental, to make a deviant condition count as a disorder, the reactions must be universal human responses, not merely the response of those in a particular society.

Although the *DSM-III*, *DSM-IV*, and *DSM-IV-TR* definition of mental disorder can be improved, it is far superior to any of the alternatives, including Wakefield's, that have been proposed to replace it. Its major achievement is its acceptance of universal values, so that values can be included in the definition of a mental disorder without thereby making a disorder relative to each individual society. That is a significant achievement.

Notes

1. *DSM-IV-TR* (2000), the most recent *DSM* volume, discusses and supplies code numbers for eight paraphilias: exhibitionism, fetishism, frotteurism, pedophilia, sexual masochism, sexual sadism, transvestic fetishism, and voyeurism. It also supplies a code number for "paraphilia not otherwise specified." Note that homosexuality is not listed as a paraphilia (see discussion below).

2. As explained in the prior chapter, we prefer the term "malady" to other "disease-terms," but the *DSM* volumes use "disorder," so we will use that term in discussing the *DSM* texts. All disorders count as maladies.

3. There have been four volumes of the *Diagnostic and Statistical Manual* issued during the past twenty-five years: *DSM-III* (1980), *DSM-III-R* (1987), *DSM-IV* (1994), and *DSM-IV-TR* (2000), the latter being the most recent volume.

4. The definition parallels closely the definition of "mental malady" that we have proposed (see Culver and Gert [1982], Gert [1992], and Gert and Culver [2004]). The parallelism is not surprising because in our *Philosophy in Medicine* we criticized the *DSM-III* definition and one of us (BG) was invited to be a consultant for *DSM-III-R*. The revised definition of a mental disorder that was developed for *DSM-III-R* differs from the *DSM-IV-TR* definition only by the addition of the words "and culturally sanctioned."

5. We think that loss of pleasure should have been included in this list.

6. See *DSM-IV-TR*, xxxi.

7. See Cohen (2003, 420).

8. See Goldman (2000, 372).

9. See Hales and Yudofsky (2004, 519).

10. See Tomb (1999, 180–181).

11. See Murphy, Cowan, and Sederer (2001, 51).

12. See Sadock and Sadock (2000, 1638).

13. See Soble (2004) for an elaboration of this point.

14. See Duggan and Gert (1967). Reprinted in *The Nature of Human Action*, edited by Miles Brand, 1970. Also see Gert and Duggan (1979). Reprinted in *Moral Responsibility*, edited by John Martin Fisher, 1986.

15. For a further discussion of voluntary abilities, see articles cited in note 14.

16. See Kendell (1986).

17. Ibid. Wakefield, like the editor of *DSM-IV*, regards the definition of mental disorder in *DSM-III* as "essentially the same as *DSM-III-R*'s" (Wakefield [1992a]). Partly, this may be due to his not knowing that Robert Spitzer responded to conceptual criticisms of the definition of mental disorder in *DSM-III* in Culver and Gert's *Philosophy in Medicine* (1982), by inviting one of us (BG) to revise the definition to make it compatible with the definition of malady that we provided in that book. See Wakefield (1992b).

18. See Wakefield (1992b). This quote is from the abstract that precedes this paper. Wakefield's view is listed as a mixed model by Christian Perring in his article "Mental Illness" for the Stanford online *Encyclopedia of Philosophy*. We have benefited from reading this article and from comments by Perring. However, we do not agree with Perring on several points.

19. It seems that on this account of dysfunction, dyslexia is not a disorder, because it is unlikely that nature designed an internal mechanism to perform the function of distinguishing between *b*'s and *d*'s.

20. See Kant, First Section, 395.

21. See Wakefield (1992b, 239).

22. See ibid., 233, where there is no mention of increased risk of suffering the universal harms.

23. See Wakefield (1992a).

24. See *DSM-IV* (1994, 523–532). In *DSM-III-R*, this criterion was not included and so there was an inconsistency between the criteria for the paraphilias and the definition of mental disorder. See Gert (1992), and also the discussion of paraphilias earlier in this chapter.

25. See Gert (2005, chapter 4, "Goods and Evils").

26. Appendix I of *DSM-IV-TR* (2000, 897–903) contains a "Glossary of Culture Bound Syndromes," but all of these that are considered disorders also involve distress, disability, or a significantly increased risk of suffering death, pain, disability, or an important loss of freedom. Wakefield (1992a, 380) says, "This list might be considered to be an operationalized approximation to the requirement that there must be harm." That he does not realize that this is a list of universal harms, not merely negative evaluations based on social norms, is confirmed by his statement on the following page. "Although a typology of harms such as that provided by *DSM-III-R* is useful, it should not be forgotten that ... the underlying reason these effects are relevant to disorder is that they are negative and this evaluative element is fundamental to our judgments about disorder." Wakefield does not realize that this list of harms provides a list of objective harms that are not dependent on the evaluative judgments of particular societies.

8

What Doctors Must Know
about Medical Practice

In recent years more and more information has become available about the underlying nature of medical practice. We now understand in a more precise way than we once did the process of diagnostic testing, for example, that the prevalence of a disease in the cohort from which a patient comes greatly affects a test's predictive accuracy, and that essentially all tests have false positives and false negatives, both of which can cause significant problems for patients. We also understand more about the outcomes of the treatments we use, for example, that a new treatment can be determined, in a randomized clinical trial, to be statistically superior to a former treatment, or to a placebo, and that it can still be entirely rational for a patient to refuse to take it because of the unlikelihood that the treatment will in fact help her (because the treatment has a high number needed to treat [NNT]; see below). We have more and more data showing that the outcome of many important medical and surgical treatments depends significantly on the frequency with which particular doctors and hospitals carry out these treatments. We also realize that there are large geographical variations within the United States in the frequency with which some treatments are administered, variations that almost certainly are only minimally related to the physical conditions or the adequately informed choices of the patients who receive them. Finally, because of the emphasis placed in recent years on evidence-based medicine, we have better information about the true efficacy of the treatments and the diagnostic and screening tests that make up the bulk of medical practice.

Three questions can be raised about this wealth of new information. (1) Why do doctors have a duty to know any of it? (2) How much of it do doctors have a duty to know?[1] and (3) a related but different question, How much of it do doctors have a duty to disclose to their patients? The answer to the first question was given in chapter 4 and concerns the special duties of doctors. A doctor has a professional duty to avoid causing any unnecessary harm to patients, including performing unnecessary medical procedures. He also has a duty not to provoke any anxiety in his patients caused by giving incorrect or misleading information. Failure to know these new kinds of information significantly increases the risk of a doctor causing his patients to suffer these unnecessary harms. This chapter discusses the second of these questions; the third question will be discussed in the next chapter. We summarize and discuss four new kinds of information that are increasingly becoming available to physicians:

1. The probabilistic nature of medical diagnosis and medical treatment.
2. The presence of strong volume/outcome relationships in medical practice.
3. The existence of significant geographical variations in the frequency with which some treatments are administered.
4. The existence of practice guidelines covering many aspects of medical practice.

The Probabilistic Nature of Medical Diagnosis and Treatment

Medical practice is inherently probabilistic. Tests almost always yield false positives and false negatives, treatments do not always help, accurate prognoses are notoriously difficult to make, and maladies sometimes improve without any treatment at all.[2] It is rare in medicine, in fact, to find any one variable that is unfailingly associated with any other variable. The presence of uncertainty is pervasive and the nature and the degree of uncertainty are factors that must be taken into account in understanding diagnostic and therapeutic phenomena and in making medical decisions.

One way of characterizing medical practice is to say that it concerns the modulation of harms. Patients suffer from maladies. A necessary part of the definition of a malady is that it is a condition that involves the suffering, or the significantly increased risk of suffering, harms.[3] Tests are meant to diagnose the presence of maladies, but tests, in addition to being imperfectly accurate, can cause the suffering of harms themselves. Finally, treatments are meant to eliminate or ameliorate the harms inherent in maladies, but virtually all treatments, in addition to sometimes being ineffective, can also cause harms themselves. Thus, the physician and the patient are operating in a matrix of possible and probable harms in which the overarching goal of decreasing the harms of maladies is complicated by the fact that diagnostic and therapeutic maneuvers aimed toward that goal don't always work as hoped for, and may cause significant harms themselves.

Except in unusual circumstances, it is patients who should make decisions about their own medical care.[4] Therefore, physicians must, during the consent process, tell patients about the nature and the degree of uncertainty that is associated with whatever factual information is being disclosed. If a physician proposes using a test, the patient should know, before agreeing to the test, about any risks associated with the test procedure itself, and also should know how helpful a positive or negative test result will be. If a physician proposes using a particular treatment, the patient should be told how likely it is the treatment will help, as well as how likely it is that any significant harms might be caused by the treatment.

However, before a physician can inform a patient about harms and benefits and about the degree of certainty that they will occur, it is clearly necessary that he or she be familiar with the information that must be disclosed. Thus, physicians need to know and understand the ways in which medical practice is probabilistic and they must be skilled at explaining this information to patients. Probabilistic phenomena in medical practice are sometimes quite straightforward, but at other times they are subtle and even counterintuitive. Close study is required to understand them and to be able to effectively communicate them to patients.

All physicians are familiar at some level with the probabilistic nature of medical practice. No physician believes that a particular pattern and time-course of abdominal pain means 100% of the time that a patient either has or does not have acute appendicitis, or believes that tricyclic antidepressant drugs always ameliorate depression, or that every suspicious area of increased density on a mammogram means that the patient has a carcinoma. But in recent years our understanding of the details of the probabilistic nature of medical practice has deepened considerably, due to the contributions of persons working in such fields as medical decision making, clinical epidemiology, and evidence-based medicine.[5] However, many physicians are unaware of this work or they understand it only superficially.

Gerd Gigerenzer gives the following example in a recent book:[6]

The probability that a woman of age 40 has breast cancer is about 1.0%. If she has breast cancer the probability that she will test positively on a screening mammogram is 90%. If she does not have breast cancer, the possibility that she will nevertheless test positively is 9%. What are the chances that a particular woman who tests positively actually has breast cancer?

The answer (about 9%) can be easily calculated from the information given. Yet when Gigerenzer asked the question of twenty-four physicians with an average of fourteen years of clinical experience, only four answered it correctly. Another four were reasonably close but the remaining sixteen were seriously in error, giving answers ranging from 50% to 90%. The median estimate of the twenty-four estimates given was 70%, a figure almost eight times too large. Gigerenzer remarks that a patient might be justifiably alarmed by this diversity of medical opinion.

Gigerenzer does not say how many of these twenty-four physicians actually worked with patients who had routine mammography, although the principles at work here are not limited to mammographic testing. They apply to all medical situations where a patient is suspected of having some disease and is given a test that is thought to have some usefulness in ruling that disease in or out. Whether the test comes back positive or negative, it is useful for both the patient and the doctor to know what the resultant likelihood is that the patient indeed has the disease. Eight of these twenty-four doctors thought the likelihood, after a positive test, was 90% while four thought it was 1%. It is difficult to see how any sensible discussion and decision making about future interventions could take place in the presence of such striking misinformation. Further, the patients of the eight doctors who thought that the likelihood, after a positive test, was that 90% of the patients had breast cancer would suffer unnecessary anxiety because they had been told that their chances of having breast cancer were ten times greater than they actually were. And the patients of the four doctors who thought the answer was only 1% might decide not to follow up.

Persons who work in bioethics, no less than physicians themselves, need to understand probabilistic phenomena. Suppose an ethics consultant is asked to comment on the *moral* justification of involuntarily hospitalizing a particular depressed patient to prevent that patient from attempting to kill himself. If the consultant wishes to give an opinion that goes beyond an intuitive hunch then she should try to establish what the likelihood is that a patient with this patient's characteristics would attempt to kill himself if he were not hospitalized, and what the sensitivity and specificity are of the predictions that psychiatrists make about the suicidality of patients.[7] None of these numbers are easy to come by with great precision, but even reasonable estimates of them will usually enable the consultant to give a more cogent answer to the question than she would otherwise be able to do.[8]

We discuss in this chapter the nature of the uncertainties associated with diagnostic tests, including screening tests, and the nature of the uncertainties associated with treatment. By convention, the term "diagnostic test" is generally used when there is a plausible reason to suspect that a patient may be suffering from the malady for whose presence one is testing. The term "screening test" is used if there is no particular reason to believe the patient has a given malady, but the patient belongs to a cohort in which the malady sometimes appears.[9] Our analysis applies similarly to the two kinds of testing although they are different enough in their particulars that we discuss them separately.

Uncertainty in Diagnostic Testing

It is common in medical practice for tests to be administered to try to determine the nature of the conditions or maladies from which patients suffer. Often these are *laboratory tests*, such as the various measurements that can be made on bodily fluids like blood, urine, spinal fluid, sputum, or semen. Genetic tests are in this category; they are increasingly common and may be expected to become even more so in the near future. Other tests are *physiological*, like the electrocardiogram or the electroencephalogram. Some tests are *behavioral*, like neuropsychological testing, or filling out a Zung depression scale, or asking a patient the four items on the Michigan Alcohol Screening Test (MAST) to try to determine whether the patient is alcohol dependent. The physical examination is filled with tests and measurements of structure and function: physicians listen for heart murmurs because their presence suggests the existence of certain valvular malfunctions, or they test for primitive reflexes because their presence suggests the existence of certain kinds of central nervous system (*CNS*) disease.

Test results in tabular form. If one is concerned about whether a particular condition or malady is present, then a test result that indicates that the condition is or may well be present is usually labeled "positive"; if the test result does not indicate the condition is or may well be present, it is labeled "negative." The simplest way to think of the relationship between a test and a condition being tested for is to assume that a positive test result means the condition is present and a negative result that the condition is absent. But positive test results rarely mean that the condition is present for certain, and negative test results do not mean that the condition is absent for certain. This state of affairs can be depicted in a simple 2×2 table (8.1):

Table 8.1

		condition	
		+	−
test	+	True +	False +
	−	False −	True −

It is conventional in constructing such tables for the term "test" to be placed to the left of the table and for the top row of the table to contain instances of positive test results and the bottom row to contain instances of negative test results. The term "condition" or "malady" is then put at the top of the table and the left column contains instances of persons who do have the malady or condition and the right column contains persons who do not have the malady or condition. By displaying data in this way it is easy to visualize the number of true positives, false positives, true negatives, and false negatives, as shown in the table.

Note that although one is displaying in the above table the extent to which a test is associated with the presence of a malady, a more general way of characterizing the table is that it shows the relationship between something that is measured (A) and some second thing (B) whose likelihood of existing now or occurring in the future is shown for both positive and negative values of A. A is often a test of some kind, but B can also be a test. For example, one can measure the accuracy of physicians' clinical impressions concerning whether persons with pharyngitis whom they examine will subsequently prove to have positive throat cultures for a streptococcal infection. Here A is a clinical prediction after an oropharyngeal and general physical examination (it is predicted that the patient will have or will not have a subsequent positive throat culture) and B is the result showing whether the throat culture subsequently does or does not grow out *streptococci*. The throat culture can be usefully used as the predicted-to "condition" even though it is realized that throat cultures themselves may be thought of as tests that have false positives and false negatives with regard to the question of whether a patient truly has a significant streptococcal infection in his or her pharynx.

Another example: B can be the number of members of a cohort of suicidal patients admitted through the emergency room with schizoaffective disorders who do or do not kill themselves over a future one-month period. A can be a considered judgment, based on whatever interview data, psychological test results, and demographic variables the examiner wishes to measure, about which patients are or are not likely to commit suicide. Here A is a balanced judgment, either impressionistic or derived from an algorithm, or some combination of the two; and B is an event. B is not a disease; all the patients have the disease. B is, rather, a behavioral event about which a prediction is being made.

Numerical examples. Here are two examples of the relationship between test performance and the existence of an underlying condition whose presence the test is intended to detect. The patients tested were those whose presenting signs and symptoms raised the possibility that they were suffering from an acute myocardial infarction (MI). The test was a blood test for the presence of a significant amount of a muscle-cell enzyme called creatinine kinase (CK), which is known to be frequently elevated in the presence of an acute MI. Data were obtained on 360 patients at the time of their admission to a cardiac care unit (CCU). At a later time, after the patients were no longer hospitalized, they were sorted in retrospect into two groups: those whose total test findings and clinical course indicated that they had suffered an acute MI and those whose data indicated they had not suffered an MI. Here are the two groups' CK test performance at the time of admission:

	MI-yes	*MI-no*	*Total*
CK positive	215	16	231
CK negative	15	114	129
Total	230	130	360

The following measures can be derived from 2×2 tables of this kind:

(1) The *sensitivity* of a test refers to the percentage of patients *with* the disorder who have a *positive* test result. In this case, of the 230 patients who were, in retrospect, believed to have been experiencing an acute MI, 215 had a positive test result, so the sensitivity was 215/230 = 93%.

(2) The *specificity* of a test refers to the percentage of patients *without* the disorder who have a *negative* test result. In this case, of the 130 patients who were, in retrospect, believed not to have been experiencing an acute MI, 114 had a negative test result so the specificity was 114/130 = 88%.

Suppose you were a physician who worked in the above CCU and after the results shown in the above table became known to you, a new patient, Mr. A, was admitted to the unit, was given the CK test, and had a positive test result. What is the chance that this new patient is having an acute MI? To answer that question you need another value:

(3) The *positive predictive value (PPV)* of a test refers to the percentage of patients with a *positive* test result who later are judged to have been suffering from the disorder. In this case, of the 231 patients who had a positive CK, 215 were having an acute MI so the PPV was 215/231 = 93%. Thus, the probability is 93% that Mr. A is having an acute MI. This is a relatively high PPV and reflects the fact that the test has relatively few false positives; only sixteen persons out of the 231 who tested positive were not having an MI.

Suppose yet another patient, Mr. B, was admitted to the CCU, but he had a negative CK test result. To estimate the probability that Mr. B was in fact not having an MI, one needs another value:

(4) The *negative predictive value (NPV)* of a test refers to the percentage of patients who have a *negative* test result who are later judged not to have been suffering from the disorder. In this case, of the 129 patients with a negative CK, 114 were indeed not having an acute MI, so the NPV was 114/129 = 88%. Thus, the probability is 88% that Mr. B is not having an acute MI. This is a reasonably high NPV and reflects the fact that there were a relatively small number of false negatives—persons who tested negatively who were, in fact, having an acute MI.

(5) The *prevalence* of actual MIs in patients admitted with the suspicion that they were having an MI can also be derived from the table: 360 patients were admitted to the CCU with the suspicion they were having an MI, and 230 of the 360 actually were having an MI, so the prevalence was 230/360 = 64%. And of course the prevalence of patients in this CCU cohort not having an acute MI was 130/360, or 36%.

Knowing the above five values (sensitivity, specificity, PPV, NPV, and prevalence) of a test given to a particular population of persons (in this case, patients admitted to this CCU) allows one to make more precise estimates of the probability that a patient is or is not having an acute MI. To illustrate: What is the probability that a patient admitted to this CCU and suspected of having an MI is actually having an MI? Without the CK test results, the probability is the same as the prevalence in this population, that is, 64%. However, if the patient has a positive CK test, the probability is raised to the PPV of 93%. If the patient has a negative CK test, the chance that he is not having an MI increases from 36% (the prevalence of patients admitted to the CCU who are not having MIs) to the NPV of 88%.

One can see why the CK test is widely used. It is an innocuous test to have performed, involving only a venipuncture to withdraw a blood sample, and it allows one to discover whether a patient admitted to this CCU cohort has a 93% or a 12% chance of currently having an MI. By combining the CK test result with other diagnostic indexes of having an acute MI (e.g., characteristic EKG changes seen frequently in persons having an MI), an even higher diagnostic accuracy can be achieved.

The effect of prevalence. A critically important feature of both the PPV and the NPV is that their values are dependent on the prevalence of the being-tested-for condition in the cohort from which a particular patient comes.[10] This phenomenon is counterintuitive to most persons. Here is an example that illustrates this prevalence specificity: Suppose that a physician, Dr. Y, was impressed with the usefulness of the CK test in the CCU population. Mindful that patients who are admitted to the hospital ostensibly for noncardiac causes occasionally prove to be suffering from MIs, Dr. Y proposes administering the CK test to all admissions to a general hospital in order to try to diagnose these occult MIs. Let us suppose that 2% of these general hospital admissions are suffering from acute MIs, although the actual number may be even lower. In order to make comparisons with the prior table, suppose Dr. Y administers the test to 360 consecutive admissions to the general hospital. We then create the following table to understand what results he would achieve.

	MI-yes	MI-no	Total
CK positive	6.7	42.3	49
CK negative	0.5	310.5	311
Total	7.2	352.8	360

How was this table created? One starts by entering 360 as the total number of patients to be tested, as was specified above. Then, since the prevalence stipulated was 2%, one calculates 2% of 360 (which is 7.2) and enters that as the total of the MI-yes column. If 7.2 persons are in the MI-yes column, then the remainder (352.8) must be the total of the MI-no column. One then apportions the MI-yes and MI-no totals into the CK positive and CK negative cells by using the sensitivity and specificity values. That is, the sensitivity of the test is 93% so 93% of the 7.2 patients (that is, 6.7) are put in the CK positive/MI-yes cell and the remaining

0.5 are put in the CK negative/MI-yes cell. The MI-no total of 352.8 is partitioned in the same way, as shown, using the specificity value of 88%.

Now, what are the PPV and NPV values? The PPV has changed considerably. It was 93% in the CCU but is now only 14% (i.e., 6.7/49). In other words, only 14% of those general hospital admissions who have a positive CK test will, in fact, have had an MI. *Eighty-six percent will be false positives.* Nothing has changed except the prevalence of the disorder, but its effect on the PPV has been dramatic: in the CCU, more than nine out of ten patients with a positive CK test will have had an MI, but in the general hospital, approximately six out of seven patients with CK positive test results will not have had an MI at all.

How could this happen? As the prevalence of the disease drops, the percentage of false positives increases significantly and the PPV inevitably decreases significantly in tandem.

Every 2×2 table showing the empirical relationship between a predictor and a predicted-to condition is necessarily based on a particular prevalence of the predicted-to condition, namely, the prevalence shown in that particular 2×2 table. This is an easily calculated value: it is the percentage of persons with the predicted-to condition (e.g., with the disease) in the entire population shown in the table. Using the usual A, B, C, and D labeling of the cells in these 2×2 tables, shown below, the prevalence $= A + C$ divided by $A + B + C + D$.

A	B
C	D

Figure 8.2

Bayes theorem. What this prevalence-PPV relationship shows is an instance of what is often called *Bayes' theorem*, namely, that the probability that an event will occur is a joint function of a test result and the event's prior probability.[11] Thus, if we are confronted with a man from the CCU, we know that the pretest probability that he has had an MI is 64%. If he has a positive CK test result, that pretest probability needs to be revised upward; if he has a negative CK test result it needs to be revised downward. The same is true of a man from the second cohort, who has a pretest probability of 2% of having had an MI. The operative equation is often expressed in this manner:

Pretest Probability + Test Result = Posttest Probability

The "+" in the equation does not literally mean that numbers are added. The equation should be understood to mean: This test result, given the pretest probability of this condition being present, suggests that there is the following posttest probability that the condition is present.

Whenever any patient is given a test, Bayes theorem can be used in interpreting the significance of the test result. To gain the maximum possible amount of information one should have some notion of what the pretest probability is of the predicted-to condition and then determine what effect the test result has on revising that probability upward or downward.

The probabilistic nature of testing. Tests are not perfect; they rarely have sensitivities and specificities of 100% and most fall far short of that figure. To the extent that their sensitivities and specificities are below 100%, the tests yield false positives and negatives. False positives and false negatives can be harmful to patients, just as true positives and negatives can often (not always) be helpful. For example, the very numerous (false) positive test results on mammography are usually followed up by surgical biopsies and the entire process causes significant anxiety in most women (see below). No test should be recommended to a patient without the physician taking into account the possible significant harms and benefits that may accrue to the patient as a function of the several possible results of the testing. In almost all cases, the physician's knowledge about the uncertainties contained in the testing process should be shared with the patient, as we discuss in the next chapter.

Uncertainty in Screening Tests

The notion of screening seems unproblematic and eminently reasonable at first glance. What could be more sensible than to administer a usually innocuous test to a large number of asymptomatic persons with the intention of occasionally discovering the existence of a significant malady at an early stage? Discovered early, the maladies might be treated in some cases with a greater expectation of cure or significant amelioration than if one had waited until symptoms were apparent. Why then is there so much discussion and disagreement about whether tests like mammography and the Prostate-Specific Antigen (PSA) should be used in screening large numbers of asymptomatic individuals?

One characteristic of screening tests that gives rise to many of the problems they cause is that the maladies for which a screening test screens are almost always rare at any given point of time in an asymptomatic population. This means that the values in the right-column 2×2 table shown above (cells B and D) will almost always be much higher than the values in the left-column cells (A and C). Thus, the PPV of a screening test, defined as $A/A + B$, will tend to be low because B will be high compared to A. The only way to avoid a high PPV if the screened-for condition is rare is for the specificity of the test to be extremely high (thus reducing the magnitude of the B cell), higher than is hardly ever the case for any diagnostic or screening test. The PPVs of screening tests are usually even lower than the 13% value shown in figure 2, because the screened-for conditions are rarer that the 2% prevalence used to generate the figure 2 values. For example, if the prevalence in figure 2 were to decrease from 2% to 1%, the PPV would drop to about 7%. Thus, ninety-three of our one hundred persons whom the test would label as positive would be, in fact, negative. This is in striking contrast to the naive but badly mistaken view that some might have about screening tests, that a positive result means that one has the condition and a negative result means that one does not.

It is sometimes possible, as in the case of mammography, to perform further testing on persons whose results are positive on screening tests; for example, open or needle biopsies may be done so that the suspicious area of breast tissue can be directly examined. If the involved tissue shows the presence of a malignancy, then such treatments as surgical excision, chemotherapy, or radiation therapy can be given. But even considering the total package of mammography plus followup tests and treatments, how effective is mammography? One concept that can be used to address that question is called the number needed to screen (NNS). The NNS asks, How many women would need to have mammography at a given frequency over a given period of time (e.g., annually for ten years) before the life of one woman, who otherwise would have died had she not had mammograms, would be saved?

There is current dispute about whether women in their forties should have regular mammograms. Even different professional medical societies have come to different conclusions. Here is the relevant NNS: about one thousand women in their forties would need to have mammography every one to two years for the decade of their forties before the life of one woman, who otherwise would have died, would be saved.[12] For 999 out of one thousand women, the five to ten mammograms (followed up for more than half of the women with one or more subsequent biopsies that show no cancer) would yield no benefit. For one woman out of one thousand the screening test would be life saving.

Would it be irrational under these circumstances for a woman to decide not to have mammography during her forties? It does not seem so. When one adds up the certain and the possible negative features associated with routine mammography (the bother and discomfort of testing; the radiation associated with frequent testing; the high percentage of tests that are positive and require subsequent biopsy; the existence of false negative results) and contrast these with the NNS of one thousand, it seems entirely rational to decline testing. The negatives are all but certain and the one in one thousand benefit is very unlikely for any given woman. Of course, a particular woman might want very much to have mammography, perhaps because she has an intense fear of developing breast cancer and would be willing to endure the negative features of the procedure in order to obtain the hoped-for negative results every one to two years.

For that woman it might be rational to choose to have frequent mammograms. Our account of rationality in chapter 2 makes it clear why, given the NNS and the possible negative features associated with routine mammography, it is rational for a woman to decide either to have routine mammography or to decline it.

If one's overriding goal were to decrease cases of breast cancer in the population as much as possible, then one would advocate that every woman be tested. Even if only one tested woman in one thousand, who otherwise would have died, would not die from breast cancer, that amounts to a great many lives saved if the millions and millions of women in this country all had mammography as they passed through their forties. Thus, our account of rationality explains why it can be entirely rational for a person to elect a course of action that, if elected by everyone, would thwart possible public health goals.

Essentially all physicians use diagnostic and screening tests. Physicians must know and understand the above numerical characteristics of these tests in order to appreciate the true meaning of positive and negative test results.[13] Without such knowledge, it seems unlikely the physician would be able to know with any precision what further steps to describe or recommend to a patient in light of his test results.

Uncertainty in Treatment

It is common knowledge that treatments are not always effective and, in some cases, not even necessary. That is, sometimes a patient is given a treatment recognized to have an effect on a disease, and yet the disease persists. At other times, a patient with a disease for which a treatment exists does not receive any treatment and yet the disease goes away "on its own." Thus, the outcomes of treatments, no less than of tests, are probabilistic in nature.

Communicating risks. Of course, almost all interventions—called "treatments"—are effective at least some of the time or they would not continue to be used and to be called "treatments." However, treatments vary a good deal in their relative efficacy. Physicians, as part of their duty to adequately inform patients during the consent process, must tell patients just what the chances are that a particular suggested intervention will actually help the malady from which the patient suffers. There are several ways in which physicians can describe the efficacy of a treatment to a patient, although some of them run the risk of being misleading.[14]

One way is simply to tell the patient that a treatment has been shown to be effective (or some analogous version of such a statement). However, it is not clear what it means simply to say that a treatment is believed to be effective. At its worst it means only that this physician has seen instances where the treatment was followed by a good result. This, of course, is a very weak kind of evidence. At its best the physician may mean that randomized clinical trials have been conducted (preferably two or more) and this treatment has been shown to be effective significantly more frequently than a placebo or than some other treatment that was formerly used. But even this latter information is relatively uninformative. If experimental studies are conducted with large groups of subjects, it is possible to achieve statistically significant differences between experimental and control groups that have relatively small mean differences. Thus, while a suggested treatment may be statistically superior to doing nothing, the degree of superiority may not be large. Whether an adequately informed patient would elect the treatment might depend on many factors: the cost and side effects of the treatment, the noxiousness of simply continuing to have the disease (e.g., some version of "watchful waiting"), and so forth.

A second common way of describing efficacy is to use relative frequency statistics. ("This drug will cut your chance of having a heart attack by 50%.") This is a kind of efficacy description used not only by some doctors but also by many journalists, perhaps because it can make a treatment sound more remarkable than in fact it is. For example, suppose a treatment is expensive and has many unpleasant side effects. Suppose further that without the treatment the patient has a one in one thousand chance of having a heart attack over the next ten years, but that with the treatment the rate is cut to one in two thousand. That would be a 50% reduction. But this reduction might not impress some patients, who might think the ten-year financial cost and the unpleasantness associated with the treatment outweigh the rather small gain the treatment confers. Thus, telling patients only about relative risk reduction gives them incomplete information and, in many cases, is actually misleading. This may lead a patient to choose the ten-year cost and unpleasantness associated with the treatment when he would not have chosen it if he had realized how small his risk reduction actually was.

There is an alternative statistic that has gained in popularity in recent years, called the number needed to treat (NNT). The NNT tells how many persons need to be subjected to a treatment before one person would benefit. The lowest possible NNT would be one, if there were a treatment that helped everyone who took it and would help no one if the person didn't take the treatment. Thus, only one person needs to be treated before one person (that person) will be helped; if that person is not treated, that person will not be helped. Some antimicrobials and some orthopedic procedures may approach an NNT of one, but very low NNTs are rare in medical or surgical practice. On the other hand, NNTs can be very large. The above-mentioned treatment that reduced the risk of a heart attack from one in one thousand to one in two thousand would have an NNT of two thousand—two thousand persons would need to be treated before one person would not have a heart attack who otherwise would have had one.

The NNT is easily calculated. Here is an example: If two out of three of all patients with a *DSM-IV-TR* diagnosis of major depressive episode improve significantly within two months of beginning to take antidepressant medication, but one out of six persons improves significantly without any medication, then:

If one hundred patients take the drug, sixty-seven will recover;
   if one hundred patients don't take the drug, then seventeen will recover;
      therefore, the drug will benefit fifty patients who would not be benefited without the drug.
   Thus, two patients need to be treated in order to benefit one patient who would not otherwise be benefited (100/50). Thus, the NNT is two.

Here is another example, based on an actual study. A group of hypertensive patients took part in a randomized clinical trial studying the effect of a particular regimen of drugs on the frequency with which they experienced either heart attacks or strokes over a subsequent three-year period. It was found that 4% of the experimental group (the patients taking drugs) experienced a heart attack or stroke, but that 9.8% of a control group (taking a placebo) had one of these maladies. What was the NNT? It can be calculated using the method shown above:

If one hundred patients take the drugs, four will have a heart attack or stroke;
   if one hundred patients don't take the drugs, ten (rounding off) will have a heart attack or stroke;
      thus, six persons will be benefited from the drugs who otherwise would not have been benefited (100/6). Thus, the NNT is about seventeen.

It would be possible for a physician, confronting a hypertensive patient, to describe these results in several ways. He might say simply, "These drugs have been shown to be effective and you should take them." Or he might use relative risk data and say, correctly, "These drugs will lower your risk of having a heart attack or stroke by 60%." (That is, going from ten to four involves a 60% reduction.) Or he might say, "These drugs can be beneficial, but not everyone is helped. If seventeen people take the drugs, one person will avoid having a stroke or heart attack who otherwise would have had one. For sixteen people it will not make any difference."

Consider the two statements, "The drugs reduce the risk by 60%," and, "Only one person in seventeen who takes the drugs will be helped." To many persons these seem, at first blush, such disparate statements that they sound incompatible, as if two different drugs were being described. The reason this is true is because of the often misleading connotations engendered by relative risk data. This misleading connotation may arise from an unreflective and false assumption that the risk of having a stroke or heart attack is 100% and that the drugs reduce the risk to 40%. That would indeed be a powerful effect, but, of course, that is a different situation than having a 10% risk that is lowered to a 4% risk. Unless the drugs were extremely unpleasant or dangerous, it might be irrational not to take them if they reduced the risk of stroke or heart attack from 100% to 40%. However, not taking drugs (for three years) with an NNT of seventeen, especially if the drugs are either expensive, or accompanied by significant unpleasant side-effects, or both, need not be irrational at all.

These days, NNTs are now rather widely available and even exist in lists that can be downloaded (and frequently updated) onto a handheld computer (PDA) that the physician can conveniently have on hand at all times. In fact, NNTs are also increasingly being reported as the key dependent variable measure in randomized clinical trials investigating the efficacy of medical treatments. For example, it might be reported that, using a standard parametric statistical test, Treatment A (a new drug) yielded a better clinical result than Treatment B (a placebo, or an older drug) at the $p > .05$ level of significance. In addition, it might be reported that the NNT for Treatment A was twenty. Patients could then be told that Treatment A has been found to be significantly better than a placebo, but that only one in twenty patients who take Treatment A achieved the better result. Patients can then decide, based on a host of factors, whether to take Treatment A or to choose some other course of action.

Do physicians have a duty to learn about NNTs? It seems that, at the very least, they have a duty to understand the phenomenon that the NNT describes: treatments, even if they yield significant group effects, may, in fact, benefit only a small minority of patients so that it would often not be irrational for the patient to decline the treatment. If a physician does not understand that principle then she is apt to convey the misleading impression that it would be irrational for a patient to decline a treatment that she is suggesting. There are many occasions when it would be irrational for a patient to decline a particular suggested treatment, but NNTs are often quite large, and alternative treatments frequently exist, so that refusing a suggested treatment is often quite rational. When a physician describes the probable effects of the treatment, she must make clear that when the NNT is large, it is rational to refuse treatment, especially when treatment involves undergoing significant harms. This requires physicians to understand both the importance of the NNT and the concept of rationality.

Volume-Outcome Studies

There has been much interest in recent years in studying the variability in outcomes associated with various medical and surgical procedures. For example, volume-outcome studies have frequently been performed in which the incidence of either in-hospital morbidity, mortality, or both associated with a particular surgical procedure or a particular surgeon is correlated with the frequency with which that hospital, surgeon, or both performs that kind of surgery.[15] Gordon, et al. note, "The relationship between volume of surgical services performed by surgeons and hospitals, and positive outcomes of care, has been well documented."[16] An illustrative study was reported by these authors[17] in which the outcomes of all 501 Whipple procedures (pancreaticoduodenectomies, a complex, fairly high-risk surgical procedure, usually carried out for cancer of the pancreas) performed in the state of Maryland between 1988 and 1993 were examined. More than half of these procedures (271, or 54.1%) were performed at Johns Hopkins Hospital (JHH) while the remainder (230, or 45.9%) were performed at thirty-eight other hospitals in the state, no one of which performed more than a total of twenty during the five and one-half years of the study.

The outcome of the procedure was significantly different between JHH and the rest of the hospitals, even after the two patient groups (JHH versus all other hospitals) were statistically matched for age, gender, race, source of payment, source of admission, and extent of comorbid processes. In-hospital mortality was more than six times higher at the low-volume hospitals than at JHH (13.5% versus 2.2%; $p < .001$).

Even among the thirty-eight low-volume hospitals there was a significant linear monotonic relationship between volume and mortality. The thirty-eight hospitals were divided into four groups based on the frequency with which they had performed the procedure. Twenty hospitals had performed a total of 1 to 5 Whipple procedures between 1988 and 1993, nine hospitals had performed 6 to 9, six hospitals had performed 11 to 15, and three hospitals had performed 16 to 20. Their respective in-hospital mortality rates were 19.1%, 14.3%, 13%, and 8.9%.

Thus, among the twenty hospitals in Maryland (more than half the total number of non-JHH hospitals) that performed only between one and five procedures, the chance of dying in the hospital was almost nine times greater than at JHH (19.1% versus 2.2%). This represents almost a one-in-five versus a one-in-fifty chance of dying. Even among the four hospitals that performed 16 to 20 procedures, the chance of dying was four times greater than at JHH (8.9% versus 2.2%).

These are substantial differences, not merely statistically significant differences of limited practical importance. Unless they had strong reasons for not doing so, any person trying to make a rational decision about treatment would choose to have the Whipple performed at JHH rather than at a local, low-volume Maryland hospital. Absent such reasons, it would be seriously irrational to choose to have the surgery in a low-volume setting. And of course there is no reason to believe that this volume-outcome relationship in performing Whipple procedures is limited to Maryland.[18]

Studies have been emerging with regularity in recent years showing similar volume-outcome relationships with respect to other surgical procedures and medical treatments.[19] These studies have been appearing so regularly in major medical journals, especially during the past decade, that it is increasingly hard to believe that any physician involved with these surgical procedures and medical treatments would be unaware of them.[20]

Do physicians have a duty to learn about volume-outcome studies? A strong argument can be made that they do. If physicians do not know about these volume-outcome studies, they may recommend that a patient be treated in a facility that it would be objectively irrational for the patient to choose. Further, except in very unusual circumstances, a physician must tell his patient about the relevant volume-outcome data.[21] However, even if a physician for some reason decides not to tell a particular patient about volume-outcome data, it is morally required for the physician to refer the patient to that treatment setting that offered the most favorable morbidity and mortality outcomes. To do otherwise would be to knowingly expose the patient to a higher risk than necessary of experiencing a poor result. And that would be immoral, clearly violating the special duties of doctors discussed in chapter 4.

Geographical Variation Studies

A related but conceptually distinct body of research has consistently shown large differences in the frequency with which certain surgical procedures and medical treatments are performed in different geographical areas of similar demographic characteristics. The phenomenon is especially apparent in the so-called "discretionary" procedures (e.g., carotid endarterectomy, radical prostatectomy, back surgery for "disc disease," and many others). Relatively "nondiscretionary" procedures (e.g., colon resection for colorectal cancer, cholecystectomy, and hip fracture repair) show less geographical variation.[22]

The magnitude of these geographical differences is often large: a fourfold to tenfold difference in incidence between closely matched areas is commonly seen. For example, small-area variation studies in New Hampshire, Maine, and Iowa showed that among different areas that were closely matched for demographic characteristics, there were broad variations. In one area only 20% of women, by the age of seventy, had had a hysterectomy; in a matched geographical area, 70% had had one by that age. Similarly, in one area, by age eighty-five, only 15% of men had had a prostatectomy; in a matched area, 60% had had one. In another study, it was found that among women with early breast cancer who, according to practice guidelines (see below), could rationally choose either to have a lumpectomy or a radical resection, there was wide geographical variation in the choices made. The extremes: in one small town, 48% of women had had lumpectomies and 52% had had radical mastectomies; in a closely matched small town, only 1.4% of women had had lumpectomies while the remaining 98.6% had had radical mastectomies.

The reasons for these geographical differences are not entirely clear. Chance variation can be shown to cause no more, at most, than a very small part of the differences observed.[23] An unlikely explanation for the discrepancies seen between different areas is that they reflect a difference in what patients in the different localities, adequately informed, would actually prefer. It seems extraordinarily unlikely that half of adequately informed women in one geographical area would opt for a breast-sparing lumpectomy while almost none of the women in a closely matched area would make the same choice. The women's "choices" are almost certainly reflections of their doctors' "recommendations."

The most likely explanation is that the differences represent different professional practice patterns that have evolved in different localities. The procedures that show the greatest variation may be those procedures for which it usually would be rational either to consent to the surgery or to refuse it (or to have a mastectomy versus a lumpectomy, etc.), as the term "discretionary" implies. However, although both choices may be rational, particular individuals, adequately informed, may nonetheless strongly prefer one to the other. It is far more likely that the doctors in the two areas provide different kinds of information and advice than that there is such a large difference in the rational choices of the women in these different areas.

Do physicians have a duty to know about geographical variation data? Perhaps not. As long as the physician discloses to a competent patient adequate information about the intervention being suggested and applies no coercion of any kind, then it may not be necessary for the physician to know whether he practices in an area that carries out this intervention more or less commonly than do other areas. It may not even be necessary for him to know whether *he* carries out the intervention more or less frequently than other physicians. However, although it might not be a duty for physicians to know this information, it would be following a moral ideal for physicians to find out which of the treatments they suggest has a high degree of geographical variation in their use. Finding out this information should alert them to carry out a particularly scrupulous consent process in such cases. These are apt to be treatments with significant possible benefits and significant possible risks, where plausible alternative treatments exist, and that it would be quite rational for the patient either to consent to or to refuse. Under these circumstances the physician must take great care to present the relevant information carefully and dispassionately.

Practice Guidelines

In recent years there have been created many medical "practice guidelines." These are sets of recommendations about the best way to manage and treat various maladies (e.g., the best way to treat an acute myocardial infarction, or a patient suffering from a manic episode). Usually the guidelines have been created by groups of specialists in a field who have relied on the best evidence that is available, especially from randomized clinical trials and from meta-analyses of randomized clinical trials, about optimal treatment strategies.

The guidelines are meant to be prescriptive. The group writing the guidelines is claiming that the particular strategy outlined has been shown to be superior in its results to any other strategy that has been tried and studied in a particular clinical situation. The guidelines are not meant to be absolute but are rather prima facie. However, frequently there is good reason, based on the circumstances of a particular case, not to follow a particular guideline, but to take some other action instead. However, the burden of proof is always on a physician who departs from a particular guideline to justify the departure. Nonetheless, departures are not only sometimes permissible, they are sometimes morally required. Departures should not be capricious or based on inexplicable hunches; the physician making the departure must be willing to argue publicly that in any future cases with relevantly similar characteristics to the case at hand, the guideline should be departed from in just this way. In fact, some future, fuller edition of the practice guidelines might say not only "Do X," but add as a corollary, "In case of Y, do not do X but instead do Z." The exception becomes a publicly defensible (sub)guideline itself.

For example, there is now excellent research evidence that patients whose depression has been successfully alleviated by the use of antidepressant medication should continue to take the medication for four to six months after their mood has improved. If patients stop the medication soon after they feel better, there is a significant and nontrivial chance they will suffer a depressive relapse and need to take the medicine for another full course.[24] This fact has been recognized for years and has been incorporated into the practice guidelines for the treatment of major depressive episodes that have been published by the American Psychiatric Association.[25] Any physician who undertakes to treat depressive episodes must be aware of this fact and must explain to patients the reason for continuing the medication. A physician who does not follow this guideline is subjecting his patients to the possibility of a good deal of avoidable future suffering, which is a clear violation of the special duties of doctors. If the physician has some reason to recommend that a patient not continue with medication for several months after the patient's depression has lifted, he must explain to the patient why he is making the recommendation that he is.[26]

One could argue that the existence of practice guidelines should be disclosed to patients, that the content of the guidelines should be an essential and central part of the information given to the patient during the consent process. Given the current existence of professionally agreed upon, evidence-based guidelines, one might expect that physicians would know about them and follow them scrupulously—unless they had good reasons for departing from them—and that patients would generally be informed of their existence. Neither expectation seems to be true.[27] In fact, practice guidelines are so commonly ignored that there is emerging a literature investigating the question of why this is so.[28]

Conclusion

New kinds of information exist about medical practice, information that would have been unavailable—in fact, not even conceptualized—only a few years ago. Strong arguments can be made that physicians have a duty to learn and to incorporate into their practices these new kinds of information. To not do so can result in patients being exposed (usually unknowingly) to a greater risk of harm than need be the case. Needlessly exposing patients to the possibility of harm is clearly immoral, violating the special duties of doctors, unless it is done with an adequate justification.

We have focused in this chapter on what we believe doctors must know about medical practice. "What doctors must know" is logically prior to "what doctors must tell patients" because doctors can't tell what they don't know. In the next chapter we discuss the important issue of what doctors have a duty to tell their patients, both about these new kinds of information and about more traditional kinds of information concerning suggested medical interventions.

Valid consent is a core concept in bioethics and health law and it is important for physicians to actually carry out the consent process in an adequate way; that they actually tell patients about the diagnostic and therapeutic interventions they are proposing. We suggest it would be at least equally useful to study how much physicians in fact know about the interventions they suggest. There are many reasons physicians may not disclose this information to patients, but prime among them may be that some physicians wouldn't know what to disclose. If that is true then the other reasons pale in importance. It would also be much easier methodologically to measure what doctors know than to measure what they tell patients in the privacy of their examining rooms.

Notes

1. We speak of "doctors" in what follows, but we believe most or all of what we say applies to allopathic and osteopathic physicians, physician assistants, podiatrists, nurse practitioners, and nurse midwives as well.

2. See, for example, Lamont and Christakis (2003).

3. See chapter 6 on maladies.

4. We discuss this topic in greater detail in the next chapter.

5. The precise boundaries of the rapidly growing discipline of clinical epidemiology are unclear and sometimes the field is referred to as clinical epidemiology and evidence-based medicine. One of us (CC) teaches a course with the latter title and finds that all of the material discussed in this chapter fits comfortably under that rubric.

6. Gigerenzer (2002, 42–44).

7. The *sensitivity* of a test refers to the percentage of persons with a malady who test positively on a test intended to detect that malady; the *specificity* of a test refers to the percentage of patients without a malady who test negatively on a test intended to detect that malady. These terms are discussed in more detail and examples are given later in the chapter.

8. See Culver (2004, 1815–1820).

9. A particular test can sometimes be in one category and sometimes in the other. For example, serum lipids can be measured in a fifty-five-year-old obese man complaining of anginal pain because the presence of hyperlipidemia is strongly suspected, but they can also be given routinely in primary care to all one's adult patients to screen for the presence of hyperlipidemia.

10. Neither the sensitivity nor the specificity of a test are affected in any important way by the prevalence of a disease in a cohort.

11. An "event," as mentioned above, can be any of several kinds of predicted-to conditions: the confirmed existence of a disease, the committing of suicide or domestic violence, and so forth.

12. For an excellent description of the significant problems associated with mammography and with cancer screening tests in general, see Welch (2004). Another well-argued discussion can be found in Malm (1999).

13. We have illustrated the usefulness of four indexes of test performance: sensitivity, specificity, and positive and negative predictive values. Interested readers may want to study the nature and the application of positive and negative likelihood ratios, which many persons in clinical epidemiology believe are even more useful measures of diagnostic test performance. For a well-written description of all of these measures, see Nicoll and Pignone (2004).

14. What follows is the letter that one of us (BG) received from his physician after his annual check-up. It shows that what we recommend is actually done by some doctors.

> Just a quick note to report your recent tests.
>
> Your total cholesterol was 255 (ideal is <200). HDL or "good cholesterol" was 65 (ideal is >35), triglycerides were 142 (goal is <250), and LDL or "bad cholesterol" was 161 (ideal is >130, mild 130–160, moderate 160–180, severe >180). This is a "mixed picture." The LDL is elevated which is a risk factor for heart disease, but the HDL is also elevated which is protective. To help put this in perspective, I ran your numbers through a cardiac risk calculator, which reports your risk of a heart attack at 13% over ten years. We know that medications to lower cholesterol reduce risk of heart attack by 30%, so treating you would reduce your risk from 13% to 9% over ten years. This is a relatively sizable benefit when looked at from a population standpoint (I would need to treat 25 patients just like you for 10 years to prevent one heart attack, and I have many more than 25 patients with similar cholesterols), but you may decide that you personally do not want to do anything about this. I think treatment at this point is optional, but certainly warranted. I should point out that your cholesterol is not worse this time than last, it's just that our threshold for treating cholesterol has dropped. I'm happy to meet and discuss, if you would like. Let me know what you'd like do, either by e-mail or through an appointment.

15. There is much anecdotal and some empirical evidence that physicians often do not even attempt to give information about efficacy, but simply "assign" a patient to a treatment. ("It looks like you have an enlarged prostate. Here's what we're going to have to do.") This manner of acting is a breach of the physician's duty to give adequate information during the consent process, as detailed in the next chapter.

16. Evidence of this kind has been accumulating for at least thirty years. For an early summary, see Luft, Bunker and Enthoven (1979). For one response to this article, emphasizing the importance of communicating volume-outcome data to patients, see Culver and Gert (1980).

17. Gordon, et al. (1995).

18. Ibid.

19. At least two other studies have found similar volume-outcome relationships with the Whipple procedure. See Birkmeyer, Warshaw, et al. (1999), and Simunovic, et al. (1999).

20. For example, see Begg, et al. (1998), Hannan, and Racz, et al. (1997), Lavernia and Guzman (1995), Tu, Austin, and Chan (2001), and many others.

21. For a recent extensive survey and summary of many of these studies, see Birkmeyer and Stukel, et al. (2003).

22. In a *New England Journal of Medicine* editorial, Kenneth Kizer (2003) comes to the same conclusion:

> Furthermore, the evidence that is now available is more than sufficient to support an insistence that informed consent for high-risk elective surgical procedures include information about the specific outcomes among patients of both the institution and the individual surgeon involved. Before undergoing procedures for which a relation between volume and outcome has been demonstrated, patients should be clearly informed that they are likely to have a reduced risk of an adverse outcome, including death, if they are cared for by providers that have demonstrated superior outcomes and, conversely, an increased risk of an adverse outcome if they are cared for by providers that have demonstrated poor outcomes. If superior outcomes cannot be demonstrated directly, then high volume can, at least for the time being, be used as a proxy for better outcomes. Of course, any referral to a provider with better outcomes should be in accordance with the patient's stated preference after he or she has been appropriately informed.

23. For an extensive summary of geographical variation data, see Center for Evaluative Clinical Sciences (1999); also see Wennberg (1999).

24. It is easy to calculate confidence intervals for the observed differences and, since most of them are based on very large groups, the probability that the difference is a chance phenomenon is extremely small. And, of course, there are many such observed differences so that the probability that all or any substantial proportion of them are due to chance is vanishingly small.

25. For a recent meta-analysis of this issue, based on thirty-one randomized clinical trials, see Geddes, et al. (2003). The average rate of relapse with continued drug treatment was 18%, versus a 41% relapse rate on placebo. Thus the NNT (the number of patients who would need to continue on the drug to avoid one relapse that otherwise would have occurred) was about four. Since, for the great majority of patients, continuing the drug for several additional months would not be particularly noxious, it seems likely that most patients, informed of these data and the NNT, would elect to continue the medication.

26. See practice guidelines at www.psych.org/.

27. The recent medical literature is filled with documented examples of large numbers of physicians not following practice guidelines, for example, failing to prescribe aspirin after a patient has suffered a myocardial infarction. See O'Connor, et al. (1999). By not prescribing an efficacious drug, a physician is unnecessarily exposing the patient to significant risks that would be avoidable.

28. One of us (cc) teaches a didactic course on evidence-based medicine to physician assistant students immediately after their twelve months of clinical rotations in area clinics, hospitals, and medical practices. Nearly all students say they have never heard the term "practice guideline" mentioned during their year-long exposure to eight to ten different physician preceptors and resident staffs.

29. See Cabana, et al. (1999).

9

Adequate Information, Competence, and Coercion

It is widely accepted in bioethics and in health law that three criteria must be satisfied in order for a patient's consent to be valid: the patient must be given adequate information about the decision she is being asked to make; the patient must be fully competent to consent to or refuse the diagnostic or therapeutic intervention that is being suggested; and coercion must not be employed in obtaining her decision. Each of these three criteria requires some explication.[1]

Adequate Information: What Doctors Must Tell Patients about Medical Practice

There is an Alice-in-Wonderland quality to the process of valid consent in medical practice. On the one hand, there is widespread deference to the concept both in bioethics and in health law. Modern codes of ethics in the medical professions all seem to require that the process of valid consent take place and many civil malpractice actions have awarded damages to plaintiffs whose physicians have been found negligent in not carrying out an adequate consent process. On the other hand, there is both empirical and abundant anecdotal evidence that the vast majority of practitioners conduct no more than a superficial consent process.[2] In fact, sometimes both treatments and diagnostic tests are apparently administered to patients with almost no accompanying information.

One reason for this apparent schism between what practitioners give lip service to and what they actually do may be a general lack of clarity about the ingredients of an adequate consent process. Though codes of ethics, which are a possible source of guidance for physicians in this area, may stipulate that a consent process should take place, they are often vague or even silent about the necessary features of that process.[3] To complicate matters further, although there is widespread agreement in bioethics and in health law that two or three particular kinds of information should essentially always be included in the consent process, there are other kinds of information (see preceding chapter and see below) that people might disagree about requiring, but that clearly could be included.

We believe it is clarifying to realize that there are some features of the consent process that are morally required and other features whose inclusion, though morally encouraged, is not morally required. Practitioners who fail to include the morally required features, unless they have clear moral justification for the omission, have acted immorally. Those who do not include the morally encouraged features have failed to act as helpfully and virtuously as they might, but they have not acted immorally. However, we believe that most physicians would want to know about and disclose information that might be critically useful to patients in making rationally optimal decisions, even if it were not always morally required that they disclose it.

It is a failing of perhaps all health care codes of ethics that they do not make a distinction between what is morally required and what is morally encouraged. This probably weakens the impact of the codes considerably because it is clear to anyone who reads them that at least some of their directives are exhortatory but not morally required.[4] If some directives are clearly only morally encouraged, who is to say, without explicit specification, which if any are morally required?[5]

Morally Required Information Disclosure

There is a general consensus in bioethics that it is morally required to disclose at least three kinds of information during the consent process. First, the patient must be told about the significant harms and benefits that may occur because of the suggested intervention. Second, the patient must be told about any plausible alternative intervention(s) that could be carried out in the current situation, and about the significant harms and benefits that might occur secondary to them. Finally, the patient must be told about the nature of the malady from which he or she suffers and, in particular, what is apt to occur if no intervention is made at all.

Treatments are not the only interventions about which pertinent information should be disclosed; as noted in the previous chapter, patients need to be told the possible significant harms and benefits associated with any diagnostic test that is being suggested. This is clearest in those situations where there can be important disagreement about the merits of testing, for example, the use of the Prostate-Specific Antigen (PSA) test to detect prostatic disease, or the use of mammography to diagnose breast cancer. Each of these tests, though they sometimes accurately detect the existence of a serious disease, is fraught with a great number of false positives (with their attendant distress) and some false negatives. If people were to add up the gains and the harms that can be caused by the testing, it can be quite rational for many or most patients not to consent to either mammography or PSA screening, although it is almost always rationally allowed for them to consent to the testing as well.

Nowhere is the need to tell patients about the possible significant harms and benefits associated with testing more imperative than in carrying out genetic testing. Testing for a variety of genetic mutations that have been found to be associated with concurrent or future disease-states is becoming increasingly possible. And there is every reason to believe such tests will be more and more available in coming years, many in over-the-counter form. The sensitivity and specificity of genetic tests[6] are often not high and, thus, it is common to encounter false positive and false negative test results.[7] For a patient to obtain genetic test results whose positive and negative predictive values are relatively low can be a mixed blessing, and no patient should consent to genetic testing who does not understand ahead of time the kind of uncertainties and anxieties that the test results may provoke. It is essential that any health care worker who suggests genetic testing to her patients understands these matters fully. It is not reassuring that a recent study, in which 177 physicians who had ordered genetic testing were interviewed, found that "in almost one third (31.6%) of the cases the physicians' interpretation of the test results was incorrect and would have led to the misinforming of the patients."[8]

Patients who know the pertinent information about a suggested intervention are in a position to make a personally optimal, rational decision about whether or not to consent to it. Without this information, it is possible they will make a different decision than the one they would make with the information, and that different decision, though rational, may lead them to experience harms they would have definitely chosen to avoid if they had been fully informed. If a particular woman with breast cancer consents to a radical mastectomy, but does not know that a lumpectomy is a plausible alternative, she may consent to the more disfiguring operation although she would definitely not do so if she were adequately informed about alternative treatments.

Doctors are widely believed to have a fiduciary duty toward their patients. A significant part of that duty is to provide patients with that information that will help them choose those courses of action that will, according to patients' own rankings of the harms and benefits involved, minimize the current harms and the future harms they may experience as a result of being ill. It follows that a doctor who gives a patient with stage 1 breast cancer full information about radical mastectomies, but fails to tell the patient anything about lumpectomies, has not done what he has a duty to do and has, therefore, acted immorally. Similarly, a doctor who suggests to a man with a moderate degree of prostatism that he have a transurethral prostatectomy, but does not tell him about the magnitude of the associated risks of subsequent impotence or urinary incontinence, has failed to do his duty and so has acted immorally. We believe this point should be clearly made: It is not just that it would be nice for a physician to disclose adequate information, or that it shows he is a splendid physician for taking the trouble to do so; rather, failure to do so is immoral professional practice and could and should be subject to professional sanctions and, when appropriate, legal redress.

Should Physicians Be Morally Required to Disclose New Kinds of Information?

It seems indisputable that each of the four kinds of information described in the preceding chapter would, on occasion, be useful to persons wishing to make a rational decision about whether or not to consent to a suggested diagnostic or therapeutic intervention. Knowing about a well-established volume-outcome relationship, or being informed about a number needed to treat (NNT) of forty, or a number needed to screen (NNS) of fifteen hundred might well cause a patient to make a decision different from the one she would have made without the new knowledge. And this different decision might result in her experiencing less harm than she would otherwise have experienced.

Although the information that doctors must give patients during the consent process is necessary to help patients make optimal rational decisions, Heather Gert has pointed out that what must be disclosed sometimes goes beyond that.[9] Consider a patient with a serious malady for which there is only one particular treatment, a surgical one. With the treatment there is a greater than 90% chance that the patient will be cured; without the treatment there is almost no possibility that the patient will experience a cure and there is a 50% chance the patient will die. This patient wants to live and, therefore, there is only one rational course of action open to him: to consent to surgery. As it happens, although the surgery will probably be curative, the postsurgical recovery period will almost certainly be accompanied by significant episodic pain for about a week and significant disability for three to four weeks. If the criterion for what there is a moral duty to disclose is limited to "that information necessary to make a rational decision," then there would be no duty to tell this patient ahead of time about the pain and disability he will almost certainly experience, because he doesn't need to know that information in order to make a rational decision. However, the patient's overall postsurgical suffering may be less if he knows about and can anticipate the recovery symptoms he will experience. Because physicians have a fiduciary duty to lessen their patients' suffering, we agree with Heather Gert that there is a duty to disclose this kind of information as well.

We believe that plausible arguments in favor of morally requiring disclosure of at least some of these new kinds of additional information can be made, but we believe it would be premature to do so at the present time. There are practical reasons for proceeding slowly (but deliberately) in this area. First, there is evidence, mentioned above, that during the consent process, only a small minority of physicians actually disclose that morally required information that a general consensus agrees must be disclosed. It is also likely true that there are many physicians who are still unfamiliar with these new kinds of information. It might, therefore, be unrealistic to stipulate that henceforth all members of the profession must include several additional kinds of information during the consent process.

We suggest a several-pronged approach to try to alter the current status of the consent process in American medicine. First, we believe that the fact that the majority of physicians does not even disclose the three basic kinds of information is alarming and morally unjustifiable. All health care codes of ethics must make clear and explicit that health care workers have a duty to disclose to patients information about the possible significant harms and benefits of suggested interventions, of plausible alternative interventions, and information about what is likely to happen without the intervention. It is not only morally required that they do so but it might also appreciably lower the number of legal actions that allege, often correctly, that physicians have inadequately disclosed important information.

The health care professions must, in their training programs and in their continued medical education efforts, acquaint health care workers with the kinds of new information about medical interventions described above. Physicians cannot disclose what they do not know, and so a first effort should focus on education.

We believe there is a ranking of importance among these new kinds of information we have described:

(1) *Volume-outcome studies* seem first in importance. There is little doubt that large numbers of patients die or are seriously harmed in this country every year because they have major volume-sensitive procedures carried out at low-volume centers where they are attended by health care workers who have much less experience in carrying out the treatments than would be the case elsewhere. For a variety of reasons, not all patients may be able to travel to high-volume centers, but they should, nevertheless, know about the relevant data so they can decide what they wish to do. Of all of the new kinds of information, this seems the most pressing to disclose, and some might wish to argue strongly that even now there is a duty to disclose it in relevant cases. It is easy information to disclose and to understand and the amount of harm that disclosure might allow patients to avoid is great. Literally, what is at stake can be a matter of life or death, and patients may be totally ignorant of that fact. Codes of ethics should be changed, in the near future, to stipulate that when treatments are suggested about which there are significant volume-outcome data, the nature of these data must be disclosed to patients.

(2) *Number needed to treat measures* seems next in importance. Medicine is pervasively probabilistic, and patients need to know how likely it is that

a suggested treatment will help, or how frequently lives will actually be saved if a certain screening test is carried out. Even if physicians do not use the NNT or related statistics, they should describe harms in terms of the absolute probability that they will occur under different conditions, and never describe the effect of a treatment only in relative frequency terms ("This drug will decrease the chance that you'll have a stroke by 50%"). Relative frequencies can be seriously misleading and, if nothing else is disclosed, they can represent a form of deception. They have nothing at all to recommend them. By contrast, absolute percentage results and the NNT kinds of measures derived from them are not deceptive.

(3) *Geographic variation data* may, in and of themselves, be less necessary to disclose, although they may be enlightening to a patient who resides in an area where the frequency of a treatment is significantly above or below the national mean. However, if a physician adequately discloses to a patient in a dispassionate way that information that he does have a moral duty to disclose, then data about the frequency with which past patients have had that intervention in that geographical area may have little effect on the decision a particular patient makes. A person wanting to make a rational decision about consenting to an intervention would probably be willing to forego learning about geographical data, so long as she was assured she had full information about the significant harms and benefits of the intervention and about plausible alternative interventions.

(4) To require that physicians disclose to patients the existence of *practice guidelines*, or any departure a physician makes from a guideline's recommendation, may be premature at present. There is a plethora of practice guidelines in some areas of medicine and occasional inconsistencies have been found among them. However, there are undoubtedly more consistencies than inconsistencies: for example, it is hard to imagine a practice guideline that would state that antidepressant medication should be stopped as soon as patients experience a symptomatic improvement. Most practice guidelines recommend clinical practices that have been found through research to result in better patient outcomes than alternative clinical practices in that situation. For the reasons stated above, rational patients would want their physicians to follow practice guidelines, when appropriate, and would want to be reassured that departures from them are adequately justified.

By saying that it might be premature to morally require at the present time that physicians disclose to patients some of these new kinds of information, we do not mean to diminish the potential importance of these new kinds of information to patients. Indeed, it is easy to imagine situations in which a particular patient's decision to consent or refuse would be more influenced by some "new" kind of information—say, of a strong volume-outcome relationship—than by some of the traditionally required consent information. But although it might be premature for a health care code of ethics to stipulate at the present time that strong volume-outcome relationships must be disclosed, it would be quite timely and laudable for them to strongly encourage their disclosure by including appropriate "should statements" in their text. Thus, a code of ethics could say, "If an intervention is suggested to a patient for which there has been demonstrated a strong volume-outcome relationship, the physician should disclose this relationship to the patient." Or, "In disclosing to patients the risks and benefits that are associated with a treatment, physicians should avoid the use of relative risk statements (for example, 'This treatment will lessen your risk of experiencing some particular outcome by 50%') and instead disclose information centered on the absolute magnitude of harms and benefits (for example, using measures like the number needed to treat)."

Competence to Consent or Refuse

"Competence" to consent to or refuse treatment is a central concept in U.S. health law and bioethics. It is widely believed that a patient must be fully competent before his consent or refusal is valid. However, despite the wide acceptance of the central role that competence plays in the consent process, there is disagreement, not only about how the term should be defined but also about its application to particular cases.

If a patient is judged to be competent to make health care decisions then, at least in general, her consent to or refusal of a suggested medical intervention is acceded to. If she has been given adequate information about the proposed intervention and no coercion has been employed during the consent process, her consent and refusal are judged to be valid and, therefore, determinative. It is regarded as legally sanctioned and morally justified for the physician to proceed with a medical intervention in the presence of a valid consent. However, it is neither legally sanctioned nor morally justified to carry out an intervention on a patient who has made a valid refusal. By contrast, if a patient who refuses an intervention is judged to be incompetent to refuse, the refusal is not valid and, under some circumstances, the physician is thought to be justified in carrying out the intervention. However, if a patient is judged to be incompetent to consent then, except in emergency situations, a physician should not carry out an intervention even if the patient has agreed to it. Rather, the physician should obtain some form of surrogate consent.

Many definitions of competence have been proposed. Although there is a high degree of agreement among them in how they would classify a random sample of competent and incompetent patients, there are occasional significant disagreements. Furthermore, these concordant classifications correlate strongly with most persons' intuitions about whether a particular patient's consent or refusal should be taken as valid. The difficult philosophical problem is to provide an account of competence that will accord with most people's considered judgments about when patients' consents or refusals should be accepted or overruled. In addition to providing a definition of competence, it is also important to provide the criteria by which, in particular cases, its relative presence or absence should be determined.[10]

The Logic of Competence

Before examining various definitions of competence, it is helpful to review some universally agreed upon features of how the term should be used. Persons are often referred to as "competent" or "incompetent," but this is a somewhat misleading shorthand locution. Competence is task-specific: a person is competent or incompetent to make a will, to perform a neurological examination, or to refuse a suggested medical intervention. It does not follow from the fact that a person is competent to do X that he is competent to do Y. For example, a somewhat confused man may be competent to eat his breakfast by himself or to tie his shoelaces but not competent to make a decision about having a radical prostatectomy. A person may even be competent to consent to a rather simple medical intervention (applying a Band-Aid to a cut finger), but not competent to consent to an intervention with a complex spectrum of risks and benefits spread out over time (having a carotid endarterectomy for transient ischemic attacks). No one is competent to do everything, although some persons (the totally unconscious) are not competent to do anything. Saying that a person is "competent" is always shorthand for "competent to do X."

In discussing the competence that is a necessary requirement for valid consent or refusal, it is crucial to have a clear and precise account of the task that a patient must be competent to perform. The standard way of describing this task is to say that the patient must be competent to consent to or refuse a medical intervention. However, this way of describing the task is both vague and ambiguous in important ways. This vagueness and ambiguity is responsible for the different definitions of competence that have been proposed. As we shall see later, specifying the task in an unambiguous way leads to a more adequate account of competence, and also makes clear what criteria should be used to determine if the patient is competent to perform that task.

Defining Competence to Consent or Refuse

The Understand and Appreciate (U + A) Definition

Various definitions of competence have much in common, but they differ in significant ways. Thus, it is possible—although it seldom happens—for a patient to be competent on one definition but incompetent on another. One thing all definitions have in common is the stipulation that one necessary element of competence be that the patient must understand at least the minimal amount of factual information that would count as adequate information for validly consenting to or refusing the medical intervention being proposed. If a patient has been given adequate information in a language that she speaks and in terms that most speakers of that language would understand, but cannot understand what she has been told (because, for example, she is significantly retarded, or because she is suffering from cognitive confusion secondary to a moderate degree of delirium), then even if she does consent or refuse, she is not regarded as competent to make that decision and her consent or refusal is not regarded as valid. Valid consents or refusals require understanding, and if a patient does not understand the minimal amount of factual information that would count as adequate information, then one necessary condition of competence has not been satisfied. To say that a patient understands indicates nothing about the content of the decision, even whether it is a consent or a refusal, that the patient actually goes on to make. What is at issue is limited to whether the patient has understood whatever adequate information he has been given.

To say that a patient appreciates what the physician tells her requires more than the patient understanding the information given to her, it requires that she appreciates that the information she has understood is indeed applicable to her at this given point in time. But, like understanding, appreciation says nothing about the content of the decision. One reason a criterion of appreciation has been added to the criterion of understanding is that, on rare occasions, patients have delusions that impinge on the consent process, and these may affect a patient's appreciation, but not her understanding. A patient, for example, can fully understand the risks that a suggested intervention carries, but also believe that he is Superman and that no harm can befall him. If he consents to a risky procedure with the false belief that he cannot be harmed by it because he is Superman, then it is plausible to say he is not competent to consent because, although he knows the risks, he falsely believes they do not apply to him. "Appreciation" could, in fact, be regarded as an additional kind of understanding; one could say that "understand" means to understand both the nature of an intervention's risks and benefits and also to understand that they do indeed apply to oneself in the current situation, although it is usually listed as a separate criterion.

"Understanding" and "appreciating" are frequently combined into a single understand-and-appreciate (U + A) criterion. It is possible to define competence to consent or refuse using these two formal criteria alone. We call this a "pure U + A" definition. An important feature of defining competence in this way, which is seen by many as its particular strength, is that the patient's actual decision does not enter into the determination of competence. Competence, as defined by U + A criteria, can, in theory—and frequently in practice—be determined before knowing whether the patient will consent to or refuse treatment. If the patient understands the adequate information she has been given, and appreciates that indeed it applies to her in the current situation, then she is competent and, absent coercion, whatever decision she makes is valid and should be respected.[11]

There are advantages to the pure U + A definition of competence that may, in part, explain its popularity. First, it fits well with the goal that many have of allowing competent patients to make any decision they want. Second, the determination of whether a patient understands and appreciates information is usually relatively easy to make (there are inevitable borderline cases) and can be investigated by briefly quizzing the patient about the content and the relevance of what she has just been told. If the patient does understand and appreciate, then the physician can simply let the patient decide and respond accordingly. It may seem far more difficult and less objective to determine whether a patient's decision is "autonomous," "rational," or "authentic," or to apply some other concept of that ilk (see below).

The Inadequacy of the Pure U + A Definition

The problem with the pure U + A definition is that it sometimes gives a result that is so counterintuitive that no responsible physician would act on it. Here is an example of such a case:

> *Case 1.* An elderly depressed woman is refractory to antidepressant drug treatment and has lost a significant amount of weight. She is very frightened about the prospect of having electroconvulsive treatment (ECT) and she cannot bring herself to consent to the procedure, either verbally or in writing. She does not disagree with her doctor's opinion that she may die without ECT, and she acknowledges that ECT would likely prevent her death, but she still cannot bring herself to consent. She did consent to have ECT when she was similarly depressed several years ago, and she remembers that ECT rather quickly alleviated her depression. She was similarly frightened of ECT on this earlier occasion, but her husband somehow pressured her to consent to the procedure. Her husband is no longer living and her two grown sons, although they very much want their mother to have ECT, have been thoroughly unsuccessful in influencing her to consent. She understands and appreciates everything her doctor has told her and disagrees with none of it, but she has an irrational fear that prevents her from consenting to ECT.

This patient clearly satisfies the U + A definition of competence.[12] Her refusal to consent was not based on any lack of ability to understand or appreciate information; it was based on the strong irrational fear that she had of the ECT procedure. And yet essentially everyone familiar with this case believed the patient should be given ECT.

Here is another example:

> *Case 2.* A severely depressed man, weakened by a cardiac disorder, refuses life-saving treatment for his eminently treatable and potentially reversible cardiac condition. Unlike some depressed patients, he manifests no cognitive delusions or distortions; he understands the relevant information about the likely sequelae of treatment versus nontreatment and appreciates that it applies to him. He refuses all treatments as well as nutrition and hydration because he wants to die. He gives, and apparently has, no reason to refuse, other than his wish to die, and there is no reason to think his life would not be satisfactory and enjoyable to him if he were to recover from his current condition. The only explanation for his refusal is that he is severely depressed.

This patient also satisfies the U + A definition of competence: he understands and appreciates all of the facts about his situation. His overwhelming desire is to die, and all of his actions (refusing cardiac treatment and refusing nutrition and hydration) are logically consistent with his goal of satisfying his desire to die.

The Irrationality of a Patient's Decision

The woman in case 1 suffers from a seriously irrational fear of ECT treatment, and the man in case 2 has a seriously irrational desire to die.[13] Most physicians believe that these patients' refusals should be overruled. Not to overrule would likely lead to the patient dying of a treatable malady in a situation in which the patient has no rational desire to die; in fact, the woman in case 1 explicitly states that she does not wish to die. However, if only incompetent patients' refusals can be overruled, and if the formal U + A criteria are used strictly and exclusively to define competence, then these patients are both competent to refuse, and the irrationality of their actual choices can play no role in determining their competence.

The U + A definition usually yields a result that coincides with physicians' judgments about which patients' refusals should be overruled, because people who make seriously irrational treatment refusals usually do so because they do not adequately understand and appreciate the facts about their situation. However, sometimes refusals are made because of irrational fears or irrational desires. Patients like the two described above can irrationally refuse treatment even though they do understand and appreciate all of the relevant information. Irrational fears (phobias) and irrational desires do not always cause the kinds of cognitive distortions that the U + A definition stipulates as the only features that make a person incompetent. If only the refusal of incompetent patients can be overruled, the U + A definition does not allow overruling the patients in cases 1 and 2. The two objectives of determining competence are (1) to prevent overruling patients whose decisions should not be overruled, but also (2) to allow overruling patients whose decisions should be overruled. It is not sufficient for the criteria defining competence to achieve only the first of these objectives.

Thus, a dilemma exists. If competent patients can make any treatment decision they want, no matter how irrational, without interference, then competence cannot be defined solely by the use of the formal criteria of U + A. Whatever formal criteria are invoked to define competence, so long as these do not specify anything about the content of the patient's actual decision, will allow for cases in which the definition is satisfied although the patient makes such a seriously irrational decision[14] that nearly everyone would favor overruling the patient.[15] It appears that using the U + A criteria requires that the rationality/irrationality of the patient's decision play some role in judgments about competence, and that both U + A and irrationality operate to some extent independently of the other.

However, there is a justifiable concern about allowing the rationality/ irrationality of the patient's decision to play any role in judgments about competence. Irrationality is often defined in such a way that any decision that deviates from the preferred decision of the doctor is labeled as irrational. When "irrational" is used in this way, the freedom of otherwise competent patients to make their own decisions about whether to accept or reject a proposed treatment is lost. However, if "rational" is used to mean "not irrational," and no decision is regarded as irrational unless (1) it would result in the patient suffering significant harm for a reason that almost no one with similar knowledge and intelligence would regard as adequate for suffering that harm, and (2) persisting in that decision would result in the person satisfying the definition for having a mental disorder, then the freedom that would be lost is not a freedom that any rational person would want to have.[16]

Modifying the U + A Definition of Competence

There are at least three ways in which the U + A criteria of competence discussed above can deal with the strong intuitions with which it sometimes conflicts. The first (A) has been discussed: competence can be defined exclusively by U + A criteria. However, within this first approach there are two opposing views about the role of (U + A) competence in determining whether to overrule a patient's decision. The first (A1) is to claim that competence defined in this way is determinative: if the patient consents, proceed with the intervention; if the patient refuses, don't proceed with the intervention. Thus, according to this view, the patients described in cases 1 and 2 above would both be regarded as competent and therefore would not be treated. Someone who held this view might acknowledge that most persons' intuitions would favor overruling the refusals in cases like these. However, the argument could be made by exponents of this view that it is better in the long run to give everyone unbridled freedom of choice, even if, as a result, some persons make seriously irrational decisions that cause them great harm.

The second alternative (A2) that can be taken is defining competence exclusively by U + A, with a finding of competence generally justifying acceding to a patient's decision, although the irrationality of the patient's decision should sometimes play an important role in determining whether to override that decision. Those who agree with this second position believe that a physician is morally justified to overrule the seriously irrational decision of a competent patient.[17] This approach has the advantage of being more congruent with people's widespread intuitions about whether to overrule in actual cases. For example, the patients in cases 1 and 2 would be labeled as competent, but their refusals would be regarded as seriously irrational, and on the basis of that serious irrationality it would be morally justified to overrule them. The disadvantage of this approach is that the notion of sometimes overruling a competent patient is at variance with the U.S. legal tradition that competent patients' decisions should never be overruled.[18]

The second position, (B), is one that can be taken to change the definition of competence so that it is no longer defined exclusively in U + A terms. Several theorists have suggested that the definition of competence be plastic and shifting so that it varies with the kind of clinical situation the patient is in.[19] Thus, if a suggested intervention holds the promise of only limited benefit and limited risk (i.e., nothing of great moment is at stake), then a patient might be deemed competent to consent or refuse simply on the basis of expressing a choice (a formal criterion). The rationality of a refusal in this situation would not be a factor in determining competence. Even if a patient's refusal were thought to be mildly irrational, that is, only minor harm would be suffered, he would be deemed competent to refuse. On the other hand, in a clinical situation in which a patient was refusing life-sustaining treatment, it would be necessary for the patient's refusal to be rational for the patient to be deemed competent.

This shifting-definition approach has problems. It is odd to have a key central theoretical term change its very meaning from situation to situation. More important, it leads to strange results. For example, two doctors can disagree about the seriousness of a patient's condition because they have a reasonable disagreement about the patient's underlying diagnosis. The patient firmly refuses further diagnostic tests but refuses to discuss his reasons for doing so. One doctor believes the malady from which the patient is suffering is minor and that there is no urgency to conduct additional diagnostic tests unless the clinical situation changes. The other doctor believes it is more probable than not that the patient is suffering from a serious occult disorder and that further tests might be clarifying and even life saving. Under the shifting-definition approach, the first doctor could claim that the patient was competent to refuse and the second doctor could claim that the patient was not competent to refuse. The two doctors' disagreement about competence would stem from the differing diagnostic inferences they have made based on the signs and symptoms they observe. But if "competence" is a mental attribute of persons, which most theorists believe, then changes in competence should vary only with changes in mental characteristics of the person, not with changes in his physical condition. The diagnostic disagreements between the two physicians should be irrelevant in determining the competence of the patient.[20] The third position, (C), will be discussed later.

Symmetry and Asymmetry of Consents and Refusals

Suppose a patient at a given time consents to a suggested intervention. Using a U + A definition of competence, she is judged to be competent to consent. Now suppose nothing about her situation is altered, but after further reflection she changes her mind and refuses the intervention. Is she, automatically, to be judged competent to refuse? Different U + A definitions of competence yield different answers to that question. Under the strict U + A definition, there is a symmetry between consent and refusal. Since competence is judged on the basis of U + A, and not on the basis of the content of the patient's decision, the patient who is competent to decide in one way—unless her U + A is somehow altered in the interim—is competent to decide in the other. For example, on the strict U + A definition, the patients in cases 1 and 2 would be judged competent no matter whether they consented to or refused treatment. However, with definition (B), patients who changed their minds and consented to treatment would be considered competent, but if they refused they would be considered incompetent. Thus, there is an asymmetry between consent and refusal.

If a definition of competence makes it possible to always determine whether a patient is competent before the patient's actual decision to consent or refuse is known, then there is symmetry and the definition is one where U + A are determinative. If a definition of competence allows the patient's actual decision to consent or refuse to sometimes determine whether a patient is competent, then there is asymmetry and irrationality or some similar normative term that is, one way or another, being included in the definition of competence. If the rationality/ irrationality of the patient's decision can affect whether the patient is judged to be competent, then it may be misleading to claim that a competent patient is free to make any decision she wants, for some decisions will result in a patient being judged to be incompetent. An important question to ask of any definition of competence is whether a patient's competence can always be determined before knowing whether the patient has consented or refused.

Any account of rationality and irrationality to be incorporated into the concept of competence must be such that no decision is regarded as irrational if any significant number of persons would regard that decision as rational. All irrational decisions must be such that they would result in the patient suffering significant harm for a reason that almost no one with similar knowledge and intelligence would regard as adequate for suffering that harm. And persisting in that decision would result in the person satisfying the definition for having a mental disorder.[21] This means that no decision based on religious beliefs that are held by any significant number of people will be irrational.

Competence as the Ability to Make a Rational Decision

The task that a patient must be competent to perform is that of making a rational decision about a proposed medical intervention. Thus, we define the kind of competence required for valid consent or refusal as (C): *competence is the ability to make a rational decision*. We noted earlier that competence was task specific. This definition is clearer about what the appropriate task is: to make a rational decision about the medical intervention being proposed. Thus, competence and rationality should not be defined independently of each other as has been done in the past, but rather they should be explicitly linked in the way the above definition indicates. This explicit linking of rationality and competence reflects the actual practice of most physicians and most courts in deciding whether a patient is competent to make a valid decision about his health care. However, without explicitly incorporating rationality into the definition of the kind of competence required to make a valid decision, it has been the practice to interpret understanding and appreciating in such a way that the patient who made a seriously irrational decision was understood to be showing that he either did not understand or did not appreciate the consequences of his decision. However, this sometimes resulted in regarding a patient as competent when he consented but as incompetent when he refused. Thus, it took away what was regarded as the primary advantage of the U + A definition, namely, that it allowed a determination of competence prior to the patient making his decision. Objections were also raised that this interpretation of U + A competence took away the symmetry that the U + A concept of competence had, by distorting the accepted meanings of "understand" or "appreciate."

Explicitly incorporating rationality into the account of the kind of competence required to make a valid decision about health care explains why the actual decision that the patient makes, or, more precisely, persists in, is sometimes decisive in determining whether the patient is competent to make a valid decision about his health care. No one who is competent to make a rational decision about his health care, or anything else, ever persists in making a seriously irrational decision about this matter. As has been recognized by many thinkers (e.g., Spinoza), freedom and rationality are closely related. Part of what this means is that no person persists in acting irrationally if he has the ability to avoid doing so. Freedom in this context does not mean absence of coercion, but rather lack of the appropriate volitional ability.[22]

Freedom as related to rationality cannot mean absence of coercion because coercion can make doing what would otherwise be an irrational decision a rational decision, for example, giving away all of one's money to someone who does not need it and whom one does not like, because he threatens to shoot you if you do not. Rather, freedom as it is related to rationality means what we prefer to call "voluntariness." No person voluntarily persists in acting irrationally. However, sometimes a person acts irrationally because he has some relevant volitional disability, for example, an addiction, compulsion, or phobia. When a person has a relevant volitional disability, he may be unable to make a rational decision even if he understands and appreciates all of the information that is adequate to make his decision an informed one.

There are several conditions that can take away a person's ability to make a rational decision. Among them are:

(a) a cognitive disability that prevents the person from understanding the information relevant to making a decision of a certain kind. In the case of medical treatment decisions, this would be the lack of ability to understand the "adequate information" given during the consent process.

(b) a cognitive disability that prevents coordinating the information in (a) above with the patient's personal rational ranking of the various goods and harms associated with the various available options, insofar as these rankings are relevant, and hence involves a failure to appreciate how that information applies to one's values.

(c) a volitional disability involving the lack of an ability to believe that prevents believing that the relevant information does indeed apply to one in one's current situation. Mood disorders, such as serious depressions, may make it impossible to believe that there are any incentives for consenting to a life-saving treatment. A volitional disability can involve the lack of the ability to believe as well as the lack of ability to act on one's beliefs. Delusions are paradigms of such a lack of the ability to believe.

(d) a volitional disability involving the lack of an ability to act on the incentives for consenting that one acknowledges make it irrational not to consent. Addictions and phobias are volitional disabilities that can interfere with a person's ability to make a rational decision.[23]

If either (a), (b), (c), or (d) is present, then the person lacks the ability to make a rational decision of the particular kind involved, which is to say that she is not competent to make a rational decision of that kind. If (a) applies, then the patient does not satisfy the understanding part of the U + A definition of competence; but if (b) applies, then the patient lacks the appreciating part of the U + A definition. If (c) applies, then the patient may be claimed to lack either the understanding part or the appreciating part of the U + A definition of competence, although these claims can be maintained only if failure to believe entails failure to understand or to appreciate. If (d) applies, then the patient would clearly satisfy the U + A definition; but if his decision was seriously irrational, he would still be regarded as incompetent by almost all doctors and judges. Our definition makes explicit that a mental disorder, for example, a mood disorder or a phobia, that involves a volitional disability that results in a seriously irrational decision is sufficient for classifying the patient as incompetent to make that decision. Thus, the ability to make a rational decision has cognitive and volitional components.

Each of the above four factors may by itself take away a patient's ability to make a particular kind of rational decision. We think this list is exhaustive and thus the absence of all four factors is sufficient to ensure that the patient is competent to make a rational decision of the kind involved. However, more than one of the factors may be present. For example, a person may suffer not only from a delirium that renders him unable to understand the relevant information but also from depression so that he would be unable to make a rational decision even if he understood the relevant information.

The vast majority of patients who make irrational treatment decisions are not competent to make rational decisions of the kind involved. Consider a middle-aged man who refuses to have an appendectomy for his acute appendicitis, even though it is in danger of rupturing and causing a possibly fatal peritonitis. It almost always is the case that (a) patients of this kind do not have the cognitive ability to understand the situation; (b) patients of this kind do not have the cognitive ability to appreciate how their choice will affect what they value; (c) patients of this kind do not have the volitional ability to believe the information that is relevant to their choice because of some delusion, which could be related to their severe depression; or (d) patients of this kind, despite their accurate cognitive understanding, do not have the ability to make this kind of rational decision because of, say, a fear of general anesthesia. Thus, this man will almost certainly be found, correctly, to be incompetent to refuse surgery. Seriously irrational decisions are seldom made by persons who have the ability to make rational decisions of the kind involved, and they are never persisted in unless the person is not competent to make that kind of decision. However, less seriously irrational decisions are sometimes made by patients who have the ability to make rational decisions. Consider a man who has a wart on the sole of his foot. He is suffering from mild to moderate chronic pain and disability; that is, he limps. The condition can almost always be totally reversed by one or another podiatric procedure, such as blunt excision, that causes only mild brief pain and is nearly risk free. Nonetheless, this man suffers from the condition for weeks or months, despite his accurate knowledge of the above facts, despite having no adequate reason for delaying treatment, and despite having no mental disorder that interferes with his ability to believe the pertinent information he has been given and to choose rationally. Thus, we could say of him that he is competent, that he has the ability to believe the information he has been given, and he has the ability to choose rationally, but that he has made an irrational choice. However, we do not think that this decision is serious enough that he should be regarded as incompetent. The seriousness of the irrational decision is determined by the seriousness of the harms that will be suffered because of the irrational decision. Only death or a significant permanent disability, without an adequate reason, will usually be serious enough for the patient to be classified as incompetent. Thus, our account of the kind of competence necessary for a patient to be competent to make a health care decision seems to track the actual practice for determining competence better than any of the alternatives.

Different definitions of competence vary in the way in which they articulate the concepts of "competence" and "rationality." The pure U + A definition of competence sharply distinguishes between competence to make a decision to consent or refuse a proposed intervention and the rationality or irrationality of the decision made. By contrast, definition (B) includes rationality/irrationality as a sometimes-important constituent of the U + A definition of competence. Definition (B) specifies that treatment refusals in high-risk clinical situations must be rational before the person can be regarded as competent to make them, but the definition does not require rational decisions in less risky settings in order to classify patients as competent. Definition (C) specifies that a person is competent to make a particular medical decision if and only if she has the ability to believe the relevant information and to make a rational decision of the particular kind involved. Being able to make a rational decision of a particular kind has constituent cognitive and volitional components.

Incorporating the rationality/irrationality of the patient's decision into the account of competence helps bridge the gap that has developed between the specified justifications for two morally similar procedures: overruling patient refusals of medical interventions, and involuntarily committing persons who are deemed dangerous to themselves or others. In most states a person can be involuntarily committed if he is suffering from a mental illness that makes him dangerous to himself or to others. There is no mention of competence, defined as U + A or in any other way, in most states' statutory criteria for commitment. The concern is solely with the probability of the person's acting dangerously because of a mental disorder. Acting in that way is exactly what we regard as acting in a seriously irrational way. A sufficient condition for incompetence should be the irrational refusal of a medical intervention because of a mental disorder.

Advantages of Definition (C)

This definition has several advantages:

(1) Everyone agrees that competence is task specific, but definition (C) seems to provide the first explicit statement of the kind of tasks that competent patients must be able to perform. Defining competence as the ability to make a rational decision explains the common intuition that a high degree of irrationality is a major factor in determining incompetence. Although continuing to distinguish between the competence of the patient and the rationality of a particular decision, this definition makes clear that determining incompetence and justifying paternalistic interventions are distinct but related. Incompetence is not determined by the seriousness of a patient's situation, but the justification for overruling a refusal is. Approaches that simply sort patients into two groups, the competent and the incompetent, seem to consider that no further justification is needed to overrule the refusals of incompetent patients, and this seems to be a mistake.

(2) Unlike the view that irrational decisions of competent patients can be overruled, this definition is consistent with the legal tradition. On definition

(C), all persons who persist in making seriously irrational decisions are correctly regarded as incompetent. This is not ad hoc, for any person who persists in making an irrational decision of any significance will satisfy the criteria for having a mental disorder.

(3) Although we define competence as the ability to make a rational decision, the incompetence of a person to make a kind of rational decision is never determined simply by the irrationality of her decision in the present case. A person is competent to make a rational decision only if both of the following are true: (1) she does not have a cognitive disability preventing her from understanding and appreciating the relevant information or coordinating that information with her own stable values; and (2) she does not have a mental disorder that takes away her ability to make a rational decision. If none of these disabilities—including having a relevant mental disorder—is present, she is competent to make a rational decision, even if she is presently making an irrational decision. Of course, persisting in a seriously irrational decision would show that the person has a mental disorder that takes away her ability to make a rational decision and, hence, she is incompetent to make that kind of decision. However, if, for example, a person overcomes a volitional disability that prevents her from consenting to ECT, and consents, she is then competent to make that kind of decision.

The ability to make a rational decision of a certain kind is what people may implicitly have had in mind when they accorded "competence" the primacy it has in the consent process. They did not realize that the bare-bones $U + A$ of the information presented could exist in the presence of mental disorders that took away from people the ability to make a rational decision of a certain kind. Definition (C) simply makes explicit what most people already hold. It is understandable that $U + A$ were initially selected as criteria for competency: they are fairly easily assessed and they usually do agree with our intuitions about particular cases. This is because the overwhelming majority of patients who lack the ability to make a kind of rational decision lack it because they don't understand and appreciate the relevant information. However, cases like 1 and 2 force us to realize that $U + A$ does not capture the full meaning of the concept of competence as the ability to make a rational decision.

Definition (C) provides the correct account of the relationship between $U + A$, the rationality/irrationality of the patient's treatment choice, and the concept of competence as an essential feature of valid consent. Neither $U + A$ by itself nor the rationality/irrationality of the patient's decision by itself provides an adequate explanation of the meaning of competence. Combining the two provides a definition of competence that (1) accords with most persons' intuitions about what should be done in particular cases, (2) is linked with a coherent theory about the paternalistic justification of overruling some patients' treatment decisions, and (3) is consistent with the prevailing legal account of the role of competence in valid consent.

Coercion

It is universally acknowledged that if a physician coerces a patient into accepting a treatment, that consent is not valid. Except when the patient is in a situation when acting paternalistically toward him is justified, a physician may not coerce a patient into consenting. To do so would be an unjustified violation of the general moral rule prohibiting depriving persons of freedom. There is nothing special about the medical situation: stating that coercion is immoral simply reminds the physician that, except when he can publicly allow such coercion, it is as immoral to coerce in the medical situation as it is in all situations.

Valid consent requires the absence of any coercion by the doctor or the medical staff. Coercion involves a threat of sufficient evil or harm that "it would be unreasonable to expect any rational man in that situation not to act on it."[24] A threat of this kind means that the person being threatened has been deprived of her freedom to choose, which is morally prohibited. Strong recommendations, even forcefully given, are not coercive. To extend the term "coercion" to include any pressure by a doctor on a patient to change a treatment decision and, hence, to require that the pressure be morally justified seems to us undesirable. In fact, sometimes it is morally praiseworthy for a physician to put pressure on a patient during the consent process, but the pressure must be limited to pointing out in a truthful manner the benefits of the treatment and the harms of not being treated. It cannot include threats to discontinue treating the patient. And it must be clear throughout the process that despite the physician's attempt to cause the patient to change his decision, in the last analysis the patient will be free to decide as he wishes.

Family coercion. On occasion, patients are coerced to choose or reject a treatment option not by the health care team, but by their family or friends. If, as is sometimes the case, the patient has not been given adequate information, or if the patient is not fully competent to make a rational choice, then on those grounds the coerced consent would not be valid. Sometimes, however, the patient has been given adequate information and is fully competent, but nonetheless consents only because of coercion from a family member.

Consider the following case: Mrs. R is a sixty-one-year-old, legally blind and chronically physically ill woman who is admitted to an inpatient psychiatric unit for treatment of a severe depression that had been poorly responsive to a series of antidepressant medications. She has had three other episodes of depression during the past ten years, each of which has similarly been poorly responsive to medication but in each case has subsequently resolved quickly with electroconvulsive therapy (ECT).

On admission to the unit, Mrs. R is reluctantly agreeable to receiving ECT. However, two days after admission she tells her psychiatrist, Dr. B, that she is actually very frightened of having ECT and is consenting only because of threats from her husband. Her husband had threatened her at the time of admission by telling her that he would not help to care for her at home if she returned without having had ECT. Because of her blindness and her compromised physical condition, she requires much assistance at home for such basic physical needs as personal hygiene, and clothing and feeding herself. There is no one on whom she can depend other than her husband. Numerous attempts by various health care professionals to contact Mr. R over the next week prove unsuccessful, but Mr. R tells his wife by telephone that he refuses to come to the hospital or talk to any staff member until she has ECT. Mrs. R asks the staff to stop trying to reach her husband. She says that she is willing to give permission for ECT, and sign a consent form, though she continues to insist to the staff that if it were up to her alone, she would not consent.

The treatment staff is unsure what to do. Mrs. R clearly regards it as impossible to return home without her husband's support. There is no one else with whom she can stay. Discharging her to a state-supported nursing home might be possible, but the psychiatric care as well as other care there is substandard, and she herself rejects this option. Should the staff proceed and give her ECT, as she is requesting?

Our view is that her consent should be viewed as valid. The physicians were not doing the coercing, and they had no control over the coercing party, her husband. We regard Mrs. R's husband's coercion as a fact-about-her-life with which she must contend, much as a victim of appendicitis must contend with her abdominal pain in deciding whether to consent to an appendectomy. In each case, the patient's decision is significantly determined by a strong negative stimulus for which the physician bears no responsibility and over which the physician has little or no control. Both the appendicitis patient and Mrs. R. may acknowledge that their decisions are being largely determined by a coercive stimulus but, on balance, wish to consent. Whether the staff believes that Mr. R's paternalistic behavior toward his wife is morally unjustified, they do not have Mrs. R's permission to intervene. We do not believe her consent is invalid, and we believe it is morally justified for her physicians to proceed with ECT. To refuse to treat would put the staff in the ironic position of refusing to give the one treatment that they themselves believe is most highly indicated.

It may seem paradoxical to regard coercion from the physician as invalidating consent, but coercion from the family as not doing so. But to see that different moral considerations apply in the two cases, consider again the example of appendicitis. When a patient's intense appendiceal pain causes her to consent to surgery, that does not invalidate her consent and it is morally justified for the surgeon to operate. The same is true when the coercive cause of consent is from a family member. However, the surgeon is acting immorally if he himself intentionally caused the painful condition that made the patient consent to surgery. Even though it might now be necessary for him to operate, he would be subject to severe penalties because he himself is the cause of the harm. The same is true if the surgeon initiates the coercive cause of consent from a family member.[25] The important point to be made is that coercion, that is, being threatened with a harm that it would be seriously irrational to refuse unless one had an adequate reason for doing so, makes a health care decision regarding treatment (that is intended to benefit the patient) invalid only if it is coercion by someone in the health care team.

Coercion When the Patient Is Not the Beneficiary

However, when the decision does not regard treating the patient, but consenting to participate in research, or donating a kidney, part of a liver, bone marrow, and so forth, then coercion from anyone—family, friends of the recipient, someone in the health care team—invalidates the decision to consent. Physicians should not be partners or accomplices to coercing a person to do something that is not designed primarily for the benefit of the person being coerced. The requirement for providing adequate information is stricter, that is, information about smaller harms and risks must be included for research and donation that are unnecessary for treatment; in addition, the requirement for absence of coercion is also stricter. Only coercion (instigated) by someone on the health care team invalidates a decision to consent to treatment; coercion by anyone invalidates a decision to consent to research or donation.

The stricter standard for absence of coercion explains why there is some controversy about whether disadvantaged populations, such as prisoners or the homeless, should be allowed to consent to research or donation. It is sometimes claimed that these people are in a situation where coercion is almost inevitable, even if no one explicitly threatens them with any harm. Their situation is such that they are already suffering sufficient harms that an offer to relieve those harms counts as coercive, that is, it would be seriously irrational to refuse unless one had an adequate reason for doing so. We are not claiming that these disadvantaged populations are necessarily being coerced, and we do not have a conclusive argument in favor of or against their being allowed to consent, but it is clear that much more care must be taken to ensure that people in these vulnerable populations are not being coerced to participate in research or donation.

Notes

1. We prefer "valid consent" to "informed consent" because the latter connotes too narrow a meaning. For example, it sounds odd to say "No coercion is to be employed if a patient's consent is to be regarded as informed," while saying "No coercion is to be employed if a patient's consent is to be regarded as valid" sounds correct.

2. See Braddock and Edwards, et al. (1999), who found that fewer than 10% of the 1,057 audiotaped consent interviews they studied met their rather modest standards for completeness.

3. For example, the American Podiatric Medical Association's code of ethics states only that "the performance of medical and surgical procedures shall be preceded by appropriate informed consent." No attempt is made to define "appropriate."

4. For example, the ethics manual of the American College of Physicians states, "The physician should help develop health policy at the local, state, and national levels by expressing views as an individual and as a professional." Suppose a physician conducts her busy practice at the highest level of professional competence and integrity, but has only minimal interest in health policy and certainly doesn't help develop it at any level of government. Has she thereby acted unethically? Almost no one would think so. Codes of ethics are filled with similar exhortatory statements.

5. The distinction between what is *morally required* and what is *morally encouraged but optional* is pervasive in moral theory and its application; see Gert (2005). It is interesting that academic accrediting agencies, like the Southern Association of Colleges and Schools (SACS), make a similar distinction in their accreditation criteria by stipulating that a rule containing the verb *must* is obligatory to satisfy, while a rule containing the verb *should* is desirable but optional. Failure to satisfy a *must* rule means a college is out of compliance; failure to satisfy *should* rules may be noted in a final evaluatory report but does not signify a punishable lack of compliance. Codes of ethics that do not make the should-must distinction are seriously defective.

6. See the preceding chapter for a discussion of sensitivity, specificity, and other parameters of diagnostic tests.

7. Some genetic tests do have a high sensitivity and specificity, especially those associated with various Mendelian disorders, like Huntington's disease, in which the mutated gene has a high degree of penetrance. However, many common disorders, like heart disease and cancer, may be associated with many genetic mutations that may independently occur in multiple genes; each of these mutations may be weakly but significantly correlated with the emergence of the disorder. Suppose finding a particular mutation were to increase a patient's likelihood of later developing some kind of cancer from 5% to 15%. A patient should consider carefully ahead of time just what that information would mean to her and how she would react to it; she should especially ponder whether there is a significant chance that after she has the information, she might wish she didn't have it. Thus, doctors need to know and disclose to patients the facts about these probabilistic relationships.

8. See Giardiello et al. (2003).

9. See Heather Gert (2002).

10. Chell (1998, 117–118) frames the definitional issue similarly: "The trick is to define [competency] so that it helps us do the job that needs to be done. The job in this context is to make decisions involving decision making. We must decide whether or not we will allow the patient to decide. Thus, what are the proper considerations we must keep in mind in making decisions? What criteria should be reflected in a proper definition?"

11. Dame Elizabeth Butler-Sloss (2002) may hold such a position. In a recent highly publicized case in England, this presiding judge wrote, quoting her own words in an earlier case, "A mentally competent patient has an absolute right to refuse to consent to medical treatment for any reason, rational or irrational, or for no reason at all." It is not clear that she is using "irrational" in the same sense that we use it, for she uses it to characterize a certain kind of reason, whereas as we use "irrational" to characterize a certain kind of action.

12. In fact, the state in which she was hospitalized (New Hampshire) had a statutory definition of competence that explicitly defined competence in terms of understanding

and appreciating, just as these criteria have been defined here. Lawyers who were familiar with the case were of the opinion that the patient should probably be classified as competent to refuse by New Hampshire standards.

13. See Gert (2005).

14. Normative terms other than "irrational" could be used: "pointless," "needlessly harmful," "dangerous," and so forth. We prefer the term "irrational" because its definition has been carefully elaborated (Gert 2005).

15. Other formal criteria could be suggested. "Expressing a choice" is sometimes mentioned; see Grisso and Appelbaum (1998). A patient, for example, might be able to understand and appreciate the relevant information, but for some neurological or psychological reason be unable to express his choice in any way, and therefore understandably be deemed "incompetent to consent or refuse." Another formal criterion sometimes mentioned is the patient's ability to reason logically in justifying her consent or refusal in terms of her general goals. However, all formal criteria have the same problem: It is possible for a patient to satisfy them and yet make a seriously irrational decision that most observers would feel should be overridden. For example, a seriously depressed patient's most important general and overriding goal may be to die and thus his refusal of treatment would be a logical extension of his goal.

16. For a full discussion of the definition of mental disorder, see chapter 7.

17. This is a position that was put forward by Culver and Gert (1982).

18. However, that legal tradition itself seems vague and confused; see Culver and Gert (1990a, 641–642).

19. This position has been advocated by Roth, Meisel, and Lidz (1977), Drane (1985), and Buchanan and Brock (1986).

20. For a lengthier analysis of shifting-definition approaches, see Culver and Gert (1990a, 632–639).

21. See chapter 2 on morality for an account of rationality and irrationality that fits this description. For a fuller discussion of this account of rationality and irrationality, see Gert (2005).

22. See chapter 7 on mental maladies for a fuller account of volitional disabilities.

23. Volitional disabilities are conditions like addictions and phobias that can interfere with a person's ability to make a rational decision. For example, a patient with a phobia about needles might not be able to consent to have her blood drawn even if she herself acknowledges that it is irrational not to consent to such a low-risk diagnostic intervention. The woman in case 1 who dreaded ECT so strongly that she was not able to consent to the one treatment that would probably save her life was suffering from a similar malady and would be judged incompetent on this definition of competence.

24. See Gert (1972).

25. See Mallary, Gert, and Culver (1986) for a more extensive discussion of this case.

10

Paternalism and
Its Justification

Paternalism may be the most pervasive moral problem in medicine. It is involved in many discussions of euthanasia, and often accounts for the failure of physicians to supply full information when attempting to obtain consent for a procedure they believe to be important. At one time, doctors thought that they were supposed to act paternalistically toward their patients; now, many of them seem to think that they should never act paternalistically. Not only is there confusion concerning whether acting paternalistically is ever justified, there is even confusion about what counts as paternalism. In this chapter we will be concerned both with the definition of paternalism and with the ethical justification of paternalistic actions.

Paternalism has an unusual combination of features; it is done to benefit another person and yet everyone agrees that it needs moral justification. These seemingly conflicting features indicate the difficulty of understanding paternalism and may explain why it is discussed so often. A discussion of paternalism is valuable for several reasons. First, it illustrates clearly that having a good motive is not sufficient for determining whether one is acting in a morally acceptable way. This is extremely important, for many people think that meaning well is all that is needed for acting morally. An examination of paternalism shows that morality requires more than good intentions, for unjustified paternalism involves good intentions as much as does justified paternalism ("The road to hell is paved with good intentions!"). Although paternalism is often unjustified, it is not always morally unacceptable. On the contrary, not only is paternalism often justified, it is sometimes even morally required so that in some situations not acting paternalistically can be immoral.

Any adequate definition of paternalism must take into account both that all paternalistic behavior is done with good intentions and that it needs to be justified in order to be morally acceptable. An adequate definition must also allow for both justified and unjustified paternalism. Since the point of providing a definition of paternalism is to enable a more useful discussion of what is commonly regarded as paternalistic behavior, the definition must include all of the clear cases, and exclude behavior that is commonly not regarded as paternalistic. It is a misuse of philosophy to offer a definition of paternalism that has the provocative result that some kind of behavior that no one considers to be paternalistic would then turn out to be so (e.g., buying one's child an educational toy), or that behavior that is taken as a clear case of paternalism (e.g., committing a suicidal patient to a mental hospital), turns out not to be so. An adequate definition can make the term somewhat more precise, so that it decides at least some cases about which there is dispute, but it should not result in a fundamental change in the way the term is used. Otherwise, the definition cannot serve the point of defining the term, which is to facilitate discussion of those cases to which the term is normally taken to refer.

The Definition of Paternalistic Behavior

We offer the following definition of paternalistic behavior:[1]

A is acting paternalistically toward S if and only if:

1. A believes that his action benefits S;
2. A recognizes (or should recognize) that his action toward S is a kind of action that needs moral justification;
3. A does not believe that his action has S's past, present, or immediately forthcoming consent; and
4. A regards S as believing he (S) can make his own decision on this matter.

From this definition, it is easy to derive accounts of paternalistic attitudes, persons, and so on. A paternalistic attitude is an attitude that indicates a willingness to act paternalistically. But an action can indicate a paternalistic attitude without itself being paternalistic (e.g., not giving money to a beggar because you believe that he will use the money to by alcohol or illegal drugs). Although this refusal indicates a paternalistic attitude, it is not, strictly speaking, a paternalistic action, for refusing to give money to a beggar does not need a moral justification.[2] A paternalistic person is one who is more inclined than most to act paternalistically. A paternalistic law is a law that is intended to benefit the person whom it deprives of freedom.

Paternalistic laws differ from paternalistic actions in that paternalistic laws almost always violate the moral rule against depriving people of freedom, whereas paternalistic actions commonly involve the violation of several different moral rules, for example, those prohibiting deceiving or causing pain, as well as the rule prohibiting depriving of freedom. A paternalistic law is one whose legislative intent is to benefit those who are being deprived of freedom by that law (e.g., seat belt laws). Taking paternalistic laws as the paradigm for paternalistic action has led some people to define paternalism as if it necessarily involved the deprivation of freedom.[3]

The four features of our definition are discussed in the following sections.

The Action Benefits S

There is no dispute about feature 1; in order for A's act to be paternalistic it must be true that A intends to benefit S. A's benefiting himself or some third party is irrelevant to classifying his action as paternalistic. Of course, A's actions can be partially paternalistic; they can be intended to benefit others, including A himself, in addition to S. But what makes A's actions toward S paternalistic is never the intended benefit to anyone other than S. Although A may be involved in self-deception, he must at least intend to benefit S (e.g., a physician may believe that she is deceiving her patient about his prognosis in order to prevent him from feeling bad, whereas the physician is actually more concerned with avoiding the unpleasantness of telling the truth to the patient). In all standard cases of paternalism, A's belief that S will benefit from her action must provide a sufficient motive for A's acting in this way.

Although doing something to S is paternalistic only if it is intended to benefit S, it need not benefit S directly. The intended benefit to S may be the intended result of benefits to those who are taking care of S. For example, a physician may give S some drug to make it easier for those taking care of S. This is done to make the caregivers less upset with S and so treat him better than they now do. If a physician gives S a drug to make it easier for the caregivers to provide S with better care in order to benefit S, giving S that drug can count as paternalistic. Although making things easier for caregivers can benefit those in their care, what is in the best interests of the caregivers is not always in the best interests of the patient.

Restraining a patient in a wheelchair may be paternalistic if done to prevent him from trying to stand and, as a result, falling. If the caregivers cannot provide the constant supervision needed, then they may regard it as in the best interest of the patient to be so restrained, and such an action can count as paternalistic. Whether this kind of paternalistic action is justified depends on the situation. However, if it is clear that the restraints are used in order to provide even less supervision with no net benefit to the patient from the restraints, and only to minimize the workload of the caregivers or to maximize the profit of the institution, then the action does not even count as paternalistic.

When one person benefits another who is not suffering any loss by providing some good for her, for example, by increasing her ability or pleasure, we call this acting on a utilitarian ideal.[4] If the person is suffering from a disability, increasing her ability counts as relieving an evil or harm. Preventing or relieving a harm, such as pain or disability, is acting on a moral ideal. Paternalistic acts can involve acting on either utilitarian or moral ideals. Paternalistically acting on a utilitarian ideal is justified only if done by parents or others in a similar role. Although medical paternalism involves acting toward patients as if they were one's children, almost all paternalistic actions that occur in medicine involve acting so as to prevent or relieve harms, which is acting on a moral ideal.

When talking about paternalism, benefiting a person does not mean doing what that person wants you to do. A physician who is acting in accord with the expressed desires of a patient is not acting paternalistically at all. Acting paternalistically involves acting to benefit a person by doing what you regard as providing a net benefit for her either when you know that she would not regard what you are doing as a net benefit or you do not know whether she would regard it as a net benefit. Normally, paternalism involves acting on one's own ranking of harms and benefits rather than that of the person toward whom one is acting paternalistically. However, even if a physician does know that a patient would regard the result of the act as a net benefit to her, if he does not know if she is willing to undergo the harm involved in order to gain the benefit, he is acting paternalistically. Even if the patient would prefer the outcome that would result from the paternalistic action, he may not want to be treated in a paternalistic way, for example, lied to for his own benefit. Some people do not want others to do anything to them without their explicit consent. Unless one knows that the patient wants to be deceived, caused pain, and so on, doing so, even for what he regards as a benefit, is acting paternalistically.

His Action toward S Is a Kind of Action That Needs Moral Justification

Feature 2, that A recognizes (or should recognize) that his action toward S is a kind of action that needs moral justification, is a key feature of paternalistic behavior. If the person does not recognize that his action is of a kind that needs moral justification, and if it is not the kind of action that he should recognize as needing justification, it is not paternalistic even if it has the other three features of paternalistic behavior. This kind of behavior is paternal or parental behavior, and it includes many of the beneficial things that parents do for their children, for example, buying them a computer or a set of encyclopedia. In chapter 2, we showed that the only kinds of actions that need moral justification are violations of moral rules, thus it is only when a moral rule is violated with regard to S that an action can be paternalistic. Killing, causing pain or disability, depriving of freedom or pleasure, deceiving, breaking a promise, and cheating can all be violated with regard to a person. All of these actions can be done to a person in order to benefit him, and thus can be paternalistic. Insofar as laws can be broken, or duties neglected, with regard to a person, these kinds of acts, if done to benefit that person, can also be paternalistic.

Our account of morality in chapter 2 shows that any kind of action that needs moral justification is prohibited by a general moral rule. Even though acting paternalistically can involve violating particular moral rules, all violations of particular moral rules also involve violations of the general moral rules. Thus, no paternalistic act is excluded by limiting paternalistic actions to violations of the general moral rules. We have, of course, not proved that no actions in addition to violations of the general moral rules need justification, but if our account in chapter 2 is correct, then the rules we list do cover all actions that need justification.

It is important to distinguish between performing the kind of action that needs justification in order to be morally acceptable (i.e., violating a moral rule), and failing to act in a way that is morally encouraged, but whose omission does not require justification (i.e., not following a moral ideal). As stated above, it is not paternalistic behavior for a person to refuse to give money to a beggar because he believes the beggar will only buy whiskey with it, which will be harmful to him. Such behavior may reveal a paternalistic attitude, for example, a willingness to act paternalistically toward the beggar if the situation arose, but it is not itself a paternalistic act. Only when one's action requires moral justification is it appropriate to call it paternalistic. There may be some disagreement concerning which acts need moral justification, but there is no disagreement that all of the clear cases involve violations of moral rules. Relieving pain is normally following a moral ideal, and a nurse sometimes has a duty to relieve the pain of her patients. If a nurse fails to act so as to relieve the pain of her patient, what needs justification is her failure to do her duty, which is a violation of a moral rule, not her failure to follow a moral ideal.

To have a justification for acting paternalistically is to have a justification for violating a moral rule. What counts as an adequate justification for violating a moral rule is discussed in detail in chapter 2 and is the account that we use in discussing the justification of paternalism. Those who have a different account of justification, however, can still accept our account of paternalism, although they may differ from us in the way in which they decide which paternalistic acts are justifiable. We recommend comparing our account of moral reasoning with that provided by others—for example, consequentialists, deontologists, contractarians, virtue theorists, principlists, or casuists—to see which is most helpful in deciding what action morally ought to be done or in explaining one's moral judgments.

We have already pointed out that those who take paternalistic laws to be the paradigm of paternalism commonly say that paternalism always involves a deprivation of freedom of the person who is being treated paternalistically. Paternalism, however, need not involve violating the moral rule prohibiting the deprivation of freedom, but can involve violating any of the moral rules mentioned in the first paragraph of this section. Paternalism involving breaking a promise is even discussed by Plato, who advocates not keeping one's promise to return a weapon to someone who has gone mad and may hurt himself. A promise to discharge a patient on a given day may be broken when the physician thinks it would not be in the patient's best interests to go home on that day, even though the patient wants to go home. In medicine, many acts of paternalism involve deception, and are often not related, except in a very indirect way, to the patient's actions at all. Rather, they are done in order to prevent the patient, at least for some time, from feeling bad because of receiving unpleasant news about her medical condition.

There can even be cases of paternalism that involve violating the rule against killing. Indeed, one of the arguments against legalizing voluntary active euthanasia is that it may lead to paternalistic nonvoluntary killing of patients, that is, killing a patient who had not explicitly requested that he be killed. This argument against legalizing voluntary active euthanasia is that some doctors who are reluctant to talk to a patient about dying may conclude that the patient would be better off dead. If the doctor acts on that belief and kills the patient, he would be acting paternalistically. Of course, many are against legalizing voluntary active euthanasia because they believe that doctors may be led to practice nonvoluntary active euthanasia for economic reasons, that is, they may act against what they take to be the best interests of their patients for what they take to be the best interest of their hospital, health care system, or society. But many also hold that legalizing voluntary active euthanasia is dangerous because some doctors may act with the best interests of their patients in mind, but do so paternalistically. This may not be a good argument, but it shows that the notion of paternalistic killing is a fairly straightforward notion.

It is easy to imagine cases of causing pain, disabling, or depriving of pleasure that would count as paternalistic. A can act toward S in any of these kinds of ways in order to prevent S from doing something that A considers dangerous. It may be more difficult to imagine paternalistic examples of cheating, but, although unusual, cheating a particular person in a card game can be paternalistic, for example, cheating because one believes that the person being cheated is too cocky and will benefit from losing the game.

It is now generally accepted that paternalism is not limited to depriving of freedom, but that there can be paternalistic deception, paternalistic causing of pain, and so forth. Paternalism requires only that A recognizes (or should recognize) that he is performing a kind of action, for example, deceiving, that requires moral justification. It does not require A to think that his particular action needs justification. A may recognize that deceiving needs justification, and he may know that he is deceiving a patient, but he may not think of his action in that way, but rather as comforting a patient. To satisfy this requirement of paternalism, all that is necessary for an act to count as paternalistic is that the person acting recognize that he is performing a kind of action, for example, deceiving, and that deceiving is the kind of action that needs justification. He need not, and usually does not, think that he is doing anything wrong, and may not even regard his particular act as needing justification. All paternalistic acts can be correctly described as violations of moral rules, but it is extremely unlikely that a person acting paternalistically will be thinking of moral rules, or of whether he is violating any of them.[5]

Some philosophers hold that some actions that are not violations of moral rules may still be paternalistic. Gerald Dworkin gives the following example: "We play tennis together and I realize that you are getting upset about the frequency with which you lose to me. So, for your own good and against your wishes I refuse to play with you."[6] Dworkin regards this as a case of paternalism, whereas we regard it only as showing a paternalistic attitude. On our account, refusing to play tennis is not paternalistic because it does not need moral justification. No violation of a moral rule need be involved in refusing to play tennis with someone. Dworkin then says, "It begins to look as if the only condition that will work is one that depends on the fact that the person who is being treated paternalistically does not wish to be treated that way." However, Dworkin realizes that this definition does not work and says that paternalism requires "a violation of a person's autonomy." He thus seems committed to the view that refusing to play tennis with someone in the situation described above is a violation of that person's autonomy.[7] He seems to take a violation of a person's autonomy to be equivalent to "an attempt to substitute one person's judgment for another's" and regards that as paternalistic when it is done "to promote the latter's benefit."[8] Dworkin clearly regards paternalistic actions as needing moral justification, but not all actions that he counts as "an attempt to substitute one person's judgment for another's" do need moral justification. Dworkin may rightly characterize his example of a person's refusing to play tennis as an attempt to substitute one person's judgment for another's, but it does not violate a moral rule and so does not need moral justification. It does, however, demonstrate a paternalistic attitude.

Dan Brock provides a similar account of paternalism. He says, "Paternalism is action by one person for another's good, but contrary to their present wishes or desires, and not justified by the other's past or present consent."[9] He explicitly states, however, that it is not intended to be a precise definition. He may be aware that refusing to give money to a beggar because you believe he will use it to harm himself by buying alcohol is not a paternalistic action, although it certainly manifests a paternalistic attitude. Thomas Beauchamp and James Childress, on the other hand, claim without any qualification: "Paternalism always involves some form of interference with or refusal to conform to another person's preferences regarding his or her own good."[10] They do not distinguish between "intentional nonacquiesence" and "intervention in another person's preferences, desires, or actions," if both are done with "the intention of either avoiding harm to or benefiting the person."[11] Childress distinguishes between active and passive paternalism: "In active paternalism an agent refuses to accept a person's wish or request that he not intervene, whereas, in passive paternalism, an agent refuses to carry out a person's wishes or choices."[12] Childress holds that active paternalism is harder to justify than passive paternalism, but seems to hold that passive paternalism still needs to be justified. Although Childress agrees that it is a feature of paternalism that it needs to be justified, it seems doubtful that passive paternalism, that is, refusing to carry out a person's wishes or choices, does need to be justified, and Childress gives no argument that it does. Dworkin and Brock also agree that paternalism needs to be justified; they disagree only with our claim that the only actions that need moral justification are violations of moral rules. They claim that some actions that are not violations of moral rules need to be justified, but they offer no persuasive examples to support this claim.

Brock, Childress, and Dworkin all hold that paternalism involves acting contrary to the wishes or choices of the person toward whom one is acting. But, as we will discuss in more detail in the chapter on euthanasia, talking about wishes and choices clouds the important distinction between requests and refusals. Unless a physician has a duty to comply with a request, he does not have to justify refusing to carry out a patient's wishes or choices. However, if a patient refuses an intervention, then a physician is depriving him of freedom if she intervenes. Although they do not have the same reasons that we do, both Brock and Dworkin agree that refusing to carry out a person's wishes or choices is not an adequate way to characterize paternalism. Although Childress recognizes that there is a difference between refusing to accept a person's request not to intervene and refusing to carry out a person's wishes or choices, he holds that both need to be justified. We claim that only when one's refusal to acquiesce to a person's wishes involves violating a moral rule does that action count as paternalistic. Normally, this refusal involves intervening, but when one has a duty to carry out those wishes, it can also involve not carrying out a person's wishes.

Further, because Beauchamp and Childress admit that a person can act paternalistically toward someone who is not acting autonomously, paternalism can no longer be characterized as a conflict between beneficence and autonomy. However, Beauchamp and Childress seem to hold that when the person toward whom one is acting paternalistically is not autonomous, then paternalism is justified. When the person is autonomous, the conditions that Beauchamp and Childress present for justifying the paternalistic action are very similar to the conditions that we offer. However, when the harms being caused and prevented are the same, we see no reason for the justifying conditions for paternalistic actions being different if the person toward whom one is acting paternalistically is not autonomous. Furthermore, even when it is clear that it is unjustified to act paternalistically, it is sometimes quite difficult to determine if a person is autonomous.

Dworkin offers the following example to show that acting paternalistically does not require violating a moral rule. "A husband who knows that his wife is suicidal hides his sleeping pills. He violates no moral rule. They are his pills and he can put them wherever he wishes."[13] Dworkin regards the husband's action as paternalistic because it interferes with the wife's self-determination and it is a violation of her autonomy. Since "self-determination" and "autonomy" are technical terms with no clear or settled meaning, no one can say whether or not the husband's action does interfere with his wife's self-determination or violates her autonomy. Regardless of whether a person who hides his own pills to prevent his wife from using them to commit suicide is violating her autonomy or not, it is clear that his action does not violate a moral rule with regard to her. Would Dworkin claim that the husband who hides his own pills from his wife because he wants to use them all himself needs to justify his action? Unless he would, Dworkin does not regard the husband hiding his own pills as needing justification. We do not regard such an action as needing justification and hence we do not regard it as paternalistic. Dworkin may be misled because he realizes that the husband certainly shows a paternalistic attitude, that is, a willingness to act paternalistically, for there seems little doubt that he would have hidden the sleeping pills even if they were his wife's and not his own.[14] However, in these circumstances it was not necessary to violate a moral rule in order to accomplish his end, preventing his wife from committing suicide. Thus, he did not act paternalistically toward her and his action needs no justification.

Suppose a very distraught patient goes to a psychiatrist and says that he feels that he is likely to harm himself in some significant way and that he would like the psychiatrist's advice about whether to be hospitalized. The psychiatrist is not acting paternalistically if he urges the patient to enter the hospital. His urging is not paternalistic not only because he has the patient's consent to give him advice but also because he is not violating any moral rule in urging the patient to enter the hospital. Urging a patient to take some action does not count as coercion (see chapter 9), and so does not count as a paternalistic act unless it involves deception, or in some other way involves the violation of a moral rule. Physicians who have come to realize that paternalistic behavior needs justification sometimes mistakenly believe that strongly supporting a treatment, even giving asked-for advice, is paternalistic. This prevents them from acting in ways that are completely appropriate, and do not need justification at all. We suspect that often when paternalism is defended as an appropriate behavior for physicians, it is not really paternalism that is being defended. Rather, it is what we call paternal or parental behavior, that is, behavior that is done for the patient's benefit but without violating any moral rule, for example, strongly advising or urging the patient to consent to treatment.[15] When this urging or advising is neither coercive nor deceptive, and is done in the appropriate manner, it does not require justification. On the contrary, it may be part of the duty of a doctor to advise and urge her patients, for example, to take their medication.

The Action Does Not Have S's Past, Present, or Immediately Forthcoming Consent

Feature 3 points out that A believes that his action with regard to S does not have S's past, present, or immediately forthcoming consent. If A has S's consent, or if A expects S's immediately forthcoming consent for his action, then an action that might otherwise be paternalistic is not so. Suppose I pull someone from the path of an oncoming car that I believe he does not see. This action needs justification because it involves touching that he didn't consent to, which is a violation of a person's freedom. If, however, I do so because I think that he would have consented to my action if I had asked him, and he will confirm this immediately after the action, my action is not paternalistic even though it may satisfy all the other conditions of paternalistic behavior. On the other hand, if I think that he is trying to commit suicide because of a temporary depression, then even if I think that he will thank me later when he recovers, my act is paternalistic, although it may be justified. It is only in situations where I cannot ask for consent prior to acting that immediately forthcoming consent prevents the act from being counted as paternalistic. Usually these are emergency situations.

Beauchamp and Childress explicitly define paternalism as "the intentional overriding of one person's known preferences or actions by another person, where the person who overrides justifies the action by the goal of benefiting or avoiding harm to the person whose preferences or actions are being overridden."[16] This definition is clearly inadequate because it is possible to act paternalistically toward someone about whom you do not know whether or not your action is contrary to his wishes. That is why we phrase feature 3 as "A does not believe that his action has S's past, present, or immediately forthcoming consent." Beauchamp and Childress present matters in a confusing way when they ask whether paternalism is justified by consent or by benefit. They cite as one of the conditions that might justify paternalism that "the beneficiary of the paternalistic actions has consented, will consent, or would, if rational, consent to the actions on his or her behalf."[17] But, as is made clear by this third feature of paternalism, if the beneficiary has consented, then the action is not paternalistic. That he would consent if rational does not prevent the action from being paternalistic, so that listing "has consented" and "would, if rational, consent" together is misleading.

One might claim that deceiving someone about a surprise party is not paternalistic, for a person cannot ask for consent to give a surprise party. Indeed, the surprise party is a very useful case for distinguishing paternalistic behavior from behavior that is not paternalistic. If you believe that the person you are deceiving loves surprise parties and will be immediately delighted when she is surprised at her party, then your deceiving her about the party is not paternalistic. Suppose, however, you do not believe—in fact, you doubt—that the person you are deceiving loves surprise parties, but you are certain that she would benefit from having one, because it would make her realize how many people care about her. You further believe that even if she is initially upset, she will, by the end of the party, be delighted. In this case, your deceiving her is paternalistic. No claims are being made here about whether either or both of these cases of deception is justified, only that the first, because of the immediately forthcoming consent, should not be regarded as paternalistic, and the second should be regarded so.

The discussion of deceiving in order to give a surprise party makes clear that the expectation of receiving consent sometime in the future, even when it is a virtual certainty, does not make an action nonpaternalistic. Consider a psychiatrist who has been treating a depressed patient for many years. Suppose, against the patient's wishes, she hospitalizes him because he is suicidal, but because she has done this several times before in the same circumstances she knows that the patient will be effusively thankful within two or three days. She is taking away the patient's freedom and even if the patient would be thankful almost immediately, that would not be sufficient to make the action nonpaternalistic. Immediately forthcoming consent does not make an action nonpaternalistic unless one believes one would have received consent beforehand if one had been able to ask for it.

Without this limitation on future consent, a clearly paternalistic injection of a fast-acting mind-altering drug would not count as paternalistic. If a physician could have asked for consent to inject the drug, but did not do so, then, given that the other conditions of paternalism are satisfied, injecting the drug is paternalistic even if he expects immediately forthcoming consent. Since it is known that some drugs change one's mood and attitude, it would be a perversion of the concept of valid consent to say that the patient's immediately forthcoming consent after taking the drug counts as the kind of consent that make the physician's action nonpaternalistic. We discuss the "thank you" theory of justifying paternalism later; here we are merely claiming that a belief, even a justified belief, that the patient will immediately thank you does not always prevent an action from being paternalistic.

Almost all non-emergency medical interventions would be paternalistic if one did not have the patient's valid consent. That is why obtaining a valid consent from a patient is so important morally. Medical interventions often involve causing pain, depriving of freedom, and so forth, and so need justification. When such actions are done for the benefit of the patient and with his valid consent, all medically appropriate treatments are strongly justified. The very same intervention with the same benefit but without the patient's consent may not be justified. One serious problem with utilitarianism—or any form of consequentialism—as a moral guide is that it may not distinguish between these two situations. If the outcome of the treatment is the same (including the patient's attitude toward the treatment after it has been done), but in one case valid consent was obtained, while in the other case it was not, then the first case is not paternalistic and the second one is. Those utilitarians who hold that only actual consequences count must hold that, morally speaking, it is not important whether a physician obtains valid consent and whether an act is paternalistic.

We have already pointed out that belief in immediately forthcoming consent does not always make an action nonpaternalistic, but there are also medical situations in which past consent does not remove A's act from the class of paternalistic acts. Consider a patient who has considerable anxiety about undergoing an operation that the doctor believes to be important for him. After considerable persuasion, the patient consents to the operation that is to be done the next morning. However, the next morning his anxiety is such that, immediately after taking the preoperative medication, he refuses to go through with it. It would clearly be paternalistic for the physician to wait for the medication to take effect and to take advantage of the patient's condition and proceed with the operation. Past consent makes an action nonpaternalistic only if it is not rescinded.

Although we say that in order for an action to be paternalistic, A must believe that his action does not have S's past, present, or immediately forthcoming consent, it is clearly present consent that is primary. Past and immediately forthcoming consent prevent an action from being paternalistic only when they are believed to be signs that one has or would have had the patient's present consent to act toward him as one did. When it is clear that the past consent does not continue into the present, or that the immediately forthcoming consent would not have been given prior to the action, then neither past consent nor immediately forthcoming consent is sufficient to make an action nonpaternalistic.

S Believes He Can Make His Own Decision on This Matter

Feature 4, A regards S as believing he can make his own decision on this matter, is presupposed in many accounts of paternalism, but rarely is made explicit. One cannot act paternalistically toward infants because infants do not believe that they can make their own decision on any matters; indeed they do not believe anything about themselves.[18] The same is true of comatose persons whose views could not be known beforehand, and for whom some action must be taken while they are still comatose. If S does not believe anything at all about himself, then it is inappropriate to regard any action with regard to him as paternalistic. One can be paternalistic toward S only if S is regarded as believing he can make his own decision on this matter.[19] This normally involves S holding that he understands at least something about what might happen to him and to have some desire about whether it is done or not. To say that A is acting paternalistically when he does not have S's consent presupposes that A regards S as at least believing that he can make his own decision on this matter.

A physician should regard S as believing he can make his own decision about treatment if S understands enough to know that the physicians want to benefit him and that this involves their doing something to him that may risk harming him. A physician need not regard S as competent to give consent, or even think that S believes that he understands enough to make his consent valid, for example, both the physician and S may realize that S does not understand the important future consequences of his decision, only the immediate consequences of it. Nonetheless, if the physician regards S as believing he understands enough to make his own decision about treatment, then if she acts on S without his consent, her action is paternalistic. When S is not competent to give valid consent, regardless of whether he believes he can make his own decision on this matter, paternalism is often justified. But even in this kind of case, it should be the patient's guardian, not the physician, who acts paternalistically.

A patient who is incompetent to make a rational decision may be regarded as deficient in two different ways. He may be regarded as not having sufficient *cognitive ability*, for example, he cannot understand enough about the benefits, or risks, or both, to be able to make a rational decision. Or he does not have sufficient information about future consequences in order to make a rational decision. Or he may not understand probabilities at all, thinking that a 5% probability of serious injury is the same as a 95% probability, both being equivalent to a 50% probability, because either the injury will happen or it will not. Children between the ages of five and nine often have sufficient cognitive ability to make rational decisions on simple matters, but do not have sufficient cognitive ability to make rational decisions on complex matters; the same is true of some adults who are mentally retarded.

A patient can have sufficient cognitive ability to understand all of the information necessary to make a rational decision concerning a certain kind of treatment, yet still be incompetent to make that decision if he cannot appreciate that this information applies to him. This lack of appreciation may be due to a mental disorder that involves delusions, for example, he may believe that his physicians are trying to kill him so that although he understands what is said about the benefits and risks of treatment, he does not believe it applies to his case. A delusion that prevents a person from making a rational decision in a certain kind of case may show that the person has a *volitional disability* that prevents him from making a rational decision in that kind of case. For as we pointed out in the chapter on mental maladies, a volitional disability may involve one lacking an ability to believe. Thus, no matter how great his cognitive abilities, and how well he understands the information presented to him, if this person has a delusion, he lacks the ability to believe regardless of the weight of the evidence, and so is not competent to make a rational decision on any matter in which his delusion affects his decision making.

A patient may also have a volitional disability with regard to making a rational decision in a kind of case if he is not appropriately affected by the incentives for and against making a decision in that kind of case. However, it is inappropriate to regard anyone who has the relevant cognitive ability as incompetent to make a rational decision unless he is suffering from some mental disorder that involves a relevant volitional disability. Addictions, phobias, and compulsions may render a person incompetent. For example, a person with a phobia of needles may irrationally refuse a life-saving injection that has no significant side effects, or a person with an irrational fear of ECT may refuse it even though he knows his fear is unfounded. People who are addicted often cannot make rational decisions concerning their addiction, even when they seem as if they are doing exactly what they want to do. Mood disorders (e.g., depression) can also make a person incompetent if the disorders are sufficiently severe. However, there are degrees of depression, from relatively mild to very severe, and even if severe depression involves a relevant volitional disability that can make one incompetent to make a rational decision, mild depression usually does not do so.

Often, whether a person is regarded as having a relevant volitional disability that makes him incompetent to make a rational decision depends on the degree of irrationality of his decision to refuse treatment. If a patient makes what is regarded as a mildly irrational decision, for example, without an adequate reason he does not take his medication or otherwise treat his moderately high blood pressure, he is not normally regarded as having a relevant volitional disability that makes him incompetent. However, if the irrational decision making persists, or if the irrational decision is more serious, for example, a person on the edge of hepatic failure refuses to stop drinking, he is more likely to be regarded as having a relevant volitional disability that makes him incompetent. If the irrational decision will soon lead to death or severe permanent injury, for example, a severely depressed person refuses to eat or drink, he will be regarded as having a relevant volitional disability that makes him incompetent by almost all.

Violating a moral rule without patients' consent, with regard to those who are incompetent to make a rational decision because of their having a relevant volitional disability, is always acting paternalistically. Similarly, violating a moral rule without patients' consent, with regard to those who are incompetent to give valid consent, but who believe that they can make their own decisions, is also acting paternalistically. Paternalistic behavior toward both of these kinds of patients is often justified, but not always. Later in this chapter we will discuss in more detail how one determines when it is justified to act paternalistically in a given case. There is only one element of feature 4—violating a moral rule without patients' consent with regard to those who are so cognitively incompetent that they do not believe that they can make their own decision concerning treatment— that is not paternalistic.

As we discussed in chapter 9, someone who lacks sufficient cognitive ability to make a rational decision about a certain kind of treatment is incompetent both to validly consent to and to validly refuse that treatment. It is his lack of sufficient cognitive ability with regard to the relevant information that renders him unable to make a rational decision, and so no decision that he makes, either to consent or to refuse, can be taken as valid. However, if someone is incompetent to make a rational decision about a certain kind of treatment because of a delusion, or some other relevant volitional disability, there may be an asymmetry between consent and refusal. If the person irrationally refuses treatment because of a mental disorder, for example, a paranoid delusion or an addiction or a phobia, then his irrational refusal shows that he is incompetent to make a rational decision in this kind of situation. However, were he to consent to treatment, this would show that, at least on this occasion, his mental disorder did not cause him to make an irrational decision and so his consent would count as valid.

Making a distinction between incompetence to make a rational decision because of lack of the relevant cognitive ability and incompetence because of a volitional disability helps resolve the dispute we have had with those who claimed that one could be competent to consent to a treatment, but incompetent to refuse the very same treatment.[20] If incompetence is the kind of incompetence based on lack of the relevant cognitive ability, which is what we assumed in our previous criticism of the legal definition of competence, then people who are competent to consent to a treatment are also competent to refuse the very same treatment. However, if incompetence is the kind of incompetence based on lack of the relevant volitional ability, which now seems to be included in the legal interpretation of incompetence, then incompetence to refuse does not imply incompetence to consent, when the former is irrational and the latter is not.[21] When a person irrationally refuses treatment because of a volitional disability, that refusal is not valid, although this does not necessarily justify overruling that refusal. However, even though the person still has the relevant volitional disability, if he changes his mind so that he makes a rational decision, his consent can count as valid. On this occasion he is regarded as having overcome the relevant volitional disability.

It is crucial not to confuse irrational decisions with unusual or unpopular ones; irrational decisions harm the decision maker without her having a rational belief about a corresponding benefit for anyone. Normally, only serious, persistent, irrational decisions raise the question of the competence of the person making the decision.[22] Since irrational decisions harm the decision maker without a corresponding benefit for anyone, it is not surprising that it is implausible that anyone knowingly and voluntarily makes an irrational decision, especially one that is seriously irrational. In all cases where a patient persistently and irrationally refuses treatment, it is appropriate to consider whether he has sufficient cognitive ability (i.e., whether he knows what he is doing), or whether he has the relevant volitional ability (i.e., whether his decision on this matter is voluntary). That a patient is incompetent because of lacking either of these kinds of abilities does not automatically justify acting paternalistically toward him, but requires further analysis.

Incompetence due to lack of sufficient cognitive ability requires a guardian to be appointed to approve both consent and refusals, whether rational or not. This guardian must consider whether it is justified to overrule both refusals and consents to treatment by considering what the patient would do if he had sufficient cognitive ability, that is, if he understood the benefits and harms involved. Unless the patient's decision is irrational, the guardian should overrule the patient's present decision only because she believes that if the patient had understood the benefits and harms involved, he would have decided differently (i.e., that given his values, his decision was unreasonable). Such paternalism, if based on genuine knowledge of the patient's preferences and rankings of harms and benefits, is usually justified.

Incompetence because of a volitional disability presents more difficulties. In these cases the patient does understand the benefits and harms involved, but still makes an irrational or unreasonable decision. Thus, the person acting paternalistically cannot say that she is overruling the patient's decision because she believes that if the patient had understood the benefits and harms involved, he would have decided differently. However, especially in cases where the decision is seriously irrational (i.e., if it involves a high risk of death or significant permanent disabilities), it may be justifiable to act paternalistically. Involuntary commitment involves this kind of paternalism and is explicitly allowed by law in all states, even though the person has sufficient cognitive ability. However, involuntary commitment requires a finding of mental disorder, so as to guarantee incompetence because of a volitional disability. In cases of involuntary commitment, serious irrational actions constitute prima facie evidence of such a mental disorder.[23]

The Justification of Paternalism

Those who hold that paternalism is never justified must both define paternalism in terms of interfering with a patient's "autonomous" choices, and claim that the choices of those who are incompetent because of lack of cognitive ability or a volitional disability are not autonomous choices. We hold that some paternalism is justified because we think it is misleading for one not to regard the act of overruling an incompetent patient's irrational decision as paternalistic when that decision is due to a volitional disability. Such overruling benefits the patient, needs justification, does not have the consent of the patient, and occurs despite the fact that the patient believes he can make his own decision on this matter. Thus, such overruling satisfies all four features of the definition of paternalistic behavior. Recognizing that overruling even incompetent patients' decisions is paternalistic forces physicians to consider whether overruling the patient's decision is justified, that is, whether the harm avoided is sufficiently greater than the harm caused by depriving the patient of freedom so that such a violation could be publicly allowed. We think that this may lead to less unjustified paternalism. A metaphysical discussion about whether a decision is "autonomous" may be more interesting to philosophers than a moral discussion about whether a doctor is justified in overruling an incompetent patient's decision, but it is less likely to have a beneficial effect.[24]

The justification of paternalism is an interesting and important topic because it provides such a clear and discriminating test of the various accounts of morality. It tests not only those accounts of moral reasoning that have some special appeal to those in bioethics (principlism, casuistry, and virtue theory) but also the two dominant general accounts of morality (consequentialism and deontology). There are, of course, many variations of consequentialism and of deontology, and it is impossible to examine all of them. We confine our examination to the clearest variation of each of these two types of theories: act consequentialism and absolutist deontology. We restrict our examination to these extreme versions because we believe that as the versions become sufficiently qualified, they turn into variations of the account of morality that we have outlined in chapter 2. As consequentialism comes to acknowledge the necessity of moral rules, it needs more than consequences to justify the violation of a rule; as absolutist deontology comes to acknowledge that some violations of moral rules are justified, it needs to determine *how* such violations are justified. Our account of morality explains how to justify violations of moral rules in a way that incorporates the insights of both consequentialism and deontology.

Because paternalism is an extremely common kind of behavior in medical contexts, the justification of paternalism has special relevance for those accounts of morality that are most widely used in bioethics, namely, principlism, casuistry, and virtue theory. We have already pointed out the inadequacies of principlism in chapter 5 so that here we limit our comments to casuistry and virtue theory. After principlism, these two kinds of accounts of moral reasoning are the most widely discussed. One critical problem with both of these accounts is that they do not explain why paternalism needs any justification. This is the result of neither of them having any concept that corresponds to what we call a moral rule, that is, they have no general concept of a kind of behavior that needs justification, but that, in particular circumstances, may turn out to be justified.

An adequate account of morality has value not merely—perhaps not even primarily—because it enables one to resolve a moral problem, for not all moral problems can be resolved. One of the most valuable features of an adequate account of morality is that it alerts one to the presence of a moral problem. This is the primary value of the moral rules. Acknowledging these rules does not enable one to resolve a moral problem, but it does enable one to know when one has a moral problem and when one does not, for example, when one's behavior is paternalistic and when it is not. When one knows that violating a moral rule needs justification, one is able to plan one's behavior so as to avoid, as far as possible, breaking any moral rules. Of course, that is not always desirable or even possible, but sometimes it will be both possible and desirable, and so our account of morality, unlike either casuistry or virtue theory, can be helpful by alerting one about when there is or will be a moral problem.

Casuistry

Casuistry,[25] properly understood, involves concentrating on a particular case and comparing it to other cases so as to determine what rules are most applicable to it, and how these rules should be interpreted when dealing with this case. Casuistry, when it does not explicitly acknowledge that it is a part of the kind of public system that was described in chapter 2, may still help to resolve problems, but it can do nothing to help avoid them. This is because casuistry, considered by itself, has no concept comparable to that of a moral rule. Of course, casuistry, properly understood, is part of the kind of moral system that we present; it is a useful method for interpreting and applying the moral system. As we pointed out in chapter 2, it is not always clear what kind of behavior counts as killing, deceiving, and so forth; casuistry helps with such interpretation. Casuistry is also helpful in determining whether the case under consideration should be viewed as a justified exception to the rule. Concentrating on the particular case and comparing it to other cases may make more salient the morally relevant features of the case. Further, this comparison of cases can also help one to see whether one would want everyone to know that this kind of violation is allowed. Divorced from the moral system, however, casuistry is of little value and simply promotes ad hoc solutions to problems.

Of course, to use casuistry successfully, one need not explicitly adopt a moral system, one need only employ it implicitly, as most of us do, in interpreting and applying that moral system. Casuistry, by calling attention to similarities with clear cases, can help in deciding whether a particular case of not telling a patient some information counts as withholding that information and thus as deception, or whether, on the other hand, there is no moral requirement to provide that information. Indeed, it is not even clear what it would be to use casuistry without using the moral system, at least implicitly. Without the moral system, casuistry seems to involve nothing more than comparing different cases and noting similarities and differences. Not only does casuistry not identify the morally relevant features, it contains no way to resolve or even understand disputes if people choose different cases as models that they claim should be used to resolve the case under consideration. Casuistry does not make clear what is causing the dispute, or why people are using different cases as models. Most important, casuistry, independent of a moral system, does not even identify what counts as a moral matter.

Although it seems to be against moral systems, casuistry has the appeal that it does because people implicitly use the moral system we have described. We do not consider casuistry as an alternative account of moral reasoning; rather, we regard it as emphasizing that morality is not a deductive system in which one simply applies absolutely clear rules to absolutely clear cases in order to determine the morally correct course of action. Although there are many cases in which everyone agrees what the morally correct course of action is, these are not the cases that anyone discusses. The cases that are most discussed are those that present unresolvable moral problems, for example, involving differing rankings of the evils. That our account of morality is intended to provide a clear and comprehensive framework for moral reasoning may explain why some have mistakenly taken us to be advocating a deductivist model of moral reasoning.[26] But our view of morality as an informal public system that involves some unresolvable moral disagreement is incompatible with such a model. On our account, individual judgment is called for in any morally controversial case.

Casuistry recognizes that the moral rules need interpretation, and that such interpretation is often essential before one can apply a rule to a particular case. Casuistry also emphasizes the need to look for all of the morally relevant features of the case when deciding whether violating a moral rule is justified, although it does not provide a list of such features. Casuistry realizes that a particular detail, for example, the relationship between the parties involved, may change the act from one that is morally unacceptable to one that is morally acceptable, although it provides no explanation of when or why this is so. Because casuistry requires a moral system, it is not an alternative to our account of morality; rather, like narrative ethics, casuistry concentrates on providing a fuller description of the particular case, focusing on the important task of helping to apply the moral system to particular cases.

Virtue Theory

We call those who believe virtue to be the fundamental concept in morality virtue theorists. A significant problem with many virtue theorists is that they usually do not distinguish the moral virtues (e.g., honesty and kindness) from the personal virtues (e.g., courage and temperance). The moral virtues are those virtues that all rational persons want other people to have. The personal virtues are those virtues that all rational persons want to have themselves. The moral virtues are directly related to the interests of others, and only indirectly related to one's own interests, while the opposite is true for the personal virtues. Understanding the personal virtues does not require understanding morality, whereas understanding the moral virtues does. We are concerned with virtue theory only insofar as it purports to provide an account of morality that believes moral virtues to be more fundamental to morality than is the moral system with moral rules and moral ideals.

Virtue theory, like casuistry, is closely related to the moral system that we have described. However, unlike casuistry, virtue theory is not a method of applying morality to a particular case, but an alternative and incomplete way of formulating the moral system. A complete account of morality must, of course, include an account of the moral virtues and vices.[27] Such an account would list the moral virtues and vices and relate them to particular moral rules and ideals. This account would describe the virtues so that those who have them could not only be identified but also would be provided a description of the way a virtuous person would act in a particular situation. Of course, this is an idealized scenario because not all virtuous persons would act in the same way in every situation, and even those who have the virtues do not always exemplify them. As Thomas Hobbes pointed out, a person is not virtuous simply because he acts morally, nor does he cease to be a virtuous person simply because he performs one morally unacceptable act.

Some virtue theorists claim to provide a useful guide to conduct by enabling virtuous persons to be identified and then used as role models. This account of virtue raises several critical questions. For example, how does one pick out a virtuous person and how does the virtuous person decide how to act? Furthermore, it is not only possible but common for a person to have some of the virtues, but not others. For virtue theorists who advocate the use of role models as basic guides, these are serious problems. If no particular person can serve as a role model for all situations, and there is general agreement that few if any can, there needs to be some way to determine what virtue is called for in a particular situation so that a role model with the relevant virtue can be selected. Even more serious, no virtuous person can be depended upon to act virtuously 100% of the time, so there has to be some independent way of determining when he is acting virtuously and when he is not. These are not new problems that we have just discovered; indeed, in a different context, Kant explicitly raised these same points.[28]

Unless it is possible to provide a description of the virtues such that one can tell in every situation what counts as a virtuous act in that situation, virtue theory is of no use to people without completely reliable role models. We have already pointed out that such role models are not available. An even more serious objection is that the notion of a completely reliable role model strongly suggests that there is complete agreement among all fully informed, impartial, rational persons on the best way to act in any moral situation. This false view plagues almost all moral theories and can lead to intolerance of differing views on particular topics, for example, people on one side of the abortion issue must view those on the other side as lacking some virtue. However, fully informed, impartial, rational persons can sometimes disagree on what is the best way to act in a particular situation. This means they can also sometimes disagree on what is the virtuous way to act in that situation. On those occasions when they do disagree, two completely reliable role models provide different models of how to act, creating a quandary for anyone who depends solely on role models to determine the morally best way of acting.

Because completely reliable role models are, at the very least, in short supply, and sometimes even disagree with one another, virtue theory, in order to be of practical use, must present some other way to determine what counts as acting virtuously in a particular situation. Common morality does provide a way to make that determination. Acting virtuously in a particular situation means one is disposed to obey the moral rules, or follow the moral ideals in that situation in the way that at least some fully informed, impartial, rational person would do. Although fully informed, impartial, rational persons do not always agree, there are always limits to their disagreement. The moral theory presented in chapter 2, by providing clear accounts of the concepts of impartiality and rationality, and by providing a clear account of the moral system (including the moral rules and ideals) does provide a way of determining what counts as a virtuous way of acting in any particular situation.

The virtue of truthfulness is not demonstrated by telling the truth when one should have remained silent. Telling the truth in such circumstances demonstrates the vice of tactlessness. Kindness is not demonstrated by withholding the truth to avoid causing unpleasant feelings when one should have told the truth. Virtue, as Aristotle points out, consists in following the rule or ideal appropriately or, as we put it, as an adequately informed, impartial, rational person would. Knowing when one should obey a rule or follow an ideal and when one should not requires judgment. That is why it is so misleading to regard any of the virtues simply as dispositions to obey the moral rules or follow the moral ideals. Having those virtues that are connected to the moral rules (e.g., truthfulness) and the moral ideals (e.g., kindness) involves knowing when it is appropriate to act on them and when it is not. Of course, having the virtue involves more than knowing how to act, it also involves regularly acting in that way, even when no one else knows how one is acting. By neglecting the question, how does one know what is the virtuous way to act? one may be led to the false claim that acting virtuously is merely acting this way because it is the virtuous way to act, that is, it is sufficient for acting virtuously that one's intention in acting is virtuous.

If the moral virtues are understood primarily as possessing the appropriate motivation for one's actions, then serious problems arise, particularly with regard to paternalistic behavior. All cases of genuine paternalism with regard to patients involve the health care worker being motivated to act for the benefit of the patient. On the motive reading of virtue theory, the doctor who acts paternalistically is necessarily a virtuous person. He is disposed to act benevolently, to try and help others, and so demonstrates the virtue of beneficence. Unfortunately, his beneficence may obscure the fact that he is also violating a moral rule, for example, the rule prohibiting deception, and so it may not even be recognized that there is a moral problem. Virtue theory not only makes one less likely to consider whether a particular paternalistic act is justified or not, it also provides no method for determining whether or not it is justified. A proper account of the moral virtues must explain not only when but why an impartial rational person should or should not violate a moral rule or follow a moral ideal in specific kinds of circumstances.

Just as with casuistry, virtue theory is valuable if it is not taken as the fundamental feature of morality. It emphasizes a dimension of moral behavior that we do not—that morality is usually concerned with a consistent pattern of behavior, and does not call for special decisions in every particular case. The virtues also provide the most powerful way to show that it is rational to be moral, for though it may be beneficial to act immorally on a particular occasion, a person is far more likely to live a satisfactory life if she has the moral virtues than if she does not. Thus, it is perfectly appropriate for parents to present morality to children as the acquiring of the moral virtues and to teach them by example. However, as a theoretical guide to behavior, the virtues are dependent on the guide provided by the moral system. Parents can teach morality by the virtues only if they appreciate the connection of the virtues to the moral system. It may be valuable to select a role model, but some way of selecting the right role model is needed, and also some way of determining if the role model is acting in the right way in a particular situation. All of this requires a clear understanding of the moral system and of how to apply it. Virtue theory is not an alternative to our account of the moral system or its foundation; rather, it is an important and practical supplement to it.

Why the Justification of Paternalism Is Interesting

Paternalistic behavior requires justification because it involves violating a moral rule. Because the violation is done in order to benefit the person toward whom the rule is violated, the consent of that person would make it a justified violation but, of course, with consent the violation is no longer paternalistic. All impartial rational persons would publicly allow violating a moral rule with regard to a person if that person gave valid consent to the violation and the violation would benefit her.[29] What makes justifying paternalism interesting is that a paternalistic act, although done to benefit a person, involves breaking a moral rule with regard to that person without her consent, when she believes she is able make her own decision. Two of the traditional philosophical accounts of morality give incompatible answers to the question of how paternalistic behavior is justified: act consequentialism says that only the consequences of one's actions are morally relevant, and strict deontology says that, without consent, only the conformity or nonconformity of one's action with a moral rule is morally relevant.

For the purpose of using paternalism as a test of various moral theories, it is convenient to discuss a common kind of paternalistic behavior such that the three theories—act consequentialism, strict deontology, and common morality—put forward answers that can be put into three categories: (1) it is always justified, (2) it is never justified, and (3) it is sometimes justified. It is even more convenient to choose a kind of paternalistic action that provides a net benefit to the person and from which no other person is harmed so that each of these theories has a plausible answer to the question of whether to act paternalistically. In such cases, act consequentialism holds that such paternalism is always justified, strict deontology holds that it is never justified, and common morality holds that it is sometimes justified. This is what makes the discussion of the justification of paternalism so important philosophically; it provides a real test of the various accounts of morality. Because the opportunity and temptation to act paternalistically are ubiquitous in the field of health care, it is of great practical value to show which theory best determines when acting paternalistically is justified.

Act Consequentialism—Always Justified

Act consequentialism is a very simple guide to conduct. It claims that an act should be done if it results in the best overall consequences. There are many sophisticated variations of this view, but in its simple form it is held by many who do not regard themselves as holding any philosophical view at all. People who hold this view often state that all that really matters is that things turn out for the best, or that as long as no one gets hurt, one can do anything she wants. It is interesting to note that when there is no alternative action that provides even greater benefits, the ethical theory of act-utilitarianism implies that all paternalistic behavior that provides a net benefit to the person toward whom one acted paternalistically (and if no other person is harmed) is justified. Of course, in many cases of paternalism it is not clear if the person gains a net benefit, for the physician may rank the harms differently than the patient does, and both rankings may be rational. Further, because there is so much self-deception, as well as so many mistakes made in predicting the outcomes of paternalistic interventions, that, even if one accepts the physician's rankings, paternalism often does not have any net benefit for the person who is being treated paternalistically.

Some act consequentialists claim that what determines the moral rightness of an act is its *actual* consequences. This view is probably the result of failing to realize that "morally right" is not a redundant phrase. Sometimes "the right act" means the same as "the act that produces the best consequences" (e.g., when picking stocks), but this is never the case when talking about what is morally right. *Actual* consequences are not even relevant when considering whether an act is *morally right*; it is the *foreseeable* consequences at the time of acting that are relevant. Those who claim that actual consequences are the relevant kind of consequences probably are contrasting them with intended consequences. These persons are right that consequences of actions that are not intended are often relevant to our moral judgments. This is shown by our making an adverse moral judgment of someone by saying that "he should have known that would happen." What this shows, however, is not that unforeseeable actual consequences are relevant to moral judgments, but that foreseeable consequences are more relevant than intended consequences.

Unforeseeable actual consequences cannot be used by anyone in deciding how to act in any moral situation, nor should they be used by anyone in making a moral judgment on the act that was performed. On the most plausible interpretation, act consequentialism holds that in any situation, a person does what is morally right by choosing that action which, given the foreseeable consequences, will produce at least as favorable a balance of benefits over harms as any other. This is the type of ethical theory that underlies what is sometimes called "situation ethics." Because this theory denies that there are any kinds of acts that need justification, that is, it denies the significance of moral rules, it denies that violations of moral rules need justification. According to act consequentialism, if the foreseeable consequences of the particular paternalistic act provide at least as favorable a balance of benefits over harms as any other act, then the act is morally right. And if the foreseeable consequences are not as favorable, then not only is there no justification for it, the act is morally wrong.

The implicit holding of this false ethical theory is probably responsible for some unjustified paternalistic behavior, especially in those cases in which the foreseen consequences are beneficial. But because the paternalistic cases may be controversial, it is best to start testing the theory with a self-interested violation of a moral rule. One may see clearly that the theory is false when one considers a case of cheating on an exam (that is not graded on a curve) in a course taken on an honor system. If the foreseeable consequences are that no one will be hurt by the particular act of cheating and the cheater will benefit by passing, act consequentialism not only says that cheating is justifiable, but that it is morally wrong not to cheat. Common morality, however, correctly judges cheating in this kind of situation as morally unacceptable, for no impartial rational person would publicly allow such a violation. Act consequentialists, however, are unconcerned with the consequences of this kind of act being publicly allowed, and consider only the foreseeable consequences of the particular act. Thus, they must make up facts about human nature, for example, given human nature, the foreseeable consequences of cheating in this kind of situation will never result in as favorable a balance of benefits over harms as not cheating. But this is playing around with hypothetical facts in order to prevent the theory from conflicting with the moral judgments that everyone would actually make.

Act consequentialism is not an accurate description of the common moral system. Although act consequentialism is sometimes presented as if it were a description of the moral system that is actually used by people in deciding how to act in moral situations or in making moral judgments, it is really an alternative guide to conduct. Although the common moral system recognizes that foreseeable consequences are morally relevant, it does not hold that only consequences are morally relevant, which is unlike act consequentialism. Common morality recognizes the moral significance of the moral rules and does not allow a rule to be broken (e.g., cheating), even when doing so has a more favorable balance of foreseeable consequences. More than the balance of benefits over harms is relevant to determining the justifiability of violating a moral rule. Further, insofar as consequences are the decisive factor in justifying the violation of a moral rule, they are not the consequences of the particular act, but the consequences of everyone knowing that this kind of violation is allowed. Many factors besides the consequences of the particular act determine the kind of violation. (See chapter 2 for a fuller discussion of justifying the violation of a moral rule.)

Strict Deontology—Never Justified

According to the strict deontological view, it is never justified to break a moral rule without the valid consent of the person toward whom you are breaking it.[30] Some hold that even valid consent does not justify violating some moral rules, for example, against disabling, so that it is even immoral to violate these moral rules with regard to oneself. This extreme position usually has a religious foundation, for example, that the moral rules were ordained by God to govern the behavior of human beings. However, this position can also have a metaphysical basis, for example, as in Kant, where reason takes the place of God as the author of the moral rules. Without such a religious or metaphysical foundation, there is no support for the view that it is never justifiable to violate a moral rule with regard to a competent person who has validly consented to allowing someone to violate the rule toward her.

Further, almost everyone who holds a deontological view holds that it is justified to violate a moral rule, sometimes even the rule prohibiting killing, with regard to someone who has himself violated a moral rule. Punishment, even capital punishment, is accepted as justified by most deontological thinkers including Kant and most religious philosophers. It is only with regard to the innocent that these thinkers and philosophers hold that it is never justified to violate a moral rule without consent. It is quite common for strict deontologists to hold that only consent can justify violating a moral rule with regard to an innocent person, and, even on this less radical account, no paternalistic behavior is justified.

Some strict deontologists, like some act consequentialists, claim that they are presenting a description of the common moral system. However, like act consequentialism, strict deontology does not provide an accurate account of common morality. Common morality sometimes justifies deception if necessary to save an innocent person's life. If the only way to prevent very serious harms is by breaking a moral rule, and the violation prevents so much greater harms than it causes that a rational person could publicly allow such a violation, common morality holds that such a violation is at least weakly justified. Common morality does not hold that in order for a violation to be justified, an impartial rational person must will that everyone act in that way; all that is necessary for justification is that a rational person can publicly allow such a violation.

Similarly, common morality may hold that paternalistic behavior is justified (e.g., paternalistic deception) if it is the only way that very serious harm to the patient can be prevented. Paternalistic deprivation of freedom, in the form of involuntary commitment, is even sanctioned by law if there is a high enough probability of the person seriously harming herself. Thus, common morality sometimes sanctions violating a moral rule with regard to an innocent person who has not given consent for such a violation. To support their view, some strict deontologists, like some act consequentialists, have put forward views of human nature that make their views sound more plausible. They have claimed that any violation of a moral rule with regard to an innocent person, without his consent, inevitably results in wholesale violations of moral rules with disastrous consequences. It is interesting that this defense of strict deontology seems to depend upon consequences, but closer inspection shows that it presupposes the view that we have put forward, that is, that the decisive factor in determining the morality of an act is the consequences of everyone knowing that the violation is allowed.

One attempt to maintain the strict deontological position with regard to paternalism has been to claim that it is never justified to violate a moral rule with regard to a *competent or autonomous* innocent person. The addition of the term "competent or autonomous" is supposed to eliminate those cases of paternalism that are generally regarded as justified. Indeed, strict deontology tries to define paternalism so that one cannot act paternalistically toward someone who is not competent to make a rational decision in this kind of situation. Those who want to hold that paternalism is never justified substitute the phrase "S is *competent or autonomous* to make a rational decision" for our fourth feature "A regards S as believing he can make his own decision on this matter." This does eliminate many cases of what we regard as justified paternalism, but not all. It often still is justified for a physician to lie to a patient with a serious heart condition if telling the truth has a high enough probability of killing him.

A more serious problem is that this way of characterizing paternalism may sometimes sanction morally unacceptable behavior toward those who are not competent to make a rational decision. Just because people are not competent to make a rational decision does not mean that it is justified to violate any moral rule with regard to them as long as they benefit from that violation. If the benefit is small, it generally is not justified for one to deceive or deprive of freedom. By making the competence of the patient a necessary feature of paternalism, strict deontologists seem to justify treating large numbers of patients in a way that would be paternalistic if they were regarded as competent. Just as extreme views of the political left and right often seem to justify violence when more moderate views do not, so act consequentialist and strict deontological views seem to justify what would be viewed by common morality as unjustified paternalistic behavior.

The act consequentialist would claim that his act is justified because there is a net benefit to the patient, while the strict deontologist would claim that his behavior is not even paternalistic because the patient is not competent. Someone who simply concentrated on the relevant behavior, however, might not be able to distinguish the strict deontologist from the act consequentialist when dealing with those patients toward whom physicians are most tempted to act paternalistically.

Another serious problem with making it true by definition that no behavior toward any incompetent person is paternalistic is that this definition transforms a genuine moral problem of justifying paternalism into a question of whether or not the action is really paternalistic. This may sound like a merely verbal dispute. However, although this is a dispute about the proper use of a word, it can have significant practical consequences. On our broad definition of paternalism, *any* violation of a moral rule toward a person who believes himself able to make his own decision, that is done for his benefit but without his consent, counts as paternalistic. Anyone who acts in this way must seriously consider whether her act is justified. Defining paternalism in a narrow way so that one can act paternalistically only toward those who are competent to make a rational decision might lead physicians to be unconcerned with justifying their violation of a moral rule with regard to someone they view as incompetent. Because many cases of medical paternalism are with regard to patients whom the physician regards as not competent, this is a serious problem.

The strict deontological proposal shifts the emphasis from the genuine moral problem of justifying violating a moral rule for a patient's benefit without his consent, to the problem of determining if the person is competent. If the patient is not competent, the interference is not paternalistic and need not be justified. On our account, even if the patient is incompetent, if he believes he can make his own decision, one still may not be justified to intervene. The harm prevented by interfering may not be great enough to justify the violation of a moral rule with regard to the patient. On the strict deontological proposal there is an absolute dichotomy between the ways the two classes of patients may be treated. No matter how great the harm prevented and how minor the violation of the moral rule, competent patients can never be interfered with for their own benefit without their consent. With regard to incompetent patients, interference does not even need to be justified. There is not such a sharp line separating competence from incompetence and, even if there were, it has not yet been reliably enough determined to allow it to play such an important role in determining whether to break a moral rule toward someone without that person's consent.

Both the strict deontologist, who holds that genuine paternalism (paternalism toward the competent) is never justified, and the act consequentialist, who holds that genuine paternalism (paternalism that has a net benefit for the patient) is always justified, have a serious problem. Neither presents us with an acceptable way of distinguishing between the particular patients who should be deceived or deprived of freedom when the foreseeable consequences are such that they would benefit from this violation of moral rules with regard to them, and those who should not. Both of these views present overly simple accounts of how physicians do and should go about determining whether or not it is justified to act paternalistically. Of course it is just these views' simplicity that makes them so attractive, for if physicians accept either of these views, they have a simple way of dealing with troublesome cases. However, those physicians who are serious about the matter have to be prepared to look at all of the morally relevant features of each case and only then decide whether or not paternalistic behavior is justified.

Common Morality—Sometimes Justified

Many writers maintain, as we do, that some paternalistic behavior is justified and some is not. However, we know of no others who use an explicit account of morality to determine when paternalism is justified. Showing how well common morality applies to cases of medical paternalism provides strong reasons for thinking that there is no special ethics for medicine. This is very important, for holding that common morality does not apply in medical situations may lead some physicians to think that they are not subject to the same moral constraints that all other people are. This may be one explanation for the many instances of unjustified paternalism in medicine.

Most philosophical discussions of the justification of paternalism oversimplify. The act consequentialist considers morally relevant only the consequences of the particular act, and the strict deontologist considers morally relevant only whether a moral rule is being broken with regard to an innocent person who has not given consent for the violation. All of these features are morally relevant, but there are also many other morally relevant features. Failure to take into account all of these features, in addition to others that may not yet have been made explicit, often leads to a failure to distinguish between cases that might differ in only one crucial respect, for example, whether that situation is an emergency. Casuistry is helpful in distinguishing between these cases, although it does not even try to provide a list of those features of a situation that are morally relevant.

For ease of reference, we repeat here the ten questions whose answers make up the morally relevant features. These were listed and discussed in chapter 2.

(1) What moral rules would be violated?

(2) What harms would be (a) avoided (not caused), (b) prevented, and (c) caused? (This means foreseeable harms and includes probabilities as well as kind and extent.)

(3) What are the relevant beliefs and desires of the people toward whom the rule is being violated? (This explains why physicians must provide adequate information about treatment and obtain their patients' consent before treating.)

(4) Does one have a relationship with the person(s) toward whom the rule is being violated such that one sometimes has a duty to violate moral rules with regard to the person(s) without his consent? (This explains why a parent or guardian may be morally allowed to make a decision about treatment that the health care team is not morally allowed to make.)

(5) What benefits would be caused? (This means foreseeable benefits and also includes probabilities, as well as kind and extent.)

(6) Is an unjustified or weakly justified violation of a moral rule being prevented? (This is usually not relevant in medical contexts, and applies more to police work and national security.)

(7) Is an unjustified or weakly justified violation of a moral rule being punished? (This is not relevant in medical contexts, and applies more to the legal system.)

(8) Are there any alternative actions that would be preferable?

(9) Is the violation being done intentionally or only knowingly?

(10) Is it an emergency situation in which a person most likely did not plan to be?

In cases of medical paternalism, some of the questions on this list have obvious answers, for example, the answer to question 7 is always no. In medical paternalism, the moral rule violation is being done to benefit the person, not to punish him. In some cases of involuntary commitment, however, there may be non-paternalistic reasons as well as paternalistic ones for justifying commitment, for example, to prevent the patient from harming another person, so that the answer to question 6 might occasionally be yes. In this kind of case, an act that may not be justified on paternalistic grounds may, nonetheless, be justified. The answer to question 9 is almost always that the violation is being done intentionally. The answer to question 10 also is usually no, for paternalism normally occurs in a situation where the physician or other health care worker has time to ask consent. Actions done in emergency situations are usually not considered paternalistic for, as discussed earlier in the chapter, when one cannot ask for consent prior to acting, immediately forthcoming consent usually prevents the act from being counted as paternalistic.

The answer given to question 4, about the duties of physicians, distinguishes our view from many others. We claim that physicians do not have a duty to violate moral rules with regard to their patients without their consent unless they are in an emergency situation, that is, the patient will suffer very serious harms if action is not taken immediately. Act consequentialism claims that all persons, including physicians, have a duty to do that act which has the most favorable balance of benefits and harms. Strict deontology defends paternalistic actions toward incompetent patients by claiming that physicians have a duty to act so as to benefit their incompetent patients, even if that involves violating moral rules with regard to them. We do not accept these claims. Except in emergency situations, a physician has no duty to achieve the best consequences for her competent patients, especially when this involves violating moral rules with regard to them without their consent. Physicians do have a duty to consult with the guardians of incompetent patients or, if an incompetent patient has no guardian, to apply to the court to obtain a guardian for the patient. Physicians also must not act against the best interests of incompetent patients.

All of the other questions—1, 2, 3, 5, and 8—are ones that need to be answered in each particular case in order to determine whether or not that paternalistic action is justified. These questions help one know what facts one should seek to discover. Everyone says, quite correctly, that finding all the relevant facts is crucial in making any moral decision. However, often no guidance is given in determining which facts are relevant. This lack can sometimes be serious, as shown by the following example. A physician wanted to perform blood tests on a fifty-year-old woman who refused to have them performed. The physician regarded these tests as necessary in order to have any chance of discovering the woman's problem and treating it appropriately. He consulted the hospital's ethics committee to ask for advice about whether it was morally acceptable to perform these tests without the woman's consent. He described the woman as sometimes delirious, so that there was some serious question about her competence. Accepting his claim that the tests were not dangerous in any way and only slightly unpleasant, the ethics committee concluded that it was morally acceptable for the physician to proceed with the tests without the woman's consent.

It was later discovered that the physician had neglected to tell the ethics committee that the woman was a devout Christian Scientist who had refused the tests because of her religious beliefs. Further, although she was sometimes delirious, her refusal was consistent and did not change when she was not delirious. She had no immediate family, but other members of her family made it clear that she had never accepted any medical treatments, even in serious situations. Thus, there was no doubt that her refusal was not due to her delirium, and that even if she were fully competent, she would have refused the tests. If the physician had been aware that it was morally required for him to consider the answers to question 3, about the patient's relevant beliefs and desires, both his presentation to the ethics committee and its advice to him would have been different.

Perhaps the most overlooked question, but one that is often the most important, is question 8, concerning alternatives. If there is a nonpaternalistic alternative that does not involve any unconsented to violation of a moral rule and does not differ significantly in the harms and benefits to the patient, then paternalistic behavior cannot be justified. This is a very significant matter, for often there is an alternative to paternalistic behavior, namely, long conversations with the patient trying to explain the benefits of accepting a treatment. Often it is one's lack of time to spend with the patient, rather than lack of alternatives, that leads to paternalistic behavior.

If lack of time does tempt some physicians into acting paternalistically, then someone else who has the time can be assigned to do what the physician does not have time to do. Giving physician assistants or nurses more of a role in talking to patients about proposed treatments, even in obtaining valid consent for treatment, is a plausible option when the physician does not have the time.

Act consequentialists claim that the answers to questions 2, 5, and 8—about harms, benefits and alternatives—are the only morally relevant features that need to be considered in determining what morally ought to be done. This claim is incorrect. Not only are there other morally relevant features that are necessary to determine the kind of violation, but determining the kind of violation is only the first step. The next step requires considering whether or not one would publicly allow that kind of violation (a violation of that rule in those kinds of circumstances). Failure to move to the next step puts one back into a kind of act consequentialism, considering only the consequences of the particular act. The function of the morally relevant features, including the foreseeable consequences, is to determine the kind of violation that, although absolutely crucial, is only the first step of a two-step procedure.

The second step of the two-step procedure is answering the morally decisive question, Would the foreseeable consequences of that kind of violation being publicly allowed, that is, of everyone knowing that they are allowed to violate the moral rule in these circumstances, be better or worse than the foreseeable consequences of that kind of violation not being publicly allowed? Consequences are crucial, but it is not the consequences of the particular act, rather, it is the consequences of that kind of act being publicly allowed that are decisive. This account of common moral reasoning incorporates the insights of both Kant and John Stuart Mill. Common morality, which has been oversimplified by previous philosophers, recognizes not only the diverse nature of the morally relevant features but also that moral reasoning involves a two-step procedure: (1) using the morally relevant features to determine the kind of violation, and (2) estimating the foreseeable consequences of that kind of violation being publicly allowed.

Disagreement about moral decisions and judgments can occur in either step. People can disagree about the kind of act, or they can disagree about whether or not they favor that kind of act being publicly allowed. Of course, one cannot even begin to decide whether one favors a kind of act being publicly allowed until the kind of act has been determined. This explains why discovering all the relevant facts is so important. It also explains why it is important for all of the morally relevant features to be recognized, for they tell one what facts to look for. Only after one determines the kind of violation, by finding all the facts indicated by the morally relevant features, can one ask the morally decisive question, Does the harm avoided or prevented by this kind of violation being publicly allowed outweigh the harm that would be caused by it being publicly allowed? If all rational persons would agree that the harm prevented by the violation being publicly allowed would be greater than the harm caused by it being publicly allowed, the violation is strongly justified; if none would agree, the violation is unjustified. If there is disagreement, we call it a weakly justified violation, and whether it should be allowed is a matter to be decided by an appropriate person or group.[31]

Our goal is not to provide a solution to every case, but rather to provide a framework that enables fruitful moral discussion of paternalistic behavior. With regard to controversial cases, this framework usually does not provide a unique answer but rather provides a range of morally acceptable answers. Further, using this explicit account of moral reasoning makes it less likely for mistakes to be made, for example, failing to consider a patient's religious beliefs. Perhaps, most important, it enables people to disagree without any party to the dispute concluding that the other party must be ill informed, partial, of perverse character, or acting irrationally or immorally. Providing limits to legitimate moral disagreement and at the same time allowing people to acknowledge that, within these limits, moral disagreements are legitimate and to be expected, provides the kind of atmosphere that is most conducive to fruitful moral discussion.

Justifying Paternalistic Behavior—Cases

In most if not all cases, in order to justify paternalistic behavior it is necessary but not sufficient that the harm prevented for S by the moral rule violation be so much greater than the harm, if any, caused to S by the violation, that it would be irrational for S not to choose having the rule violated with regard to himself.[32] When this is not the case, then the behavior cannot be justified on paternalistic grounds. If it is not irrational (or unreasonable) for S to choose suffering the harm rather than having the moral rule violated with regard to himself, then no rational person can publicly allow the violation of the rule in the same circumstances, for that is the same as publicly allowing someone to force her own rational ranking of harms on someone else who has a different rational ranking. No rational person wants this kind of violation to be publicly allowed.

We now consider situations in which there are different combinations of morally relevant features. The most interesting set of cases is where the violation of different moral rules is involved (so that there are different answers to question 1), but the amount of harm caused, avoided (not caused), and prevented, and the benefits caused (the answers to questions 2 and 5) are very similar. This set of cases provides a test of whether our two-step procedure of justification provides a more adequate account of moral reasoning than does act utilitarianism in those difficult cases where the two accounts give different answers. We begin by applying this moral framework, that is, the morally relevant features and the two-step justification procedure, to two cases of paternalistic behavior, one justified and one not.[33]

> *Case 1.* Mr. K was brought to the emergency room by his wife and a police officer. Mrs. K had confessed to her husband earlier that evening that she was having an affair with one of his colleagues. He became acutely agitated and depressed and, after several hours of mounting tension, told her he was going to kill himself so "you'll have the freedom to have all the lovers you want." She became frightened and called the police because there were loaded guns in the house and she knew her husband was an impulsive man.
>
> In the emergency room, Mr. K would do little more than glower at Dr. T, his wife, and the officer. He seemed extremely tense and agitated. Dr. T decided that for Mr. K's own protection he should be hospitalized, but Mr. K refused. Dr. T therefore committed Mr. K to the hospital for a seventy-two-hour emergency detention.

Using the above moral framework, Dr. T could attempt to justify his paternalistic commitment of Mr. K by claiming that by depriving Mr. K of his freedom for a very limited time, there was a great likelihood that he was preventing the occurrence of a much greater harm: Mr. K's death or serious injury. Dr. T need not claim that self-inflicted death is a harm of such magnitude that paternalistic intervention to prevent it is always justified. Rather, he could claim that it is justified in Mr. K's case on several counts. First, Mr. K's desire to kill himself seems irrational, for he appears to have no reason at all, let alone an adequate reason, for killing himself. An adequate reason would be a belief on his part that his death would result in the avoiding of great harm(s) or the attaining of great goods for himself or others. His statement to his wife, "You'll have the freedom to have all the lovers you want," is not intended as an altruistic reason, but is merely a sarcastic expression that, even if taken literally, would not be an adequate reason for his suicide.

Second, there is evidence that Mr. K suffers from a condition that is well known to be transient. Dr. T can support this conclusion by noting that in his professional experience that the majority of persons in Mr. K's condition who were hospitalized subsequently recovered from their state of agitated depression within seventy-two hours and then acknowledged the irrational character of their former suicidal desires.

Third, the deprivation of freedom that Dr. T has imposed on Mr. K is a much lesser harm than the harm (death) that Mr. K may perpetrate on himself, even taking into account that the former is certain and the latter is only somewhat probable. Of course, Dr. T must have a justified belief that the probability of suicide is high enough (e.g., more than 10%) that it would be irrational to choose the risk of death over the loss of three days of freedom, and the psychological suffering involved.

It is, however, not sufficient justification for Dr. T merely to show that the harms prevented for Mr. K by his paternalistic action outweigh the harms caused to Mr. K; he must also be willing to publicly allow the deprivation of freedom of anyone in these circumstances, that is, he must be willing for everyone to know that in these circumstances any person may be deprived of his freedom for a limited period of time. In this case, because Dr. T actually supports the law allowing exactly this kind of action, it is clear that he does advocate publicly allowing it. If the case is filled out such that all of Dr. T's beliefs are well supported, Dr. T's action could be regarded as strongly justified. However, if there is some disagreement about the facts, and the probability of Mr. K harming himself is taken to be lower (e.g., less than 5%), then Dr. T's behavior might be regarded as only weakly justified or not justified at all.[34]

> *Case 2.* Mrs. R, a twenty-nine-year-old mother, is hospitalized with symptoms of abdominal pain, weight loss, weakness, and swelling of the ankles. An extensive medical workup is inconclusive, and exploratory abdominal surgery is carried out, which reveals a primary ovarian cancer with extensive spread to other abdominal organs. Her condition is judged to be too far advanced for surgical relief, and her life expectancy is estimated to be, at most, a few months. Despite her oft-repeated request to be told "exactly where I stand and what I face," Dr. E tells both the patient and her husband that the diagnosis is still unclear but that he will see her weekly as an outpatient. At the time of discharge she is feeling somewhat better than at admission, and Dr. E hopes that the family will have a few happy days or weeks together before her condition worsens and they must be told the truth.

Dr. E could attempt to justify his paternalistic deception by claiming that the harm, namely, the psychological suffering, he hoped to prevent by his deception is significantly greater than the harm, if any, he caused by lying. While this might be true in the short run in this particular case, it is by no means certain. By his deception, Dr. E is depriving Mrs. R and her family of the opportunity to make those plans that would enable her and her family to deal more adequately with her death. In the circumstances of this case as described, Mrs. R's desire to know the truth is a rational one; in fact, there is no evidence of any irrational behavior or desires on her part. This contrasts sharply with Mr. K's desire to kill himself, which is clearly irrational.

In this case, Dr. E is violating the rule against deception in circumstances in which there is a high probability that he is preventing psychological suffering for several days or weeks, and at least an equally high probability that he is depriving the patient and her family of the opportunity to make the most appropriate plans for her future. The person affected by the deception has a rational desire to know the truth about her condition. Given this description of the kind of violation, would a rational person publicly allow it, that is, be willing for everyone to know that they are allowed to deceive in the circumstances described? The following discussion shows that no rational person would publicly allow such a violation.

Suppose someone ranks one harm (e.g., unpleasant feelings for several weeks) as greater than another (e.g., the loss of some opportunity to plan for the future), but another person ranks them differently.[35] If both rankings are rational, should the first person be allowed to deceive the second, if his deception results in the second person suffering what the deceiver regards as the lesser harm? Would any rational person hold that such deception be publicly allowed, that is, be willing for everyone to know that they are allowed to deceive in these circumstances? Because publicly allowing this amounts to allowing deception in order to impose one's own ranking of harms on others who have an alternative rational ranking, no rational person would publicly allow such a violation. Not only would publicly allowing deception in such circumstances allow persons to impose their own ranking on others, it would clearly have the most disastrous consequences on one's trust in the words of others. Thus, this kind of violation being publicly allowed would have far worse consequences than it not being publicly allowed. This analysis shows that Dr. E's deception, though clearly done with benevolent motives, is an unjustified paternalistic act.

> *Case 3a.* Mrs. V is in extremely critical condition after an automobile accident that has taken the life of one of her four children and severely injured another. Mrs. V is about to go into surgery and Dr. H believes that her very tenuous hold on life might be weakened by the shock of hearing about her children's conditions, so he decides not to give her that information until she has had the operation and recovered sufficiently.
>
> *Case 3b.* Mrs. V is in extremely critical condition after an automobile accident that has taken the life of one of her four children and severely injured another. Mrs. V is about to go into surgery and asks Dr. H how her children are. He believes that her very tenuous hold on life might be weakened by the shock of hearing of her children's conditions, so he decides to deceive her by simply telling her that they are concerned about her. He plans to tell her the truth about her children after she has had the operation and recovered sufficiently.

In case 3a, Dr. H. is not deceiving by withholding information, so he is not acting paternalistically. A physician's withholding information is deceiving when he has a duty to provide that information, as in case 2. A physician has a duty to provide the diagnosis and prognosis to a patient unless he can justify not doing so. A physician has no duty to provide nonmedical information that is irrelevant to the treatment that he is providing, so that not telling the mother about her children is not even withholding information, it is simply not providing it. Dr. H. may be demonstrating a paternalistic attitude by not telling her that information, that is, he may be demonstrating that he would act paternalistically if deception were required to keep the information from Mrs. V. This is the situation in case 3b, where Dr. H's answer to Mrs. V.'s question is deceptive, even if it is not clearly a lie.

Dr. H. is acting paternalistically in case 3b. This is, however, an example of justified paternalism. This assessment depends upon one accepting that telling Mrs. V. that one of her children died would increase significantly her own chances of dying, for example, by more than 1%. It also depends upon Mrs. V. not being in a situation where she is being deprived of any significant opportunity to make appropriate plans or decisions. She is going to be operated on immediately and so is not able to make any plans, even if plans need to be made.

Anyone acting rationally who had to choose between a loved one (1) being deceived for a short period of time, when this would have (almost) no effect on her planning for the future, and (2) being fully informed but thereby significantly increasing her chance of dying would choose the former. If, in this situation, Mrs. V said that she wanted to know now, it would be assumed that she did not realize that knowing the truth now would increase her chances of dying during the operation. (We are assuming that she wants to live and there are no other morally relevant features, such as religious beliefs, that would make knowing now especially significant.) In these circumstances, deception significantly decreases the chance of death and causes no significant harm. Would a rational person publicly allow this kind of violation? What would be the effect of publicly allowing this kind of violation? There might be some loss of trust, but whatever loss might occur would seem to be more than balanced by the number of lives that would be saved. Thus, we hold that deceiving in this case is at least weakly justified, and may even be strongly justified.

Those cases of paternalistic actions in which the two-step procedure and act consequentialism yield the same answer are those in which there is usually no question about how one should act. Many of the problem cases are those in which considering other morally relevant features in addition to the consequences and applying the two-step justification procedure yields a different answer than act consequentialism yields. These later kinds of cases make the inadequacy of act consequentialism apparent. Part of the standard philosophical literature against act consequentialism consists of examples in which it is inadequate to consider only the foreseeable consequences of a particular act. Consider a particular example of a situation discussed earlier. A medical student who has always been in the middle of his class, but who, for fairly trivial reasons, has not studied during the weeks preceding the state medical examinations, is now taking those exams. He has good reason to believe himself to be adequately qualified for the practice of medicine. He therefore cheats in order to increase his chance of qualifying for the practice of medicine now and thereby preventing the unpleasant feelings to himself and his parents that would accompany failure. His cheating has not caused harm to anyone (the exam is not graded on a curve) and on a simple, negative, act consequentialist view he would therefore be morally justified—perhaps even morally required—to cheat.

Now consider the consequences of everyone knowing that they are allowed to cheat for the purpose of decreasing unpleasant feelings if they have good reason to believe that no one will be hurt by their particular act. Included in their belief that no one will be hurt is their belief that they either have or do not need the qualifications that the test is designed to measure. People have limited knowledge and are fallible. If everyone knows that cheating is allowed in these circumstances, it is very likely that some individuals, who believe themselves qualified when they are not, will cheat and thereby pass. Further, if everyone knows that everyone is allowed to cheat in these circumstances, this destroys the value of these tests on which people rely to determine who is qualified, for example, for medical practice. If, contrary to fact, the tests were not changed to prevent cheating, the consequences of everyone knowing that they are allowed to cheat might result in some people having positions, for example, as doctors, for which they are not qualified. This might result in an increased risk of the population's suffering greater harms, such as pain and disability. In counting the anxiety caused to everyone—especially patients, who know that cheating is allowed—it seems clear that this anxiety outweighs the occasional suffering caused to those who cannot qualify without cheating.[36] Using the two-step procedure yields the judgment that is intuitively obvious: cheating in these circumstances is morally unjustified. Act consequentialism tries to avoid the conclusion that cheating in these circumstances is justified, if not morally required, by invoking very implausible features of human nature, for example, anyone who cheats once will continue cheating forever and so will cause great harm eventually.

Further Examples of the Justification Procedure

All of the above cases involve the balancing of great harms, such as dying, deception about terminal illness, and the infliction of severe pain. The paternalistic interventions described have been obvious and often dramatic: commitment to a mental hospital or lying to a mother about the death of her child. The health care professionals making the decisions were all physicians, and in most of the cases (though we have not mentioned this feature) the possibility of legal intervention was present, in the form of suits for negligence or battery, or injunctions to stop treatment. However, the vast majority of paternalistic interventions in medicine take place on a smaller scale. The following case not only illustrates a much more common type of paternalism, it also provides an excellent example of the value of using all of the morally relevant features and the two-step procedure that are essential to moral reasoning.

Paternalistic acts committed by physicians may involve the violation of many different moral rules, but the three most common violations seem to be depriving of freedom, deceiving, and causing pain or suffering. Each of these three kinds of violations can be either justified or unjustified paternalistic acts. The examples of depriving of freedom in case 1 (Mr. K), and of deception in case 3b (Mrs. V), are justified, and the example of deception in case 2 (Mrs. R) is not. In order to show how what may seem like minor changes in the facts can affect the final moral judgment reached, we present the following case of medical paternalism. Agreement on the facts is crucial.

Case 4. Mr. J is a fifty-year-old patient in a rehabilitation ward who is recovering from the effects of a stroke. A major part of his treatment consists of daily visits to the physical therapy unit, where he is given repetitive exercises to increase the strength and mobility of his partially paralyzed left arm and leg. He was initially cooperative with Ms. Y, his physical therapist, but soon became bored with the monotony of the daily sessions and frustrated by his very slow progress in regaining his ability to move his partially paralyzed limbs adequately. He told Ms. Y that he did not wish to attend the remaining three weeks of daily sessions. Ms. Y knew that patients like Mr. J rarely regress, that is, become worse than they presently are, if they stop exercising. But her experience showed that if patients like Mr. J stopped the sessions early, they did not receive the full therapeutic benefit possible and might suffer for the remainder of their lives from a significantly more disabled arm and leg than would be the case if they exercised now in this critical, early poststroke period. Accordingly, she first tried to persuade him to continue exercising. When that was not effective, she became rather stern and scolded and chastised him for two days. He then relented and began exercising again, but it was necessary for Ms. Y to chastise him sternly almost daily to obtain his continued participation over the ensuing three weeks.

Ms. Y's scolding and chastising was paternalistic behavior on our account: she caused Mr. J some psychological pain and discomfort without his consent for what she believed to be his benefit, and she knew that Mr. J believed himself competent to make his own decision about physical therapy.

Had Ms. Y attempted to justify her action by claiming that the relatively minor amount of harm she inflicted by chastising Mr. J to exercise was so much less than the relatively greater harm Mr. J would suffer by being significantly more disabled than necessary for the rest of his life, it would have been irrational for one to rank these harms in the opposite way. We agree that the kind of violation engaged in by Ms. Y was inflicting a mild degree of suffering on Mr. J (through her chastising and his resumed exercising) by imposing her rational ranking of harms on Mr. J, whose ranking was not rational. A rational person could publicly allow this kind of violation, and we conclude that Ms. Y's paternalistic behavior was at least weakly justified.

This case involves the balancing of harms that, while significant, are not of the intensity of our earlier cases. Refusing three weeks of exercising versus greater lifelong disability seems irrational, although it is quite likely that Mr. J did not believe the facts or, at least, did not appreciate that they applied to him. The amount of harm associated with the possibility of Mr. J's needlessly greater lifelong disability seems significant enough to at least weakly justify causing him a mild to moderate degree of transient suffering without his consent. However, there are some kinds of violations that would not have been justified in Mr. J's case. It would have been unjustified to inflict intense physical pain on him to force him to exercise. The amount of harm associated with the possibility of his increased disability was not great enough that a rational person could publicly allow that kind of violation.

Philosophically, the most interesting alternative to consider is Ms. Y's deceiving Mr. J. Suppose Ms. Y told him that if he continued to exercise, he might not only improve but, more important, she could guarantee that he would not regress to the point that he might be unable to walk at all. She would thus be strongly suggesting that unless he continued to exercise for three more weeks he might regress and end up not being able to walk at all. Thus, Ms. Y did not quite lie, but she clearly intended to deceive Mr. J. Suppose that deceiving in this way has the same probability of getting Mr. J to resume exercising as daily chastising. In addition, such deception causes Mr. J less total suffering than daily chastising, for he now is not bothered by his slow progress, but, on the contrary, is pleased by what he perceives as his successfully preventing any regression, especially a complete inability to walk. Two questions now seem to arise: (1) Is this paternalistic deception justified? and (2) Is this kind of deception morally preferable to daily chastising?

Using a simple negative act consequentialist method of calculation, it might seem that if chastisement were justifiable paternalism, this kind of deception would be even more strongly justifiable. This is not a case of deceiving in order to impose one person's rational ranking of the harms on another person's different rational ranking, but rather deceiving in order to substitute a rational ranking for an irrational one. It is deception that results in a temporary (three weeks), mild, physical discomfort (of physical therapy) in order to prevent the possibility of a permanent (twenty or thirty years), moderate amount of disability. Mr. J does not want to be deceived and Ms. Y does not have a duty to deceive him, but, nonetheless, she does intentionally do so. The situation is not an emergency situation, although that might be disputed by some, for some action must be taken now to prevent the increased level of disability.

Would a rational person publicly allow deceiving in these circumstances? Allowing deceiving in a situation where trust is extremely important, for example, in medical situations, in order to prevent a harm significant enough that it is irrational not to avoid it (the high probability of permanent, moderate disability) is an issue on which rational persons can disagree. The erosion of trust that would follow from everyone knowing that deceiving is allowed in these circumstances might have such harmful consequences (e.g., legitimate warnings might come to be disregarded) that it is not clear that even preventing a significant number of persons from suffering permanent moderate disability is enough to counterbalance these consequences. If deceiving were the only method whereby Ms. Y could get Mr. J to continue his treatment, and deceiving has a high probability of being successful in doing so, rational persons might disagree; some might publicly allow this kind of violation, some might not. However, if there is an alternative to deceiving, namely, the method of chastising and scolding, then deceiving would not be justified.

We believe that when presented with these alternative methods of getting Mr. J to continue treatment, rational people would, after careful consideration, regard chastising and scolding as morally preferable to deceiving, and some would regard intentional deception as completely morally unacceptable. Simple negative utilitarianism cannot account for this result because, in this particular case, deceiving results in no more and probably less overall suffering than chastising and scolding. The method of justification that we have been presenting, however, accounts for these moral intuitions quite easily. The two alternatives differ *only* in two morally relevant features: (1) the moral rules violated—causing pain (the unpleasantness caused by the scolding) versus deception—and (2) the harms caused, for it seems that more unpleasantness is caused to Mr. J. by the scolding than by deceiving. We have assumed that the harm prevented, including probabilities, is the same: permanent, moderate disability in both cases; and that Mr. J. has the same relevant beliefs and desires in both cases. Because it is clear that the two alternatives do not differ in any other morally relevant feature, it is primarily the difference in which moral rule is violated that determines the kind of violation. Taking the second step and determining the consequences of publicly allowing these two kinds of violations makes clear that the consequences of publicly allowing deceiving has worse consequences than publicly allowing scolding and chastising. Consider which hospital you would choose to go to if you knew that one allowed paternalistic deception and the other allowed paternalistic harassment. This result accounts for the moral intuitions that thoughtful people have about this case.

The key morally relevant feature is the presence of the alternative of scolding and chastising, which, by hypothesis, has the same probability of getting Mr. J to continue his exercising as deceiving him does. Without this alternative, deceiving prevents a harm significant enough that it is irrational not to avoid it (the high probability of permanent, moderate disability). With the alternative of chastising and scolding, deceiving only prevents three weeks of mental discomfort caused by chastising and scolding. When one considers the harmful consequences of everyone knowing that they are allowed to deceive in order to prevent the amount of harm caused by three weeks of chastising and scolding, it becomes clear that no rational person would publicly allow such deception. The amount of harm, that is, the suffering due to the scolding and chastising, that might be prevented by everyone knowing that deception is allowed seems far less than the amount of harm that would be caused by the loss of trust.[37]

Lying Versus Other Forms of Deception

Suppose that instead of deceiving Mr. J in the way described, namely, guaranteeing Mr. J that if he continued exercising he would not fall below his present level of ability to function, and in particular would never become completely unable to walk, Ms. Y simply lied to him and said that unless he continues to exercise for three more weeks he would regress and might end up unable to walk at all. She knew that this was not true because stroke victims are at their worst right after the stroke and never get worse later, even if they do not exercise at all. In both cases, the deception and the lying, she knew that Mr. J would think that it was the exercise that guaranteed that he would get no worse, and so would believe that if he did not exercise he might get considerably worse. Would violation of the rule against deception by lying be publicly allowed? Is lying worse than the previously described intentional deception?

It is commonly believed that lying is a more serious form of deception than withholding or misleading in other ways. Insofar as intentionally breaking a moral rule is worse than doing so only knowingly (morally relevant feature 9), intentionally deceiving is worse than only knowingly deceiving. Because lying is necessarily intentionally deceiving, whereas withholding information and misleadingly communicating may sometimes involve only knowingly deceiving, lying does seem worse than other forms of deception. However, if it is clear that the deception is intentional, it does not seem to make much difference if it is done by lying or in some other way. The loss of trust that would arise from everyone knowing that deception is allowed in these circumstances would have the same, or nearly the same, harmful consequences as publicly allowing lying. Theoretically, the consequences may seem not quite so bad because patients presumably could ask questions that would prevent them from being deceived if they knew they would not be lied to, but we think the difference in loss of trust would be negligible at best.

The above case is typical of a multitude of everyday situations in medicine in which doctors, nurses, and other health care workers act or are tempted to act paternalistically toward patients. For example, consider the problems presented by the patient with emphysema who continues to smoke, by the alcoholic with liver damage who refuses to enter any treatment program, or by the diabetic or hypertensive patient who exacerbates his disease by paying little heed to dietary precautions. Each of these patients is apt to stimulate paternalistic acts by a variety of health care professionals (as well as members of his own family). Before acting, it is crucial for health care workers to determine all of the morally relevant features of the situation, including the feasibility of alternatives. A clear and full account of the kind of situation involved is essential for deciding which paternalistic acts are justifiable and which are not.

Another Theory of Justification

One approach to justification that some physicians and philosophers have cited and used deserves brief discussion: the "thank-you" test. According to this test, one may justifiably act paternalistically if one is certain that at some later time one will be thanked by the person (patient) toward whom one is acting. Alan Stone's "thank you theory of civil commitment" is a variation of this approach.[38] John Rawls has similarly written: "We must be able to argue that with the development or the recovery of his rational powers the individual in question will accept our decision on his behalf and agree with us that we did the best thing for him."[39] James F. Childress has labeled these approaches "ratification theories," though it is not clear whether he wholly agrees with them.[40]

The simplicity of these theories makes them seem attractive. However, while the recipients of justified paternalistic acts are often subsequently grateful, thank-you theories are inadequate accounts of the justification procedure. That obtaining future thanks or ratification is neither necessary nor sufficient to justify paternalistic acts can be seen by imagining a case in which one is certain a patient will be thankful (and thus the act will be justifiable according to this test), and then imagine that the patient, a rather grudging person, is not thankful. No one would say that the action had turned out to be unjustified after all. It is never actual consequences, only foreseeable ones, that determine the morality of an act. Moreover, foreseeable future thanks do not provide sufficient justification either. It may be true that some physicians know that some patients are so obeisant toward them that the patients forgive the physicians and even thank them for a variety of what appear to be unconsented-to violations of the moral rules with regard to them. Patient obeisance is not sufficient justification for particular paternalistic acts. What the justification depends on is not the patient's actual or foreseeable thanks but knowing, rather, whether one could publicly allow the violation based solely on the factors known at the time one decided to act paternalistically.[41]

If a physician has paternalistically deceived her patient and it would be counterproductive to reveal the deception, the patient may never know that his physician has acted paternalistically toward him. The thank-you theory seems inapplicable in such a case. It is tempting to say that the patient would thank the physician if it were possible to let the patient know what had actually happened. This shows that whether one will later be thanked is not important. It seems important because it is related to the morally relevant features of a given case at the time that one decides to act paternalistically. These features, which determine the kind of violation, and the consequences of publicly allowing that kind of violation, are what count. Thank-you theories have an illusory simplicity, but they do not allow one to avoid the task of isolating the actual criteria for justified paternalism. The plausibility of these theories comes from the fact that doctors usually judge whether a patient will say "thank you," at least implicitly, by using the criteria we have developed in our account of the justification of paternalism. It is a mistake to think there is some special theory of moral justification for paternalistic interventions in medicine.

Notes

1. Throughout our analysis we assume that A's beliefs are at least rational, though they need not be true. If A's beliefs are irrational, for example, if he thinks flowers are competent

to give consent, it is implausible to maintain that he is acting paternalistically toward the flowers when he waters them though he believes that they would prefer to remain dry. We are indebted to Timothy Duggan for calling our attention to this latter point.

2. Those who do not make a distinction between moral ideals and moral rules may hold that refusing to give money to a beggar does need justification. In chapter 2 we show why this is a mistake.

3. Gerald Dworkin (1972) seems to make this mistake in an important article entitled "Paternalism": "By paternalism I shall understand roughly the interference with a person's liberty of action justified by reasons referring exclusively to the welfare, good, happiness, needs, interests, or values of the person being coerced" (20). Dworkin's view that paternalism always involves the restriction of liberty used to be the standard one. See, for example, Bayles (1974) and Regan (1974). However, partly in response to criticisms that we made, Dworkin had second thoughts, and in an article entitled "Paternalism: Some Second Thoughts" (1983, 105–111) he admits that a broader definition is needed. Indeed, he now holds that "the attempt to broaden the notion [of paternalistic behavior] by including any violation of a moral rule is too restrictive" (106). He now thinks, "There must be a violation of the person's autonomy (which I conceive as distinct from that of liberty), for one to treat another paternalistically. There must be usurpation of decision-making, either by preventing people from doing what they have decided or by interfering with the way in which they arrive at their decisions" (107). However, Dworkin seems to agree that something like our feature 2, in which A recognizes that his action toward S is a kind of action that needs moral justification, is a feature of paternalism. Thus our only disagreement with Dworkin seems to be on what kinds of actions need moral justification. However, this will result in our classifying some cases in different ways than Dworkin. See the discussion later in this chapter.

4. See chapter 2.

5. Paternalistic acts can also be described as violations of rights. Those who prefer the language of rights to that of moral rules might plausibly hold that all paternalistic behavior involves the violation of a person's rights. Confusion between rights and liberties may then partly explain the widely held but mistaken view that paternalism always involves the restriction of liberty of action. For example, paternalistic behavior involving deception may sometimes be taken as violating the person's right to know when it cannot be taken as restricting his liberty of action. But violating a person's rights is always the same as violating a moral rule with regard to that person who has not given his consent. Since we find the terminology of moral rules to be clearer than that of rights, we have presented our analysis of paternalism solely in terms of violating a moral rule. See Gert (2005, 174–177).

6. See Dworkin (1983, 106).

7. This is another example of why "autonomy" is a term that is best avoided. One author of *Principles of Biomedical Ethics* (Beauchamp and Childress [2001]) also prefers the conception that "all paternalistic actions restrict autonomous choice," but the authors recognize that this is not "the current mainstream of the literature on paternalism" (178).

8. Dworkin (1983, 107).

9. See Brock (1983, 238).

10. See Beauchamp and Childress (2001, 178).

11. Ibid.

12. See Childress (1982, 241).

13. See Dworkin (1983, 106). This example is a very slightly revised version of a case that we provide in Culver and Gert (1982, 128). However, the slight revision is quite

significant, for in that case, the husband removes all of the sleeping pills, and it is not clear whether he is removing only his own pills, or also those of his wife. See note 5 above for further discussion of the implication of this unclarity. Dworkin's example makes clear that it is only his own pills that he hid.

14. The issue here is whether, by hiding the pills, he is depriving his wife of the opportunity to take the pills, hence, breaking a moral rule. Since they were his own pills, we would say that he was not depriving his wife of opportunity. For further discussion of what counts as depriving, see Gert (2005, 111–112).

15. We do not intend this statement to be taken as a complete account of paternal or parental behavior. We recognize that the term "paternalistic" is often used to describe behavior that we think is more appropriately described as parental, but we do not think this significantly affects our analysis. (In a similar way, an analysis of jealousy is not significantly affected by the fact that "jealousy" is often used to refer to an emotion that is more appropriately referred to as "envy.")

16. See Beauchamp and Childress (2001, 178).

17. Ibid., 183.

18. Feature 4 seems to be suspended in one very unusual kind of case: killing a severely defective neonate in order to prevent it from the great suffering it will experience due to its severe defects. It does not seem paternalistic to take action to save the life of the neonate even if this involves causing considerable pain. Killing the neonate to prevent his pain seems paternalistic, whereas causing him pain to prevent his death does not, because the former prevents the neonate from ever becoming a person, whereas the latter does not. Thus, the only time one can be paternalistic toward someone who does not even believe he is competent to give consent is when one's act prevents that being from developing into a person who would believe himself competent to give consent. It may be paternalistic even if it is known that he would never develop into such a person. These are very special cases, and we shall not consider them any further here.

19. Thus, acting for the mildly retarded without their consent, if it meets the other elements of the definition, is clearly paternalistic. See Wikler (1979).

20. See particularly Buchanan and Brock (1986, 1990), and Drane (1985).

21. See Culver and Gert (1990a).

22. An unreasonable action, that is, one that is rationally allowed but conflicts with the rankings of harms and benefits of the person acting, can also raise the question of competence. In these cases it must be clear that the rankings of harms and benefits are not merely those that the patient had in the past, but are those that he continues to have at present, even though his decision conflicts with those rankings. Most of these cases are those in which the patient is regarded as incompetent because of his inability to understand or to appreciate the information provided, but they can also be the result of a volitional disability that the patient himself regards as unreasonable. Sometimes these can be serious enough that the patient can be regarded as incompetent.

23. See chapter 7, on mental maladies, and Gert and Culver (2004).

24. Compare with the discussion of autonomy in Beauchamp and Childress (2001).

25. The most prominent defense of casuistry is *The Abuse of Casuistry* by Al Jonsen and Stephen Toulmin (1988), but, as with principlism, we are primarily concerned with the general approach of casuistry, not any particular version of it.

26. Al Jonsen has a favorite analogy that he uses to contrast casuistry with a theoretical account of morality like ours. Casuistry is compared to a bicycle and a moral theory is compared to a hot air balloon. Supposedly, the person on a bicycle has a better view of what is going on at the ground level (real cases) than does the person in the hot-air

balloon. However, it is quite clear that both persons would do better if there were constant communication between them. The person in the hot-air balloon can provide better information about traffic patterns (e.g., as helicopters are used to give traffic reports at rush hours), and the person on the bicycle can provide detailed information about particular problems. See Jonsen and Toulmin (1988).

27. That account is provided in Gert (2005), but we do not discuss the virtues in chapter 2 of this book because we do not consider them to be useful in helping to explain or resolve the moral problems that arise in medicine.

28. See Kant, 408–409 (Hackett Publishing Co., 1981, 20–21).

29. The only possible exception is killing, where, because of the special characteristics of death, there may be some disagreement. See chapter 12 on euthanasia for fuller discussion.

30. The person must also be innocent, for strict deontologists usually do not think punishment of the guilty is unjustified. See the next paragraph in the text.

31. See chapter 2 for a fuller discussion. Because some disagreement is unavoidable in many cases, having a public policy about who makes the decision is essential. Further, whenever possible, we think that in cases of bioethical disagreement, there should be a public policy that involves consulting some experienced advisory body, for example, an ethics committee.

32. Throughout this chapter when we say "that it would be irrational for S not to choose having the rule violated with regard to himself" we mean, it would be objectively irrational, that is, irrational if he knew all of the relevant information. Thus, we are not claiming that S's decision is personally irrational, only that it would be personally irrational if he knew all of the relevant information. Thus, we use irrational decisions to refer to objectively irrational decisions, which include those that are seriously mistaken, as well as those that are personally irrational. Also, if S's rankings are reliably known, it might be justified to act paternalistically if S's decision is unreasonable rather than irrational, and in what follows this should be taken into account.

33. This framework is presented in chapter 2 and more fully described in Gert (2004 and 2005).

34. See Culver (2004).

35. The particular harms being ranked make no difference; completely different harms could be used, for example, prolonged severe pain versus an earlier death. See chapter 12 on euthanasia for a fuller discussion when these latter harms are involved.

36. It is this limited knowledge and fallibility of persons, their inability to know all the consequences of their actions, that explains not only why no rational person would publicly allow cheating simply on the grounds that no one would be hurt by it but also why moral rules are even needed. The nature and justifiability of a violation cannot be determined after one sees how things actually turn out; rather, it must be determined when the violation is being contemplated or carried out. Only then does the limited knowledge of persons and their fallibility play its proper role. See chapter 2.

37. Considering the consequences of this kind of deception being publicly allowed alerts one to the far greater harm that is risked by deception even in the particular case, that is, the loss of trust, and not only by Mr. J. If Mr. J finds out about the deception, he is extremely likely to tell other patients that they should not trust what their therapists say. Although there might be a very small chance of Mr. J finding out that he had been deceived, if he does find it out, the consequences could be very great. Similarly, the chances of any particular house being burned down are very small, yet almost everyone regards it as imprudent not to spend their money in order to buy fire insurance.

38. See Stone (1975, 70).
39. See Rawls (1971).
40. See Childress (1979, 26).
41. Childress acknowledges this point in a footnote: "Since many individuals who are subject to paternalistic interventions in health care will never regain rational powers, the ratification theory often takes a hypothetical form: what individuals would consent to if they *could* consent. This version of the ratification theory, of course, appeals to some vision of what rational individuals do and should desire" (26). Even in this form, ratification theories are still too simple.

11

Death

Definitions

Definitions of words are often not merely verbal matters. Some words are so closely related to a concept that is part of social and legal practices that knowing whether or not that word is correctly applied determines whether or not it is appropriate to initiate or terminate those practices. The word "dead," with all of its close relatives, for example, "die" and "death," is so closely related to the concept of death that when it is correct to refer to a person as dead, it is appropriate to terminate all medical care and to initiate funeral proceedings. Many other social and legal practices are initiated when a person is declared dead, for example, if he is president of the country, someone else immediately takes over that office. Insurance policies, Social Security benefits, and many other legal matters are affected. Failure to recognize how many practices are dependent on the correct application of the term "dead" has led some physicians to think that the determination of the time of death affects only medical practices. The time at which a person is declared dead has many practical consequences and only a small number of them have anything to do with medical practice. For most of these practices, it is usually not important to determine the time of death with split-second accuracy, but it is often important to determine it within a day or two, if not within an hour or two.

One new reason for trying to determine the time of death with some greater precision is due to advances in medical technology. It is often expensive to keep someone on life-support systems; being able to determine the time of death more precisely may prevent a serious waste of medical resources. But for many, what now seems the most important reason for determining the time of death with greater precision concerns the transplantation of organs. The sooner after death that organs can be removed for transplantation, the greater the likelihood that the transplanted organ will function properly in a new body. Indeed, some physicians are so concerned about assuring that the organs to be transplanted are in the best possible condition that they want to change the definition of death to further that end.[1] But changing the meaning of a word that plays such a significant role in so many important social and legal practices is a dangerous thing to do. This is especially true when a person does not recognize that the definition is being changed, but thinks that new scientific information is simply being brought to bear on the question of how the word is best defined.

When it is very important that a word have a clear and precise meaning, ordinary use is often supplemented by law in order to eliminate any troubling vagueness. When a word is very widely used, as the word "death" is, it is important that any legal definition of it not result in any significant changes in the way that word is ordinarily used; otherwise, there will be widespread confusion about the proper use of the term. When a term plays an important part in social and legal practices, as "death" does, then the greater the change in the meaning of the term, the greater the likelihood that there will be significant social and legal problems. Any attempt to make a term clearer and more precise than it is in ordinary use necessarily results in some people being bothered by what they perceive to be a change in its use. This perception of change cannot always be avoided, but it is important that any change be a reduction in vagueness. There should be no cases where, in ordinary use, it is clear that the term "dead" correctly applies, but according to the new definition, "dead" does not apply. Even more important, there should be no cases where in ordinary use it is clear the term "dead" does not correctly apply, but according to the new definition "dead" does apply. When a precise definition is needed, the overriding goal should be to change ordinary use as little as possible.

As one can easily see by looking at any dictionary, a definition of a "referring term" (e.g., "table" or "rectangular") consists of a description of the essential features of that which is referred to by the term. In defining a referring term like "dead," which plays a significant part in important social and legal practices and is very widely used, the features included in a description of what is referred to by that term should not conflict with what people ordinarily think. The only time that it is necessary to conflict with what is ordinarily thought is when advances in knowledge, usually scientific or technical knowledge, show that mistakes are embedded in the ordinary use of the term. The meaning of the term "atom" had to be changed when it was shown that what was referred to by that term, contrary to earlier belief, could be split. Atoms ceased to be the ultimate building blocks of the universe. But the term "atom" played no significant role in any social or legal practice, so that changing its meaning had no disturbing practical effects.

In biology and medicine, the definitions of terms change not only when new knowledge shows that the ordinary use of the term depends on false assumptions but also when new classification schemes are adopted, for example, whales ceased to be fish when a new scientific classification scheme was adopted. Insofar as this changed the meaning of the ordinary word, "fish," and that word played a role in some social and legal practices, some adjustments had to be made. But most scientific terms do not play significant roles in social or legal practices, and most are not widely used by the general public. When a term is widely and appropriately used by the general public, and plays a significant role in medical, social, and legal practices, even strong practical reasons for changing some of those medical practices are not sufficient for defining the term in ways that conflict with ordinary use. It is, nevertheless, understandable that physicians, who are primarily concerned with medical practices, should think only of the benefits of changing those practices when proposing changing the meaning of a term like "dead."

Changing the meaning of a term confuses people and creates general distrust of those proposing the change in meaning. Thus, when a term plays a significant role in so many social and legal practices, as "dead" does, rather than trying to bring about a change in some medical practice by changing the meaning of a key term involved in that practice, it is preferable to argue explicitly for changing that particular practice. It is almost impossible to describe a situation in which it is appropriate to redefine a term with widespread ordinary use in order to change any particular medical (or even social or legal) practice, in which that term plays a significant role. George Orwell has shown the bad consequences of redefining ordinary words in order to serve the political purposes of those in power. But even when the purposes to be served are worthwhile, changing the meaning of ordinary words is not the appropriate way to bring about those changes.

Proposed Definitions of Death

Death as a Process or an Event

A prominent and influential example of a physician neglecting the ordinary use of the term "dead" is Robert Morison's claim that death is a process rather than an event (1971). He supports this claim by citing the following scientific facts about dying. He correctly notes that a standard series of degenerative and destructive changes occur in the tissues of an organism, usually following but sometimes preceding the irreversible cessation of spontaneous ventilation and circulation. These changes include necrosis of brain cells, necrosis of other vital organ cells, cooling, rigor mortis, dependent lividity, and putrefaction. This process actually persists for years, even centuries, until the skeletal remains have disintegrated, and could even be viewed as beginning with the failure of certain organ systems during life. Because these changes occur in a fairly regular and ineluctable fashion, he seems to claim that the stipulation of any particular point in this process as the moment of death is arbitrary.

Although the biological facts cited in the previous paragraph are correct, they are not relevant to determining the definition of "death." The use of many terms, for example, many of the common color words, is even more arbitrary, from a scientific point of view, than the use of the term "dead." Even though pink is related to red as pastel blue is related to blue, it is misguided to say that pink is really pastel red. The following considerations show some serious problems confronting any definition that makes death a process. If death is regarded as a process, then either (1) the process starts when the person is still living, which confuses the process of death with the process of dying, for everyone regards someone who is dying as not yet dead, or (2) the process of death starts when the person is no longer alive, which confuses the process of death with the process of disintegration. Although there is some inevitable vagueness in determining the precise instant of death, this vagueness is no greater than that involved in determining the precise instant of other important events, for example, birth and marriage. In ordinary use, the word "death" refers not to a process but to the event that separates the process of dying from the process of disintegration.

A physician writing on this matter admits that, "the reigning view has assumed that life and death are nonoverlapping dichotomous states."[2] Unfortunately, she seems to think that this view reigns only among philosophers and physicians, that is, that it is a technical view about the biological processes that accompany dying. However, as stated before, "death" is not a technical term but one that is used by ordinary people. It is they, as well as almost all philosophers and physicians, who use "dead" as a term that cannot be correctly applied at the same instant to the same organism to whom the term "alive" is correctly applied. This is what makes life and death "nonoverlapping dichotomous states." In ordinary language, "dead" is used of someone only when it is appropriate to have a funeral for him, that is, to bury or cremate him.

As Ludwig Wittgenstein pointed out, philosophical problems often arise from a misunderstanding of ordinary language. It is a failure to understand ordinary language that leads to the following kind of remark, "To say 'she is dead' is meaningless because 'she is' is not compatible with 'dead'."[3] Consider a daughter concerned about her dying mother who asks the doctor how her mother is doing. The doctor replies, "She is dead." Only someone overcome by metaphysical arguments could regard the doctor's statement as meaningless. A decent respect for the ordinary use of language requires that a definition of "death" be provided that fits with its use in ordinary language.

It is very tempting, however, to give a technical sense to ordinary words without realizing what one is doing. When *Philosophy in Medicine* was translated

into Japanese, the translators were physicians. In a note discussing our introduction of the term "malady" as a technical term, they denied our claim that there
was no ordinary word in any language that referred to both diseases and injuries.
They claimed there was a word in Japanese that did refer to both diseases and
injuries.[4] Upon investigation, it turned out that ordinary speakers of Japanese
never use that term to refer to a broken arm or leg. The Japanese translators had
done something similar to what American doctors sometimes do: they had taken
an ordinary Japanese term, analogous to the English word "disease," and had not
realized that they had enlarged it so that it no longer had its ordinary use (see
chapter 6). A similar process seems at work among those who propose new and
more elaborate definitions of death, definitions that are "a more descriptively
accurate model of life's progressive cessation."[5]

On a practical level, regarding death as a process makes it impossible to declare
the time of death with the level of precision that already has been achieved. As we
mentioned earlier, this is not a trivial issue. There are not only pressing medical
reasons to regard death as an event (e.g., deciding when to cease treatment), there
are also serious legal, social, and religious reasons for declaring death as having
occurred at some fairly precise time. These include burial times and procedures,
mourning times, and the reading of wills. There are no countervailing practical or
theoretical reasons for regarding death as a process rather than as an event in
formulating a definition of "death."

Nor are there adequate reasons to introduce several senses of the term "death,"
each of which is used in a different medical practice, for example, one for ceasing
treatment and one for retrieving organs. Imagine a situation in which someone is
told that a spouse has died, and then has to ask, in what sense, in the normal sense
when it is appropriate to have funeral services, or only in one of the newer senses,
when various medical treatments can be stopped, or organs removed. It may not
always be appropriate to use the time of death, in the normal sense of that term, to
determine the appropriateness of stopping or starting some particular medical
procedures; however, it is not necessary to change the ordinary meaning of
"death" or to introduce new senses of "death" in order to change the timing of
these procedures. It is both possible and preferable to use new precisely defined
technical terms or phrases, for example, "in a persistent vegetative state," in
order to devise a policy for when it is morally acceptable to discontinue any life
support, retrieve organs, and so forth.[6] To use the same term, "death," for all of
these different stages is to invite confusion, mistrust, and abuse.

Ordinary Features of Death

The definition of death must capture our ordinary use of the term, for "death" is
a word used by everyone, and is not primarily a medical or legal term. In this
ordinary and literal use, certain facts are assumed, for example, that all and only

living organisms can die, that the living can usually be distinguished from the dead with complete reliability, that the time when an organism leaves the former state and enters the latter can be determined with a fairly high degree of precision, and that death is permanent.[7] Recent advances in science have not called into question any of these assumptions, but they have made plausible some scenarios that were formerly regarded as limited to science fiction. It now seems that an animal can be kept alive for a significant time even when its head has been severed from its body, so that the organism is no longer functioning as a whole. To insist that the animal is dead, even though its head responds to sounds and sights, has little or no plausibility and is incompatible with our ordinary understanding of death.[8] Therefore, it is important that our definition apply to some plausible science fiction speculations, for example, about brains continuing to function independently of the rest of the organism.[9]

Some who believe in what is called "life after death" believe that after the organism dies, the person who was that organism, or the soul that inhabited that organism, continues to be conscious. However, both those who believe in life after death and those who do not do agree in their ordinary application of the term "dead." Those who believe in life after death do not believe that the organism that has permanently ceased to function is still conscious, but only that something that had been closely related to that biological organism is still conscious. No matter what view is taken about the plausibility of a belief in life after death, this belief has no relevance to determining the meaning of the word "dead." Regardless of what one believes concerning life after death, there is no dispute about the permanence of the death of the organism that used to be a living organism.

In the literal use of the term "die," which is also the medical use of that term, all and only living organisms can die. In this same literal sense, death is permanent. Some people may claim to have been dead for several minutes and then to have returned to life, but this is only a dramatic way of saying that both consciousness and most observable functioning of the organism as a whole was temporarily lost (e.g., because of a brief episode of cardiac arrest). But a temporary loss of consciousness and a temporary loss of all observable functioning of the organism as a whole is not sufficient for what is meant by "death." These losses must be permanent; when they are, even those with the relevant religious beliefs do not doubt that the organism has died. In fact, when the facts are not in dispute, there is almost no disagreement in ordinary life about whether and when someone has died.

In its basic sense, the terms "alive" and "dead" normally apply only to whole organisms, for example, a cat, a dog, a mosquito, or a tree. The tail of a cat or dog, or the wings of a mosquito are not said to be either alive or dead. Nor is the fruit of a tree said to be either alive or dead. However, people do talk about dead branches of a tree, and some people talk about keeping parts of a body alive, so that they can be transplanted. If only part of the organism is kept alive, normally the organism is regarded as dead, but if the part of the organism that is alive is sufficiently important, the organism may be regarded as alive. If any part of a human organism retains consciousness, that organism would be regarded as still being alive. Thus, the presence of consciousness is sufficient to establish that the human organism is not dead. It was formerly assumed that consciousness depended on the functioning of the organism as a whole, but recent scientific studies have cast some doubt on this assumption.

From the moral point of view, killing someone does not seem any worse than causing him to be permanently unconscious, and in this context it may not be important to distinguish between having caused the death of an organism and having caused the permanent loss of consciousness of the person who was that organism.[10] In other contexts, however, this distinction may be important, for example, only after the death of the organism is burial or cremation appropriate. But purely from the point of view of the victim, and apart from some unusual religious or metaphysical beliefs, it does not seem to make any difference whether one has been killed or simply caused to be permanently unconscious. However, the use of the term "dead" is not determined from the point of view of the victim; rather, "dead" is used by conscious living persons to describe someone who can be buried, whose will can be probated, and so forth. This common use of "dead" is the one that plays the most significant role in medical practice as well as in a wide variety of legal and social practices.

Definitions, Criteria, and Tests

Much of the confusion arising from the current brain death controversy is due to the failure to distinguish among three distinct elements: (1) the definition of death, which should be determined so as to capture most accurately the ordinary use of the term "dead" and related terms, (2) the medical criterion for determining that death has occurred (which must stay current with changes in our scientific understanding of the organism), and (3) the tests, which often change with improvements in medical technology, to prove that the criterion has been satisfied.[11] We concentrate on defining death in a way that makes its ordinary meaning explicit. We use our present scientific understanding of the organism to provide a criterion of death. When there is any doubt about whether a person is dead, this scientific understanding is the criterion that is used to determine whether the definition of death has been satisfied. Because the tests to prove that the criterion is satisfied change as technology improves, we simply mention some past tests that have demonstrated perfect validity in determining that the criterion of death is satisfied.

It is a source of some confusion that both the "definitions" of death that appear in legal dictionaries and the new "statutory definitions" of death are not actually attempts to provide a definition of the term "death," that is, attempts to describe what the term means in ordinary usage. Rather, these "definitions" are actually statements of the criteria by which physicians should legally determine when death has occurred. Because "death" is not a technical term but a common term in everyday use, a proper understanding of the ordinary meaning of this word or concept must be achieved before a medical criterion is chosen. A definition of death must make explicit what is ordinarily meant by "death" before physicians can decide how to medically determine it. Agreement on both the definition and medical criterion of death is literally a life-and-death matter.

Whether a spontaneously breathing patient in a persistent vegetative state is classified as alive or dead depends on whether one accepts a definition of death that makes explicit its ordinary meaning, or thinks that a new definition is required. The definition that we propose makes explicit the ordinary meaning of "death." However, more than a definition is needed. A definition, by itself, does not completely determine the status of a patient with a totally and permanently nonfunctioning brain who is being maintained on a ventilator. That determination depends on the criterion of death employed. Defining death is primarily a philosophical task. Providing the criterion of death is primarily a medical matter. But it must be recognized that the criterion of death is a criterion for the definition being satisfied, and so depends upon what that definition is. Choosing the tests to prove that the criterion is satisfied is solely a medical matter. In this chapter we concentrate our discussion on the definition of death, but also say something about the criterion of death. We say very little about the tests that are used to determine whether the criterion has been satisfied.

The Definition of Death

The definition of death that we provide describes and explains the ordinary use of "death" and related words. Explicit use of this definition allows those who are aware of all the relevant facts to describe as dead all and only those whom they ordinarily describe as dead. We are providing an ordinary dictionary definition, only slightly more detailed than most dictionary definitions, and perhaps one that makes the term slightly more precise. Its correctness is determined by seeing if there is any clear case where use of this definition is in conflict with the ordinary use of the term "death." The following is our definition: death is the permanent cessation of all observable natural functioning of the organism as a whole, and the permanent absence of consciousness in the organism as a whole, and in any part of that organism.

By the organism as a whole, we do not mean the whole organism, that is, the sum of its tissue and organ parts, but rather the highly complex interaction of all or most of its organ subsystems. The organism need not be whole or complete—it may have lost a limb or an organ (such as the spleen)—but it still remains an organism. By the observable natural functioning of the organism as a whole, we mean a sufficient amount of natural spontaneous and innate activities of integration of most subsystems, and at least limited response to the environment, that results in observable activity. It is not necessary that all of the subsystems be integrated with one another. Individual subsystems may be replaced (e.g., by pacemakers, ventilators, or presser drugs) without changing the status of the organism as a whole. Even if almost all parts of the organism have been replaced by nonliving mechanisms, if these mechanisms have been integrated into the organism by the natural brain stem, and manifest observable functioning, the organism is still alive. We include the word "natural" in our definition because it now seems possible that nanotechnology may allow for implants in the brain stem that will keep the organism, as a whole, functioning even though the whole brain has completely ceased to function. If this occurs, and there is no consciousness, on our definition the organism is dead.

It is possible for individual subsystems to function for a time after the organism as a whole has permanently ceased all observable natural functioning. Spontaneous ventilation—as well as temperature regulation, it seems—ceases either immediately after or just before the permanent cessation of natural functioning of the organism as a whole, but spontaneous circulation, with the assistance of artificial ventilation, may persist for several months after the organism as a whole has ceased to function naturally. The control of this complex process is located in certain neuroendocrine cells in the hypothalamus and the process is important for normal maintenance of all cellular processes. These neuroendocrine cells usually, but not always, cease functioning when the organism as a whole has permanently ceased all observable natural functioning. However, even if these cells do not completely cease functioning, if there is a permanent absence of consciousness in the organism as a whole and in any part of that organism, and if the organism as a whole has permanently ceased all observable natural functions, the patient is still dead.[12]

If science develops replacement parts for every part of the organism, such as the whole brain including the cortex, that will force a change in our concept of death. Such a scientific development would also force a change in our concept of personal identity. Indeed, it is hard to predict what would be correct to say about the death of a person, or about who counts as the same person at two different points in time if enough of our present beliefs about those organisms that are persons change.[13] We are attempting to describe the present concept of death, one that is based on acceptance of present facts about those organisms that are persons. We are not making metaphysical claims about death, that is, those that hold in all possible worlds; our aim is to clarify our present concept, that which accounts for the ordinary use of the term "dead." An important practical benefit of clearly defining the present concept of death is that it enables the evaluation of the various criteria of death that have been proposed.

Including as part of the definition of death "the permanent absence of consciousness in the organism as a whole and in any part of that organism" is compatible with "death" meaning the same for all animals, including those that were never conscious. Although death is a biological phenomenon common to members of all species, criteria for the death of a plant are not as precise as the criteria for the death of a conscious animal. Furthermore, because plants and some animals have no consciousness, it is only the permanent natural cessation of the functioning of the organism as a whole that is used to decide whether a nonconscious animal or a plant has died. The death of a conscious animal, especially human beings, usually must be determined with some precision, whereas that of a nonconscious animal or a plant need not. It is relatively unimportant whether a plant is very sick or dead, whereas this is a crucial distinction for conscious animals, especially human beings. The importance of consciousness to a conscious organism has no counterpart in nonconscious animals or plants. Thus, it is not inappropriate for the definition to acknowledge the importance of consciousness in the life of conscious animals. Indeed, this seems especially true as technology advances and if, as now seems likely, it becomes possible for a part of the organism to remain conscious while the organism as a whole ceases to function.

Consciousness is not limited to human beings. All mammals are conscious to some degree, and other animals and birds seem to be conscious as well.[14] Although consciousness is usually manifested only by an organism that is functioning as a whole, it now seems possible to sever an animal's head from its body and for that severed head to manifest consciousness, for example, to respond appropriately to external stimuli. Given that death requires both a permanent natural cessation of the organism functioning as a whole and the permanent absence of consciousness in the organism as a whole and in any part of that organism, a dog, whose head has been separated from its body, does not count as dead if that head continues to manifest consciousness.[15] Even though there has been a permanent natural cessation of the functioning of the organism as a whole, an identifiable part of that organism continues to be conscious. An adequate criterion of death must allow for consciousness of any part of the organism to be sufficient for that organism to count as still living.

Previously we had held that permanent cessation of the functioning of the organism as a whole was sufficient for death.[16] We did not realize that an identifiable part of an organism might continue to be conscious even though the organism as a whole had permanently ceased to function. This was simply a mistake on our part. Our recognition of this new fact made clear that we had not accurately described the present concept of death. However, as previously unknown facts are discovered, our concept of death may have to change. However, even if these new facts require a change in our concept of death, they do not allow the concept to be changed without significant constraints. The concept must accommodate the newly discovered facts, but it should be changed as little as possible. Indeed, it may turn out that, as we mentioned above, the new fact simply makes it clear that our previous description of the concept was mistaken. This possibility explains why it is sometimes useful to consider science fiction examples. Contemplating the possibility that these examples might be facts can sometimes make clear the inadequacy of previous accounts.

We now recognize that our previous definition of the concept of death was inadequate. The chapter on death in *Philosophy in Medicine* contained the following paragraph:

> We believe that the permanent cessation of the functioning of the organism as a whole is what has traditionally been meant by death. This definition retains death as a biological occurrence which is not unique to human beings; the same definition applies to other higher animals. We believe that death is a biological phenomenon and should apply equally to related species. When we talk of the death of a human being, we mean the same thing as we do when we talk of the death of a dog or a cat. This is supported by our ordinary use of the term *death*, and by law and tradition. It is also in accord with social and religious practices and is not likely to be affected by future changes in technology.[17]

Most of what we said in that paragraph remains correct, but we would now rewrite that first sentence as follows. "We believe that the permanent cessation of all observable natural functioning of the organism as a whole, the permanent absence of consciousness in the organism as a whole, and in any part of that organism is what has traditionally been meant by death." It is both interesting and important to note that this change in the first sentence does not require any changes in the rest of the paragraph. Improvements in technology have made clear that there can be laboratory-determined functioning of cells responsible for the function of the organism as a whole, even though there has been a permanent cessation of all observable natural functioning of the organism as a whole. Developments in biology seem to have established that a part of the organism can remain conscious even though the organism as a whole has ceased to function. Consciousness, even of a part of the organism, is always sufficient to establish that the organism is alive. However, when the whole natural brain has permanently ceased to function, the patient is permanently unconscious, and there is no observable natural functioning of the organism as a whole, the person is dead even if nanochips implanted in the brain stem take over the functions of the brain stem and the organism as a whole is functioning artificially.

In our previous account, we recognized the importance of consciousness, claiming that "consciousness and cognition are sufficient to show the functioning of the organism as a whole in higher animals, but they are not necessary."[18] If we had taken science fiction more seriously, we might have anticipated the recent research that has demonstrated that consciousness of a part of the organism is possible independent of the functioning of the organism as a whole. In these science fiction stories, it is quite clear that the organism as a whole has ceased to function, although a part of the organism remains conscious. We now realize that when consciousness is maintained in a part of the organism, even though that part, namely, the head or the brain, has been separated from the rest of the organism, the organism has not died.

We erred in not recognizing consciousness as a sufficient condition for life, independent of the functioning of the organism as a whole. The opposite error was made by those who claimed that permanent loss of consciousness was a sufficient condition of death. Both of these errors arose from a desire to frame a simple definition of death. We defined death as the permanent cessation of functioning of the organism as a whole, whereas others defined it as the permanent loss of consciousness. Both views were partly right; death does require the permanent cessation of all observable natural functioning of the organism as a whole, and it does require the permanent absence of consciousness. Both sides were also partly wrong, each holding that what was a necessary condition for death was also a sufficient condition. Both wanted one feature to be both a necessary and sufficient condition for death. Although it would be far more elegant if either side had been correct, the concept of death, like many of the concepts in our ordinary language, is more complex than philosophers and others have usually portrayed it. Death requires both the permanent cessation of all observable natural functioning of the organism as a whole and the permanent absence of consciousness in the organism as a whole, as well as in any part of that organism. Attempts to eliminate either component result in a distortion of the concept.

We now realize that even when the organism as a whole has permanently ceased to have any observable natural functioning, consciousness and cognition in any part of that organism are sufficient to show that the organism has not died. Unlike those who maintain that consciousness, or the possibility of future consciousness, is necessary for an organism to be alive, we maintain only that it is sufficient. Even when higher organisms, including human beings, are comatose, evidence of any observable natural functioning of the organism as a whole is sufficient to show that the organism is still living. Both the permanent cessation of the organism's natural functioning as a whole and the permanent absence of consciousness in the organism as a whole, as well as in any part of that organism, for example, the head of an organism, are necessary before that organism can correctly be said to have died.

A definition that took permanent absence of consciousness to be sufficient for death was proposed by Robert Veatch (1976) and has attracted some support. This definition does not mention consciousness, but defines death as the irreversible loss of that which is essentially significant to the nature of persons. Although this definition may initially seem very attractive, it does not state what is ordinarily meant by death. It is not self-contradictory to say that a person has lost that which is essentially significant to the nature of a person, but is still alive. Many human beings have lost sufficient mental function so that they have lost that which is essentially significant to the nature of a person, but everyone acknowledges that they are not dead. Indeed, it is often regarded as a blessing for such persons if they were to die very quickly. Permanently comatose patients in persistent vegetative states are extreme examples of this kind of human being, but they are still considered to be living.[19]

The patients described by Multi-Society Task Force on PVS are in this category.[20] These patients have complete neocortical destruction with preservation of the brain stem and diencephalic (posterior brain) structures. They have isoelectric (flat) electroencephalograms (EEGs) and are permanently comatose (indicating neocortical death), although they have normal spontaneous breathing and brain stem reflexes. They retain many of the vital functions of the organism as a whole, including neuroendocrine control (i.e., homeostatic interrelationships between the brain and various hormonal glands) and spontaneous circulation and breathing. They are in a persistent vegetative state.

The definition of death as the irreversible loss of that which is essentially significant to the nature of a person, or as the permanent loss of consciousness, actually states what it means to cease to be a person rather than what it means for that person to die. "Person" is not a biological concept but rather a concept defined, not only in terms of certain kinds of abilities and qualities of awareness but also in terms of the attitudes it is appropriate to take toward it. Because death is a biological concept, "death," in a literal sense, applies directly only to biological organisms and not to persons. Of course, it is perfectly ordinary to talk about the "death of a person," but this phrase in common usage actually means the death of the organism that was the person. For example, one might overhear in the hospital wards, "The person in room 612 died last night." In this common usage, one is referring to the death of the organism that was a person. We think that Veatch and others have not appreciated that the phrase "death of a person" is normally applied to an organism that was a person and has died, not to an organism that has ceased to be a person but has not died.

A patient in a persistent vegetative state is usually regarded as living in only the most basic biological sense, but this basic biological sense is just what our definition of death makes explicit. The death of an organism that was a person must not be confused with an organism ceasing to be a person. The loss of personhood in persistent vegetative patients makes it inappropriate to continue treating them as if they were persons. Consciousness and cognition are essential human attributes. If they are lost, life has lost its meaning. Unless there are religious reasons to the contrary, we recommend that nothing be done to keep such patients alive. This alternative is preferable to considering these persistent vegetative patients as already dead. No one favors burying or cremating a patient who is still breathing spontaneously. Unless one favors "killing" such patients, it is still necessary to wait for the organism as a whole to permanently cease to function. In most cases there is no practical advantage to regarding such patients as dead rather than regarding them as having ceased to be persons, and thus discontinuing all treatment.

The only cases in which there might be a practical advantage in regarding patients who have ceased to be persons as dead is in the procurement of organs for transplantation. Waiting until the organism as a whole has ceased to function may sometimes reduce the chances of a successful transplant. However, changing the definition of death in order to gain some practical advantage in transplantation is exactly the kind of maneuver that concerns many people. Changing the ordinary meaning of such important words as "death" for practical advantage is very dangerous. If people know that the definition of death has been changed to obtain better quality organs for transplantation, their distrust of the medical profession is bound to increase. Changing the meaning of ordinary words for practical advantage is far too likely to be mistrusted and misused for it to confer any overall practical advantage.[21] It is better to explicitly argue in favor of removing organs from living but permanently unconscious patients than to change the meaning of the word "death" in order to accomplish the same goal.

Apart from obtaining more viable organs, considering permanent loss of consciousness and cognition as what it means for an organism to be dead rather than for an organism to cease to be a person does not seem to have any practical advantages. It is far less troubling to argue for nonvoluntary cessation of life support for the permanently comatose than to claim that the patient is already dead. The justification of nonvoluntary passive euthanasia, as well as the justification of obtaining organs for transplantation, must be kept strictly separate from the definition of death. Most people would prefer to die when they cease to be persons, but few think that this should be accomplished simply by redefining "death" so that when they cease to be persons, they have died.

Organisms that are no longer persons have no claim to be treated as persons. However, just as human corpses are treated with respect, even more so living organisms that were persons should be treated with respect. Treating these organisms with respect does not mean that one should strive to keep them alive. No one benefits by doing this; on the contrary, given the care needed to keep such organisms alive, it is an extravagant waste of both economic and human resources to attempt to do so. On the other hand, allowing—let alone requiring—anyone to kill these living organisms creates serious practical problems. Even though these organisms are no longer persons, they still look like persons, indeed, are almost indistinguishable from persons who are asleep. Because these patients are not suffering in any way, ceasing to provide any medical care, including artificial hydration and nutrition, is completely appropriate. There is no good reason for killing them; on the contrary, because killing them might weaken the prohibition against killing, there are good reasons for not doing so.

It is important to note that because these patients have permanently lost all consciousness and cognition, they do not suffer from lack of care. Any patient who retains even the slightest capacity to suffer pain or discomfort of any kind remains a person and must be treated as such.[22] Of course, all patients should be encouraged to make out advance directives in order to make clear whether or not they want to be allowed to die if they were to become permanently comatose. In the absence of any advance directive to the contrary, we propose that the legal guardian or next of kin be allowed to direct that all treatments, including food and fluids, be discontinued and the patient be allowed to die. The fact that discontinuing all treatment, including food and fluids, for such patients causes no pain and results in death in two weeks or less makes it unnecessary to kill them. We put this proposal forward here because we think that its adoption significantly reduces the temptation to change the definition of death from its ordinary biological sense to that of an organism that has ceased to be a person.[23]

The Criterion of Death

We have argued that the correct definition of death is "the permanent cessation of all observable natural functioning of the organism as a whole, the permanent absence of consciousness in the organism as a whole, and in any part of that organism." In order for this definition to be applied to actual cases of death, there must be a criterion that is taken as establishing with complete certainty that the definition has been satisfied. Four criteria of death have been put forward: (1) the permanent loss of cardiopulmonary functioning, (2) the total and permanent loss of functioning of the cortex, (3) the total and permanent loss of functioning of the brain stem, and (4) the total and permanent loss of functioning of the whole brain. Only one of these four proposed criteria is completely compatible with the above definition of death, namely, the fourth criterion: "the total and permanent loss of functioning of the whole brain." Thus, it is the only acceptable criterion of death. In the following sections we point out the inadequacies of the other three proposed criteria.

Characteristics of Optimum Criteria and Tests

A criterion of death yields a false positive if it is satisfied, and yet it is still possible that there will be observable natural functioning of the organism as a whole, or that any part of it will be conscious. An essential requirement for a criterion of death is that it yield no false positives. Indeed, because the criterion of death serves as the legal definition of death, it cannot have any exceptions. It is not sufficient that the criterion be correct 99.99% of the time. Although it is most important that the criterion yield no false positives, it should also yield no false negatives. A criterion of death yields a false negative if it is not satisfied at the time there is permanent cessation of all observable natural functioning of the organism as a whole, and a permanent absence of consciousness in every part of the organism. Yielding false negatives, while not as dangerous as yielding false positives, does result in a significant waste of resources.

Of course, physicians often determine death without explicitly using the criterion, but it can never be that the criterion is satisfied and yet the person is not dead, or that the criterion is not satisfied and the person is dead. This is why it is so easy to mistakenly regard the criterion as a real definition, rather than solely the legal definition. The criterion serves as the legal definition because it is what is used by the medical profession in declaring death whenever there is any doubt about the matter. Often, however, there is no doubt about the matter, and it is not necessary to directly establish that the criterion is satisfied. Often, the circumstances are such that it is absolutely certain that the person is dead, for example, most cases of terminally ill patients not on artificial life support, whose hearts have stopped beating and who are no longer breathing. In less clear cases, when there is some doubt about whether the criterion is satisfied, this determination is provided by validated tests that show whether or not the criterion is satisfied.

Permanent Loss of Cardiopulmonary Functioning

Permanent termination of all heart and lung function seems to have been used as a criterion of death throughout history. Even the ancients observed that all other bodily functions ceased shortly after cessation of these vital functions, and the irreversible process of bodily disintegration inevitably followed. Permanent loss of spontaneous cardiopulmonary function was a perfect predictor of permanent cessation of all observable natural functioning of the organism as a whole, as well as permanent absence of consciousness in all parts of the organism. There were no false positives. Furthermore, if the loss of spontaneous cardiopulmonary function was not permanent, the organism as a whole could continue to function naturally even if that loss caused a permanent absence of consciousness in all parts of the organism. Thus, there were no false negatives. For a very long time, the permanent loss of spontaneous cardiopulmonary function served as an adequate criterion of death.

Times have changed. Current ventilatory/circulatory technology now means that permanent loss of spontaneous cardiopulmonary functioning is no longer a perfect predictor of permanent cessation of all observable natural functioning of the organism as a whole. Even more clearly, it is not predictive of permanent absence of consciousness in all parts of the organism. Consider the case of a conscious, talking patient who is unable to breathe because of poliomyelitis and who requires an iron lung (thus having permanent loss of spontaneous pulmonary function), who has also developed asystole (loss of spontaneous heartbeat) requiring a permanent pacemaker (thus having permanent loss of spontaneous cardiac function). It is absurd to regard such a person as dead.

It is now quite clear that the permanent loss of *spontaneous* cardiopulmonary function is not the criterion of death. Even though it does not result in any false negatives, it does what is far worse: it results in false positives. To eliminate the false positives, some physicians have proposed to change the cardiopulmonary criterion from the permanent loss of *spontaneous* cardiopulmonary function to the permanent loss of *all* cardiopulmonary function, whether spontaneous or artificially supported. However, now that ventilation and circulation can be mechanically maintained, an organism with permanent loss of whole-brain functioning can have permanently lost all observable natural functioning of the organism as a whole, and all parts of the organism may have permanently lost consciousness, weeks or months or more before the heart and lungs cease to function with artificial support. Thus, this revised cardiopulmonary criterion is not satisfied, yet the person is dead. The revised cardiopulmonary criterion eliminates the false positives, but it produces false negatives.

The cardiopulmonary criterion can continue to be put forward only if the ambiguity involved is not noticed. The cardiopulmonary criterion of death cannot be permanent loss of *spontaneous* cardiopulmonary functioning nor can it be permanent loss of *artificially supported* cardiopulmonary functioning. Permanent loss of spontaneous cardiopulmonary functioning is no longer perfectly correlated with death, and continued artificially supported cardiopulmonary function is no longer perfectly correlated with life. Loss of cardiopulmonary functioning now seems to have no straightforward relationship either to the permanent loss of all observable natural functioning of the organism as a whole, or to the permanent absence of consciousness in the organism as a whole, and in any part of that organism.

Total and Permanent Loss of Functioning of the Cortex

Total and permanent loss of functioning of the cortex does not provide an adequate criterion of death on the definition of death provided above. Even its supporters acknowledge that total and permanent loss of functioning of the higher brain or cortex is an adequate criterion of death only if one defines death as the permanent absence of consciousness in the organism as a whole, and in any part of that organism. We have already given our arguments against accepting this definition of death, so there is no need to provide new arguments against accepting loss of all higher brain functions as the criterion of death. Everyone acknowledges that a human organism can continue to function naturally as a whole even if the entire cortex has ceased to function. On the definition of death that we have provided, this proposed criterion of death continually produces false positives; people would be declared dead who do not satisfy the definition. Nonetheless, because some people have supported permanent loss of consciousness of all parts of the organism as the definition of death, this criterion has some supporters.[24]

Total and Permanent Loss of Functioning of the Brain Stem

Total and permanent loss of functioning of the brain stem is, except for purely theoretical considerations, a good criterion of death. Permanent loss of all observable natural functioning of the organism as a whole inevitably accompanies total and permanent loss of functioning of the brain stem. If permanent loss of all observable natural functioning of the organism as a whole always results in permanent loss of consciousness in the organism as a whole, and in all of the parts of the organism, total and permanent loss of all natural functioning of the brain stem provides an adequate criterion of death. However, it now seems possible, at least theoretically, for there to be total and permanent loss of all natural functioning of the brain stem and yet for consciousness to remain in one part of the body, the cortex.[25] This possibility may never be realized, but sufficient work has been done with the higher brain that it cannot be completely ruled out. Patients suffering from locked-in syndrome have been able to manipulate electrical devices by pure thought, that is, by increasing or decreasing the amount of electrical energy given off by their brains. If such devices were attached to a person's cortex and he continued to operate them even after total and permanent loss of all natural functioning of his brain stem, it would clearly be a mistake for one to declare that patient dead.

As we pointed out above, the essential requirement for a criterion of death is that it yield no false positives. If the brain stem criterion has even a remote possibility of yielding a false positive, it is not an adequate criterion of death. It does seem possible for someone who is still conscious to have total and permanent loss of all natural brain stem function. Therefore, the brain stem criterion cannot be accepted as the criterion of death. Further, there seems to be minimal practical gain in accepting permanent loss of brain stem functioning over permanent loss of whole-brain functioning as the criterion. Except in extremely unusual cases, the tests that are adequate to show that the one criterion is satisfied are also adequate to show that the other criterion is satisfied. Indeed, the cortex is more sensitive to loss of oxygen than is the brain stem. This is why so many patients in a persistent vegetative state are those who have been resuscitated after a period of cerebral anoxia; the brain stem has survived but the cortex has not. The main difference between the brain stem criterion and the whole-brain criterion is theoretical. The former allows for the possibility of a part of the organism being conscious even though the organism as a whole has ceased all observable natural function, while the latter does not allow for this possibility.

New nanotechnology may make total and permanent loss of brain stem function ambiguous in the same way that total and permanent loss of cardiopulmonary function was made ambiguous by new technology. If it is possible for there to be total and permanent loss of all natural functioning of the brain stem, although implanted brain chips continue to perform all the necessary functions of the brain stem, it would be absurd to regard a person as dead who is not only conscious but talking to us. However, if the implanted brain chips perform all of the functions of the brain stem, but the person has permanently lost consciousness because his cortex has been totally destroyed, the person is dead. The person now satisfies the definition of death: the permanent cessation of all observable natural functioning of the organism as a whole, the permanent absence of consciousness in the organism as a whole, and in any part of that organism. Although the implanted brain chips continue to allow the observable functioning of the organism as a whole, there is a cessation of any natural functioning. Consciousness, whether natural or artificially supported, is sufficient for a person to be alive; functioning of the organism as a whole is sufficient for life only if it is not totally dependent on artificial support. This fact would be apparent if the machines that performed the function of the implanted brain chips were outside of the body rather than inside.

Total and Permanent Loss of Whole-Brain Functioning

The criterion for the permanent cessation of all observable natural functioning of the organism as a whole, the permanent absence of consciousness in the organism as a whole, and in any part of that organism is the permanent loss of natural functioning of the entire brain.[26] This criterion is perfectly correlated with the permanent cessation of all observable natural functioning of the organism as a whole because it is the brain stem, which is part of the entire brain, that is necessary for all observable natural functioning of the organism as a whole. The brainstem integrates, generates, interrelates, and controls complex bodily activities. A patient on a ventilator with a totally destroyed brain stem is merely a collection of artificially maintained subsystems because the organism as a whole has ceased to function naturally. This criterion also correlates perfectly with the permanent absence of consciousness in the organism as a whole and in any part of that organism, because the cortex, which is part of the "entire brain," is the seat of consciousness, and if it has permanently ceased to function, then no part of the organism can be conscious. The permanent loss of whole–brain natural functioning entails the permanent loss of natural function of both the brain stem and the cortex. Using the permanent loss of whole–brain natural functioning as a criterion of death yields no false negatives or false positives, and thus is completely adequate as a criterion.

Using permanent loss of natural functioning of the whole brain as the criterion for death is also consistent with tradition; it is not a new departure. Throughout history, whenever a physician was called to ascertain the occurrence of death, his examination included the following important signs indicative of permanent loss of natural functioning of the whole brain: unresponsivity; lack of spontaneous movements, including breathing; and absence of pupillary light response. Only one important sign, lack of heartbeat, was not directly indicative of whole-brain destruction. But because the heartbeat stops within several minutes of cessation of breathing, permanent absence of the vital signs is an important sign of permanent loss of whole–brain, natural functioning. Thus, in an important sense, permanent loss of whole–brain, natural functioning has always been the underlying criterion of death.

The Tests of Death

Having provided both the definition of death (viz., the permanent cessation of all observable natural functioning of the organism as a whole, the permanent absence of consciousness in the organism as a whole, and in any part of that organism) and the criterion of death (viz., the total and irreversible cessation of natural functioning of the whole brain), we now briefly discuss the available tests of death. The tests must never yield a false positive result, that is, result in someone who does not meet the definition of death being declared dead. It would be ideal if no test ever yielded a false negative, that is, someone who meets the definition of death yet is claimed to be still living. Unlike the criterion of death, however, a test can remain acceptable if it results in a very few and relatively brief false negatives.

Cessation of Heartbeat and Ventilation

Although permanent loss of spontaneous cardiopulmonary function is not the criterion of death, in the vast majority of deaths not complicated by artificial ventilation, it is a completely valid and reliable test for determining that the criterion is satisfied. The physical findings of permanent absence of heartbeat and respiration show that the criterion of death has been satisfied because, in the absence of artificial ventilation, the absence of heartbeat and respiration always quickly produces permanent loss of natural functioning of the whole brain. However, when mechanical ventilation is being used, these tests lose most of their utility due to the production of numerous false negatives, which can occur for as long as two months or more. It has become almost common for the death of the organism to occur while the circulatory-ventilatory subsystems are still intact. Although the circulatory-ventilatory tests suffice in the overwhelming majority of deaths, in cases where there is artificial maintenance of circulation or ventilation, special tests for permanent cessation of whole–brain natural functioning are needed.

Tests for Irreversible Cessation of Whole-Brain Functioning

Numerous formalized sets of tests have been established to determine that the criterion of permanent loss of whole-brain functioning has been met.[27] What we call tests has sometimes been called "criteria," but it is important to distinguish these "second-level criteria" or tests from the criterion of death itself. While the criteria for the death of the organism must be understandable by the layman, the (second-level criteria) tests to determine the permanent loss of natural functioning of the whole brain need not be understandable by anyone except qualified clinicians. To avoid confusion, we prefer to use the designation "tests" for the "second-level criteria."

All the proposed tests require total and permanent absence of all natural functioning of the brain stem and both hemispheres of the brain. They vary slightly from one set to another, but all require unresponsivity (deep coma), absent pupillary light reflexes, apnea (inability to breathe), and absent brain stem reflexes. They also require the absence of drug intoxication and low body temperature, and the newer sets require the demonstration that a lesion of the brain exists. Isoelectric (flat) EEGs are generally required, and tests disclosing the absence of cerebral blood flow are of confirmatory value. All tests require the given loss of function to be present for a particular time interval, which in the case of the absence of cerebral blood flow may be as short as thirty minutes.

Current tests of irreversible loss of whole-brain function may produce many false negatives of a sort during the thirty-minute to twenty-four-hour interval between the successive neurological examinations that different tests require. Certain sets of tests, particularly those requiring electrocerebral silence by EEG, may produce false negatives if an EEG artifact is present and cannot confidently be distinguished from brain wave activity. Generally, a few brief false negatives are tolerable and even inevitable, because tests must be delineated conservatively in order to eliminate any possibility of false positives. When a physician properly performs and interprets the validated tests for loss of whole-brain function outlined in the 1981 report of the medical consultants to the President's Commission, he can be confident that the loss of whole–brain natural functioning is permanent.[28]

A Legal Definition of Death

In July 1981, the President's Commission for the Study of Ethical Problems in Medicine and Biomedical and Behavioral Research published its report, "'Defining Death,' a Report on the Medical, Legal, and Ethical Issues in the Determination of Death." In this report, the Commission proposed a statute, the Uniform Determination of Death Act (UDDA), which provides a criterion of death that is to serve as the legal definition of death.

An individual who has sustained either (1) irreversible cessation of circulatory and respiratory functions, or (2) irreversible cessation of all functions of the entire brain, including the brain stem, is dead. A determination of death must be made in accordance with accepted medical standards.[29]

This statute or an equivalent, which has been adopted by almost all state legislatures, has given rise to the view that there are two criteria of death: irreversible cessation of circulatory and respiratory functions, and irreversible cessation of all functions of the entire brain, including the brain stem. However, as we pointed out earlier, the first of these supposed criteria, irreversible cessation of circulatory and respiratory functions, is not properly regarded as a criterion at all; it is, at most, a test to show that the second supposed (and actual) criterion, irreversible cessation of all functions of the entire brain, including the brain stem, has been satisfied. The statute has to be interpreted not as proposing two distinct criteria for death, but rather as proposing a complex two-part criterion. Otherwise, it is subject to the criticism that we pointed out earlier, that the first supposed criterion, irreversible cessation of circulatory and respiratory functions, is ambiguous, not distinguishing between spontaneous and artificially supported circulatory and respiratory functions.

The wording of the UDDA statute of death promotes the idea that there are two kinds of death: heart death and brain death. Because heart death is most well known, and most easily determined, brain death is thought of as a new form of death, one that applies only to those who are on some form of artificial life support. Some have considered that brain death is not really death at all, but merely a legal maneuver to stop life-support systems. Hans Jonas (1974) has asked, "Why are they alive if the heart, etc., works naturally but not alive when it works artificially?" We think that it reduces confusion to make clear that there is only one criterion of death, the irreversible cessation of all natural functions of the entire brain, including the brain stem. That should be the legal definition of death and it should be made clear that the other part of the proposed criterion of death, irreversible cessation of *spontaneous* (our addition) circulatory and respiratory functions, is only a test that the real criterion has been satisfied.

We have revised the UDDA statute of death with these points in mind:

An individual who has sustained irreversible cessation of all natural functions of the entire brain, including the brain stem, is dead.

(a) In the absence of artificial means of cardiopulmonary support, death (the irreversible cessation of all natural brain functions) can be determined by the prolonged absence of spontaneous circulatory and respiratory functions.

(b) In the presence of artificial means of cardiopulmonary support, death must be determined by tests of natural brain function.

In both situations, the determination of death must be made in accordance with accepted medical standards.[30]

By using the irreversible cessation of spontaneous circulatory and respiratory functions as a test for irreversible loss of whole-brain natural function, our proposed statute allows us to answer the question raised by Jonas, "Why are they alive if the heart, etc., works naturally but not alive when it works artificially?" Our proposed statute makes clear that spontaneous circulation and ventilation show that at least part of the brain continues to function, whereas artificial support does not show this. Thus, in the latter case one must directly test if the whole brain has permanently ceased to function naturally.

Finally, our statute makes explicit that it is the brain, not the heart and lungs, that is essential both for any observable natural functioning of the organism as a whole, and for any part of the organism to be conscious. Our statute allows for new technological advances, such as a totally implantable artificial heart, which may continue to function after the entire brain has permanently ceased to function, or for implanted brain chips, which may continue to perform the functions of the brain stem even though it has permanently ceased to function naturally.

A statutory definition of death should include as a criterion of death only the irreversible cessation of total, natural brain functions, for only that criterion always satisfies the ordinary definition of death: the permanent cessation of all observable natural functioning of the organism as a whole, and the permanent absence of consciousness in the organism as a whole, and in any part of that organism. Irreversible cessation of spontaneous ventilation and circulation can continue as the usual method for determining death, but this method should not be elevated to the status of a criterion of death. Rather, it should be explicitly noted that the cessation of these functions is only the most common test for determining that the true criterion of death—irreversible, total cessation of whole–brain natural functioning—has been satisfied.

Conclusion

We have shown that the meaning of a common word like "death," which is an integral part of many social and legal practices, cannot be separated from its use in those practices. Attempts to use a better understanding of the biological facts concerning death to revise what is meant by "death" are based on a misunderstanding of how the meaning of such a word is determined. Although death is a biological phenomenon, it is not an esoteric event but one with which the vast majority of humanity has had experience. From prehistoric times until the end of humankind, death has been and will be a familiar experience. People have killed animals for food, children have seen their pets die, and wars, famine, and maladies have resulted in death for countless people. Throughout all of this time, there have been almost no problems in determining who had died and who was still living. There have been some problems; some people have been buried who were not yet dead but only in a profound coma. However, these problems have been rare and with increasing medical sophistication it has become possible to determine who is dead with 100% accuracy.

This increasing medical sophistication, however, has also brought with it pressure to determine the time of death with greater speed. This speed is desired not merely to prevent pointless use of expensive medical treatment but, most important, to allow the harvesting of organs while they are in the best possible condition, thereby improving the chances for a successful transplant. This increasing medical sophistication and these goals also prompted a reconsideration of the concept of death. In many cases, this medical sophistication has made it impossible to determine death in the way that it had been usually determined throughout the history of humankind, that is, by noting when the person stopped breathing and his heart stopped beating. Techniques and machines have become available that can maintain breathing and heart functioning even though the person is dead. The goals of avoiding useless care and obtaining organs in better shape for transplantation made it desirable for a person to be declared dead even though these techniques and machines were maintaining heart and lung function.

A closer examination of the concept of death makes it clear that the absence of heart and lung function was historically such a reliable test of death because absence of breathing and absence of circulation inevitably lead to the permanent loss of natural functioning of the entire brain. The complete and permanent loss of whole-brain function inevitably results *in the permanent cessation of all observable natural functioning of the organism as a whole, the permanent absence of consciousness in the organism as a whole, and in any part of that organism.* It was this permanent cessation of natural functioning of the organism as a whole, and the permanent absence of consciousness that was always understood, although not explicitly, as death. One may see this by looking at stories in which either natural functioning of the organism as a whole or consciousness is present. In these cases, it is universally held that the person is not dead.

Not surprisingly, before it became clear what was meant by death, there was some disagreement about what should serve as the criterion of death, and what should serve as appropriate tests to determine that the criterion was satisfied. Prior to the advent of modern medicine, it was not necessary to distinguish clearly between the tests of death, the criterion of death, and the definition of death. If, for a significant period of time, a person stopped breathing and his heart stopped beating, he was dead. But with the advent of modern medicine, with so many people dying in the hospital while attached to so many machines, it is necessary to be more precise about what is meant by death. What is the medical criterion on the basis of which a person is declared dead? And what are the tests to determine that the criterion is satisfied? In the beginning of this discussion, there was more concentration on the criterion of death than on the definition of death. In fact, because the criterion of death was the legal definition of death, many people were not always clear whether they were discussing the medical criterion of death or the definition of death. Thus, for a long time, it seemed as if people thought that providing a definition of death was a matter to be determined on medical grounds.

Only relatively recently has it been recognized that an account of the ordinary meaning of the term "death" must be provided before one could settle on the appropriate criterion of death. For the criterion of death is that state of the organism on the basis of which medical personnel determine that the organism satisfies the definition of death, that is, the organism is dead. The two main proposals for a definition of death are that death means the permanent loss of all features of personhood, namely, the permanent loss of consciousness, and that death means the permanent loss of all observable natural functioning of the organism as a whole. However, it is clear that neither of these proposals, by itself, is adequate and that the loss of both of these features is necessary for death.

Once one recognizes that both features are necessary, it is clear which of the various proposed criteria of death—permanent loss of natural functioning of (1) the cortex, (2) the brain stem, (3) the whole brain, and (4) heart and lungs—is correct. Only the third criterion, the loss of whole-brain natural functioning, is perfectly correlated both with loss of all observable natural functioning of the organism as a whole, and with total absence of consciousness. The fourth criterion turns out to be ambiguous, for it can mean either (4a) loss of spontaneous heart and lung functioning, or (4b) loss of all heart and lung functioning, either spontaneous or artificially supported. Criterion 4a can be used as a test when the person is not on a heart-lung machine, for then it is clear that the criterion—the whole brain having permanently stopped natural functioning—must be satisfied. Criterion 4b, however, cannot be used as a test, for even if a person does not meet this criterion, although his lungs continue to breathe and his heart continues to beat (albeit only because he is on a heart-lung machine), the correct criterion of death might still be satisfied, and he might still be dead.

Notes

1. For similar reasons, some physicians have adopted controversial tests of death so as to facilitate faster harvesting of organs. If there is the slightest chance that these tests would ever yield a false positive, that is, result in someone being declared dead who is not dead according to the accepted definition and criteria of death, these tests should not be allowed. We discuss the criterion and tests of death later in this chapter.

2. See Linda Emmanuel (1995, 27).

3. Ibid.

4. See Culver and Gert (1982).

5. See Linda Emmanuel (1995, 27).

6. See chapter 12 on euthanasia for a discussion of a proposal for dealing with those in a persistent vegetative state.

7. "Death" can be applied in a metaphorical way to companies, projects, feelings, and so on, but almost everyone recognizes that this is not using "dead" in the basic or literal sense.

8. See White, Wolin, Verdura, et al. (1971) and O'Shea (1990).

9. See Gert (1967, 1971).

10. See Gert (2005, 47).

11. Parts of this section are adapted from Bernat, Culver, and Gert (1981).

12. Patients who have been determined by the laboratory to still have some functioning neuroendocrine cells have been declared dead and will continue to be declared dead; this determination is completely appropriate. It is not necessary to perform tests on patients to see if there are any functioning cells remaining before they are declared dead, as long as it is certain that there is a permanent absence of consciousness in the organism as a whole, and in any part of that organism and the cells have permanently ceased all observable functions of the organism as a whole.

13. See Gert (1971).

14. Establishing a criterion for consciousness is very difficult; however, normal human social behavior is a paradigm of conscious behavior and any animal behavior that is sufficiently similar to normal human social behavior is usually regarded as manifesting consciousness, for example, social behavior among mammals. A criterion of consciousness is a display of a learned response to artificial stimuli, for example, a dog sitting up in response to the word "beg." An even clearer criterion is the restraining of a natural response because of learning, for example, a dog not attacking another dog because of the word "stay."

15. See Gert (1971).

16. See Culver and Gert (1982, 182).

17. Ibid.

18. Ibid.

19. See Jennett and Plum (1972).

20. See Multi-Society Task Force on PVS (1994).

21. See, for example, two works by George Orwell: *Animal Farm* (1945) and *1984* (1949).

22. As we understand the concept of a person, it is at least partly historic. If an organism was a person, it remains a person as long as there is any possibility of any future consciousness. This means that any actual consciousness, even if it is only of pain, entails that the patient remains a person and must be treated as such.

23. See chapter 12 on euthanasia for a more detailed account of our proposal for dealing with patients in a persistent vegetative state who have not filled out an advance directive.

24. See Bernat (2002, 273–274n24).

25. See ibid., 251–252.

26. See ibid., 249.

27. Report of the Medical Consultants on the Diagnoses of Death to the President's Commission for the Study of Ethical Problems in Medicine and Biomedical and Behavioral Research (1981).

28. Ibid.

29. Ibid.

30. This statute is similar to one proposed by the Law Reform Commission of Canada (1979).

12

Euthanasia

A Moral Dilemma for Physicians

In the developed countries, the benefits of public health measures and new drugs had, until the AIDS epidemic, dramatically reduced deaths due to infectious disease. This had resulted in a significant increase in the number of older people suffering from chronic diseases that are often progressive, incapacitating, and terminal. Coincidentally, AIDS is, in these respects, very similar to the chronic diseases of the elderly, and what we say about elderly patients also applies to patients with AIDS. Patients with terminal illnesses that are accompanied by considerable pain and suffering often do not wish their disease to be treated aggressively. All want the pain and suffering to be minimized, but many, at least at some stage, do not want their lives prolonged. In fact, many actually want their lives shortened; they want to die sooner than they would if they simply waited for the disease to run its natural course.

This has put a considerable burden on physicians, whose culture, tradition, and instincts are devoted to the prolonging of life, not to the shortening of it. Of course, physicians also consider their profession to be devoted to the relieving of pain and suffering, but in the past these two goals were not usually seen as conflicting with each other; treatments that relieved pain and suffering were also generally life preserving. The increase in the number of elderly patients with chronic diseases, for whom death is the only way to avoid significant pain and suffering, has increased the frequency of conflict between two of the acknowledged goals of medicine: prolonging life, and relieving pain and suffering. Physicians faced with this conflict are often unsure how to respond in a morally acceptable way. One the one hand, if they stop treating patients, not only do they fear they may be violating the rule against killing but also that they will be violating what many take to be the most important duty of a physician: to preserve life. On the other hand, if they do not abide by the patients' wish to die, not only may they be depriving patients of the freedom to make their own decisions, they may also be violating another important duty of physicians: to relieve pain and suffering.[1] This has created for many physicians what seems like an unresolvable moral dilemma.

In actual practice, far too many physicians do not provide sufficient relief for the pain and suffering of those who are suffering from chronic diseases or are terminally ill. Inadequate palliative care is one of the significant reasons patients seek to die. Everyone agrees that adequate palliative care should be provided to those terminally ill patients who could benefit from it. The only questions are practical ones, for example, how does one train physicians to take the pain and suffering of terminally ill patients more seriously and to provide adequate palliative care? We think that if such care were universally provided, the question of euthanasia would arise far less frequently.[2] We are concerned that some proposals under discussion, for example, legalizing physician-assisted suicide and even active euthanasia, are likely to perpetuate the failure to provide adequate palliative care. Nonetheless, there still are some situations where palliative care is not sufficient and patients want to die sooner than they would if either life-prolonging treatment were continued or if they simply waited for the disease to run its natural course. In these situations, providing palliative care does not resolve the doctors' dilemma.

Active and Passive Euthanasia

In order to help resolve this dilemma, a distinction has traditionally been made between active and passive euthanasia. Active euthanasia is considered killing and, even if requested by the patient, is prohibited by the American Medical Association and by all state laws. Passive euthanasia is considered "allowing to die" and, if requested by the patient, is permitted. What is the difference between active and passive euthanasia? The following are the standard ways of making the distinction: (1) acts versus omissions, (2) stopping treatment (withdrawing) versus not starting treatment (withholding), (3) ordinary care versus extraordinary care, and (4) whether or not the death is due to natural causes. However, none of these ways of distinguishing between active and passive euthanasia has any clear moral significance. It is worthwhile to show their inadequacies before presenting a morally significant way of distinguishing between active and passive euthanasia.

Our concern in this chapter is only with voluntary euthanasia, those cases in which a competent patient has explicitly expressed his rational desire to die. Euthanasia with regard to incompetent patients presents even more difficult problems, but we believe that until it is completely clear what to do with competent patients, it will be impossible to become clear about what to do with incompetent patients. A clear example of euthanasia for incompetent patients being parasitic on euthanasia for competent patients is when the incompetent patient has an advance directive. Insofar as possible, the advance directive of the formerly competent patient should be followed just as if the patient were still competent. The most difficult cases are those of nonvoluntary euthanasia, in which the patient is permanently incompetent and has never expressed his desires on the matter. Later in this chapter, we suggest how to avoid some of these difficulties and propose a long-term procedure for dealing with the remaining problems.

The point of distinguishing between active and passive euthanasia is to help physicians resolve the moral dilemma caused by caring for patients for whom death seems a rational way to relieve their pain and suffering. Many physicians believe it is morally unacceptable to kill a patient, even at a competent patient's rational request, and yet they recognize the pointlessness of keeping a patient alive when the primary result is more pain and suffering. Physicians hope to resolve the dilemma by distinguishing between active and passive euthanasia, counting only the former as killing and the latter as allowing to die. This distinction is intended to allow physicians to continue to hold that it is morally unacceptable to kill a patient, but at the same time to maintain that it may sometimes be morally acceptable to allow a patient to die. This immediately raises the question, Is there a morally relevant distinction between killing and allowing to die, and if so, how should it be made?[3] Our examination of four above-stated ways of making this distinction will show that none of them provide a way of making a morally relevant distinction between killing and allowing to die.

Acts Versus Omissions

The philosophical distinction between acts and omissions initially seems a natural way to distinguish between killing and allowing to die. According to this approach, if a physician *does* something, performs an action, for example, injects an overdose of morphine or turns off the respirator, it counts as active euthanasia; it is considered killing, and is prohibited. If the physician does nothing, but rather simply fails to do something, for example, does not turn on the respirator, does not provide essential antibiotics, or does not do CPR, that is an omission; it counts as passive euthanasia, and is considered allowing to die, and is permitted. This way of distinguishing between killing and letting die requires that there be a significant moral distinction between a physician turning off an intravenous solution container (an act) and not replacing it when it is empty (an omission). Since it has not been shown that there is such a moral distinction (i.e., that the act is morally prohibited, but omission is morally allowed), some have claimed that the standard medical and legal practice, which permits allowing to die and does not permit killing, should be given up.[4]

Further, the distinction between acts and omissions is a difficult one to make. Some acts do not even require any bodily movement at all, for example, standing at attention. How could such a subtle philosophical distinction be essential for making a fairly common moral decision? The discussion in chapter 2 showed that morality is a public system that applies to all rational persons and, hence, must be understandable by all of them. The subtle distinction between acts and omissions is not even well understood by philosophers, hence it cannot be an essential feature of morality. Moreover, if a physician has a duty to prolong the life of her patients, then even if the distinction between acts and omissions were clear, it would not have any moral significance. If a physician has such a duty, then her failing to do so is clearly morally unacceptable, even if that failing is an omission on any plausible account of acts and omissions. No one would hold that a physician is morally allowed to neglect her duty if she does so by omissions rather than acts.[5]

Not Starting Versus Stopping (Withholding Versus Withdrawing)

Another proposal that has great appeal for some doctors is the distinction between not starting a treatment and stopping it (withholding a treatment versus withdrawing it). These doctors maintain that if the patient does not want treatment, physicians do not have a duty to start it. Once treatment is started, however, physicians have a duty to continue it if discontinuing it would lead to the patient's death. They are not required to force a patient to go on a respirator if the patient refuses, but once the patient has gone on the respirator, doctors have a duty to keep him on it, even contrary to the patient's wishes, if taking him off would result in his death.

Accepting this way of making the distinction between active and passive euthanasia creates serious practical problems. Some physicians are hesitant to put seriously ill patients on respirators if they think the patients have poor prognoses and are likely to become respirator dependent. This hesitancy may be due to the prospect of being required to continue a pointless treatment that only prolongs the pain and suffering of patients. One result is that a patient who has a very small but finite chance of recovering may sometimes not be put on the respirator because once put on, it is mistakenly believed that he cannot be taken off. Thus, this attempt to resolve the moral dilemma creates additional problems of its own.[6]

Further, it has not been shown that there is any morally significant difference between stopping a treatment and not starting it. Consider two patients who have been in an accident, identical twins with identical presenting diagnoses and prognoses. When they arrive at the hospital, everyone agrees that they are unlikely to survive. One twin is conscious and refuses to be put on a respirator; the other twin is put on a respirator while still unconscious. If one were to use the distinction between not starting and stopping in order to make the distinction between active and passive euthanasia, the second twin, if he becomes conscious several minutes after he is put on the respirator, cannot be taken off even if he requests it. This follows, even though—except for the fact that he is already on the respirator—he is identical to the twin who has refused to be put on a respirator. Both patients want to die, and without the respirator both would die. Why should the fact that treatment has been started, perhaps mistakenly, make it morally wrong to stop it, when it would have been morally acceptable not to start it? It is psychologically harder to withdraw treatment than withhold it, but recognizing that there is no moral difference between withholding and withdrawing may help to ease the physician's psychological burden.

Ordinary Care Versus Extraordinary Care

The next ad hoc attempt to explain the distinction between active and passive euthanasia employs a distinction between ordinary care and extraordinary care. If, given the condition of the patient and the facilities and resources available, the care counts as ordinary, according to this way of making the distinction, not only is a physician required to continue it, she is required to start it (e.g., a course of antibiotics for an easily curable infection). However, if the care counts as extraordinary (e.g., difficult to obtain or very expensive), she is neither morally required to start it, nor is she morally required to continue it. A very significant implication of this way of making the active-passive distinction is that it is almost always morally wrong not to provide food and fluids; providing food and fluids, in all normal situations, counts as ordinary care. On this account, the line between ordinary and extraordinary care not only changes over time but may also be different in different places. Whether a treatment is ordinary or extraordinary can be a function of the available level of technology, for example, changes in the availability of dialysis machines and improvements in transplant surgery. Although it may have some moral significance, this way of distinguishing between ordinary and extraordinary treatment does not seem to distinguish between killing and allowing to die.[7]

The original way of making the ordinary and extraordinary distinction, namely, comparing the burden imposed on the patient with the benefit to be gained by him, has clear moral significance. If this comparison shows the burden to be "extraordinary," that is, much greater than the likely benefit, treatment can be stopped, or not started; if the burden is "ordinary," that is, small relative to the likely benefit, it cannot be stopped once started. This interpretation raises the question, Who determines if the burden is ordinary or extraordinary, the physician or the patient? If it is the physician, there is a great danger of unjustified paternalism. If it is the patient, then, as we argue below, when he is competent and his decision is not irrational, what he says determines the matter. If he chooses to die rather than continue with treatment, it is morally unacceptable to continue, whether the burden is ordinary or extraordinary according to any other standard. However, suppose the patient determines that simply continuing to live is an extraordinary burden and requests the physician to shorten his time of living. What should the physician do? The ordinary-extraordinary distinction, no matter how it is made, does not provide an answer to this question.

Whether Death Is Due to Natural Causes

Euthanasia is sometimes regarded as passive if death is due to natural causes. Thus, stopping or not starting a course of antibiotics is often regarded as passive euthanasia because the patient's death is due to his infection, a natural cause. On the other hand, providing a patient with pills that will kill him, or more clearly, injecting the patient with some drug that kills him, is active euthanasia, for the patient's death is not due to natural causes, but rather to the physician injecting a drug. Because in stopping or not starting a course of antibiotics, the death is caused by the disease process, no person is assigned responsibility for the death. This freedom from responsibility for the patient's death is psychologically helpful to the physician. To make some state laws authorizing advance directives more acceptable to the public and to physicians they have even been labeled "natural death acts."

When death rezsults from lack of food and fluids, however, it is less plausible to say that the death is due to natural causes. Thus, someone must be assigned responsibility for the patient's death, and many physicians wish to avoid this responsibility. A partial explanation for the overuse of technology to unjustifiably prolong dying may be an attempt by physicians to avoid responsibility for a patient's death. But if the refusal of food and fluids is rational and made by a competent patient, then the patient is responsible for his own death. Physicians who recognize that patients have the authority to refuse any treatment, including hydration and nutrition, are more likely to avoid unjustified feelings of responsibility for their deaths.[8] However, even holding a patient responsible for his own death is more troubling than assigning the responsibility to natural causes such as the underlying disease process. It is far easier to view stopping or not starting the respirator as allowing the underlying disease process to take its course. Withholding or withdrawing food and fluids, especially if the patient can eat and drink in the normal way, creates a new malady, dehydration, which becomes the cause of death. Thus, withholding or withdrawing food and fluids has been regarded by some as more like killing than not starting or stopping a specific life-prolonging treatment.[9]

If one accepts the view that passive euthanasia requires that the death be due to natural causes, but nevertheless regards allowing patients to refuse food and fluids as morally acceptable, one can take advantage of the fact that the term "natural" is open to many interpretations. To reconcile these two positions, one must hold the view that patients can refuse intravenous feeding tubes because they are not natural, and that the patient is dying from his inability to eat or drink in a natural way. However, this interpretation has the disturbing implication that patients who can eat and drink in the natural way are not allowed to refuse food and fluids, even if they are competent and their refusals are rational.

"Natural" is often used as a word of praise, or more generally, as a way of condoning something that otherwise would be considered unacceptable.[10] However, the condoning or condemning of something is not, in fact, determined by whether it is natural; rather, if it is condemned, it is often called unnatural, and if it is condoned, it is labeled as natural. But, just as it is erroneous to think that the distinction between acts and omissions has any moral relevance, it is also erroneous to think that anything morally significant turns on the use of the term "natural" or the phrase "due to natural causes." If a competent patient has rationally refused food and fluids, we will argue below that it is morally and legally unacceptable to overrule that refusal, whether or not the food and fluids are administered in a natural way, or only intravenously.

Using the Common Moral System

The above four ad hoc distinctions mistakenly focus on what the physician does or does not do, or with the medical context in which the physician acts or does not act, but they do not adequately consider the decisions of the patient. It is the failure to appreciate the moral significance of the kind of decision the patient makes, that is, whether it is a request or a refusal, that leads to the mistaken conclusion that there is no morally significant distinction between active and passive euthanasia. A careful investigation of the duties of physicians is necessary before one can resolve the moral dilemma caused by having patients who believe that death is the best way to relieve their pain and suffering. Clarifying the duties of physicians requires using the standard medical distinction between requests and refusals. Overlooking this distinction made it impossible to solve this dilemma.

First, a terminological matter needs to be clarified. In the earlier sections of this chapter, we ourselves have used the term "request" when we were talking about refusals. It is perfectly standard English to say as we did that a patient requests that a treatment be stopped, for example, to be taken off of a respirator, when one is actually talking about refusals, for example, the patient is, in fact, refusing to continue to use the respirator. Unfortunately, this perfectly correct and common way of talking obscures the crucial distinction between refusals and requests. When combined with the use of the terms "choice" and "decision" to cover both requests and refusals, it fosters the false conclusion that all patient decisions or choices, whether refusals or requests, generate the same obligation on physicians.

This confusion is compounded because the most common use of the terms "decision" and "choice" with regard to a patient involves neither refusals nor requests, but rather the patient's picking one of the options that his physician has presented to him. However, when dealing with patients who want to die, this most common use of "decision" or "choice" is not relevant. Rather, a patient is either (1) refusing treatment, (2) requesting the physician to kill him (voluntary active euthanasia), or (3) requesting the physician to provide the medical means for the patient to kill himself (physician-assisted suicide). Thus, talking of a patient's decision or choice to die can be extremely misleading. Refusals of treatment and requests for treatment, whether or not death is a foreseeable result, are very different in their moral and legal implications.[11]

Physicians, as mentioned above, are troubled because they seem to have two irreconcilable duties: (1) to prolong the lives of their patients, and (2) to relieve patients' pain and suffering. Further, even if physicians do not believe that they always have a duty to prolong the lives of their patients, they still have a dilemma, for it seems to some physicians that the only way to relieve the pain and suffering of some of their patients is to kill them; but many physicians think that it is completely inappropriate for physicians to kill. In order to resolve this dilemma, the duties of physicians must first be determined. Then a morally significant way to make the distinction between active and passive euthanasia, or between killing and allowing to die, must be provided. The moral acceptability of physician-assisted suicide, a practice that is more than allowing to die, but less than killing, must also be considered.

The Duties of Physicians

It is important to determine what the duties of physicians are because neglecting one's duty needs to be morally justified, that is, there is a moral rule that requires doing one's duty. How are the duties of physicians determined? Partly, it is by looking at the society in which the physicians are practicing their profession. It cannot be assumed that physicians in every country have exactly the same duties, although substantial similarities should be expected. The duties that are involved in any job or profession are largely determined by the function of that job or profession in the society. The function of medicine is similar in every society, so one would expect physicians in all societies to have similar duties.

Some differences in the relative importance of different duties, however, should also be expected; for example, some societies place greater weight on duties to the individual patient while others place greater weight on duties to protect the health of the society as a whole.

However, the concept of duty is not completely equivalent to "what one is required to do by one's job or profession," so that anthropological investigation of a society does not completely determine what one's duties are. Duties must be compatible with what an impartial rational person can publicly allow. If no impartial rational person can advocate that a given kind of violation be publicly allowed, having a job or belonging to a profession cannot provide a duty to perform that violation. A "professional" pickpocket does not have a duty to steal, even if he is being paid to do so by his employer. Indeed, it is hard even to imagine a profession in which there is a duty to do what is morally unacceptable, although there are some who mistakenly view lawyers as sometimes having a duty to act in a morally unacceptable way if it is necessary to defend their clients. By showing that a kind of action that some have claimed that doctors have a duty to do involves an unjustified violation of a moral rule illustrates that physicians do not have a duty to do that kind of action. Thus, it may be possible to rule out as mistaken some claims about the duties of physicians without doing any anthropological investigations.

Paternalism and Patient Refusal

Physicians often violate the moral rule against causing pain with regard to their patients, because many treatments involve causing some pain. In most of these cases, however, the physicians are not only acting to prevent greater pain, or to prevent death, they are doing so with the valid consent of their patients. The patient usually has a rational desire that the physician cause him pain, for he prefers to have that pain inflicted rather than suffer the harms that he would suffer if the doctor did not administer the painful treatment. Causing pain to a patient with his valid consent in order to prevent greater harms or to promote compensating benefits is strongly justified, that is, all impartial rational persons would advocate that such violations be publicly allowed. This explains why it is morally significant to obtain valid consent, that is, uncoerced consent, by a competent patient who has been given adequate information. Having valid consent makes most medical treatments morally unproblematic.

Some patients prefer to suffer the harms that are likely to come from not being treated to the harms of being treated. If they do not fully understand the extent of the harms that they will suffer without treatment, then, of course, the physician has a duty to inform them of the consequences of not being treated. Sometimes, however, a patient who does fully understand the consequences of not being treated ranks the harms of treatment as worse than the harms of not being treated, and so does not want to be treated.[12] The physician who has suggested the treatment obviously ranks the harms differently. Whose ranking should determine whether the patient should be treated? Assuming that the physician's rankings are rational, there are two possibilities: (1) the patient's rankings are also rational, and (2) the patient's rankings are irrational. We have already pointed out that rational persons can rank the harms differently, so it should not be surprising that two rational persons can disagree on whether or not to undergo a given treatment.

Suppose the patient's rankings are both informed and rational. Would any rational person publicly allow a violation of the moral rule against causing pain when the person toward whom the rule is being violated rationally desires that it not be violated? Does it make any difference that the person doing the violating would want the rule violated with regard to herself, given the same harms being caused, avoided, and prevented? An indication of the morally misleading character of the Golden Rule, "Do unto others as you would have them do unto you," is that it allows an interpretation that advises violating a moral rule in these circumstances. If a patient is fully informed, and it is rational—that is, rationally allowed—to prefer the harms of not being treated to the harms of being treated, then in all normal cases, it is irrelevant what anyone else's preferences are, including those of family members or the physician; the patient's refusal should not be overruled. However, if the refusal is irrational or if it is clear that given the patient's values, it is unreasonable for him to prefer no treatment to forced treatment, then rational persons may favor publicly allowing that kind of violation. No impartial rational person would advocate that the violation of a moral rule be publicly allowed when the victim of the violation has a rational desire that it not be violated and there are no other countervailing morally relevant facts. Chapter 10 on paternalism provided more detailed arguments.

If the rankings of the patient are irrational, would impartial rational persons differ in whether they would advocate that physicians be prohibited from forcing treatment? It depends upon how seriously irrational the rankings are. If the balance of the harms of not being treated versus the harms of being treated is such that with the loss of freedom being added to the harms of being treated, it would no longer be irrational to prefer not being treated, then it still seems as if no impartial rational persons would advocate that such a violation be publicly allowed. (This is especially so when one appreciates that the harms of treatment are certain, whereas the benefits of treatment are usually only probable.) To allow such a violation would be to advocate that a violation of the rules be publicly allowed without the consent of the person, when the harm to be avoided or prevented by the violation is no greater than the harm to be caused. No impartial, rational person would favor publicly allowing overruling an irrational treatment refusal in those cases in which adding deprivation of freedom to the harms of treatment would make it rational to rank the total harm as worse than the harms of nontreatment. Publicly allowing such overruling would increase the chances of people suffering unwanted violations of the rules without any decrease in the amount of harm being suffered.

Finally, let us suppose that the rankings of the patient are so seriously irrational that even if one adds the loss of freedom that results from having one's decision overruled, it would still be irrational to prefer the harms of not being treated to the harms of being treated. Then, at least some impartial, rational persons would favor that kind of violation being publicly allowed, and so it would be at least weakly justified. It may not be strongly justified if the difference between the harms caused and the harms prevented is not great. In this kind of case, one might hold that publicly allowing such violations would result in enough mistakes and abuses that more overall harm would be suffered if that kind of violation were publicly allowed. However, if the harms prevented are serious enough and the harms caused trivial enough, all rational persons would favor that kind of violation being publicly allowed, and it would be strongly justified. In these kinds of cases, not only is the desire not to have treatment irrational, there is also no doubt that less harm will be suffered because of the violation, even if everyone knows such violations are allowed.

For the overruling of a refusal to be even weakly justified, the harms to be avoided or prevented by the violation must be serious. If the loss of freedom suffered from having one's refusal overruled counts as a greater harm than the harm that would be prevented or relieved, then that harm is a minor harm and forcing treatment to prevent this kind of minor harm would never be publicly allowed. However, often there is disagreement about the seriousness of the harms caused and the harms prevented, even when all agree the patient's refusal is irrational. When members of the health care team disagree as to whether the patient's refusal is irrational, or whether, given the patient's rational rankings, the refusal is unreasonable, overruling the refusal is not justified. Publicly allowing such overruling would increase the chances of people suffering unwanted violations of the rules when there is rational disagreement about whether there is any decrease in the amount of harm being suffered.

It should be noted that the conclusions reached in this section simply exemplify the points made in our earlier general discussion of the justification of paternalism. Contrary to the popular practice, we are not presenting an ad hoc discussion of when one should abide by a patient's refusal of treatment, including life-sustaining treatment, but rather are showing how our systematic account of rationality and morality informs and clarifies this discussion.

Refusal of Treatment and the Duties of a Physician

Overruling a competent informed patient's rational refusal of treatment, including life-preserving treatment, always involves depriving the patient of freedom, and usually involves causing him pain. We have just shown that no rational person would advocate that these kinds of paternalistic violations of moral rules be publicly allowed. Since it is morally prohibited to overrule the rational refusal of a competent, informed patient, it cannot be the duty of a physician to do so, for no one can have a duty to do what is morally unacceptable. Theoretically, the situation does not change when lack of treatment will result in the patient's death, but, as a practical matter, it does make a difference. Death is such a serious harm that it is never irrational to choose any other harm in order to prevent death. Even though it is sometimes rational to choose death over other harms, choosing death may be, and often is, irrational. People are usually ambivalent about choosing death, often changing their minds several times. But death is permanent, and once it occurs, no further change of mind is possible.

The seriousness of death requires physicians to make certain that patients recognize that death will result from lack of treatment. It also requires physicians to make sure that the harms patients are suffering cannot be relieved by adequate palliative care and that patients' continuing suffering is sufficient to make it rational for them to prefer death to continuing to live. The physician also must make sure that patients' desires to die and, hence, their requests to die, are not merely the result of a treatable depression. When patients are suffering from terminal diseases, however, it is generally the case that when they want to die, it is rational for them to choose death.[13] Further, although there is often some ambivalence, in our experience, patients' desire to die usually remains their dominant desire. When a competent, informed patient makes a rational decision to stop life-prolonging treatment, a physician cannot have a duty to overrule his refusal of treatment, even though treating him counts as trying to prevent his death.

We have shown that physicians cannot have a duty to preserve the lives of their competent patients when those patients want to die and their desires are informed and rational. When following the moral ideal of preserving life requires unjustifiably violating a moral rule, following the ideal is not only not morally good, it is not morally acceptable. We have thus established that physicians do not and cannot have a duty to prolong the lives of their patients when their patients have a rational desire to die. We are not suggesting that whenever a patient with a terminal illness makes any tentative suggestion that treatment be stopped, the physician should, with no question, immediately do so. It is part of the duty of a physician to make sure both that the refusal is rational and that it is the informed and considered preference of the patient. When, however, it is clear that a patient is competent, really does want to die, and the refusal is rational, then the physician is morally prohibited from treating him.

A Case of Overruling a Refusal of Treatment

Mr. L is a twenty-six-year-old, single, male patient with a past history of intense participation in physical activities and sports, who has suffered severe third-degree burns over two-thirds of his body. Both of his eyes are blinded due to corneal damage. His body is badly disfigured, and he is almost completely unable to move. For the past nine months he has undergone multiple surgical procedures (skin grafting, the eventual removal of his right eyeball, and amputation of the distal parts of the fingers on both hands). He has also required very painful daily bathings and bandage changings in order to prevent skin infections from developing over the burned areas of his body. The future he now looks forward to includes months or years of further painful treatment, many additional operations, and an existence as an at least moderately crippled and mostly (or totally) blind person. From the day of his accident, he has persistently stated that he does not want to live. He has been interviewed by a medical center psychiatrist and found to be bright, articulate, logical, and coherent. He is firm in his insistence that treatment be discontinued and that he be allowed to die. Nonetheless, his physicians are continuing to treat him.[14]

According to our definition, Mr. L's doctors are acting paternalistically: they believe that saving Mr. L's life benefits him; they know they are causing him great physical and psychological pain without his consent; and they know that Mr. L. believes that he can make his own decision on this matter. Mr. L's physicians could claim that they are acting as they are because they believe that the pain they are causing him by continuing treatment is a lesser harm than the death that would occur should they stop. Most burn victims share that ranking and consent to treatment. It is certainly a rational ranking on their part. If Mr. L agreed, then, although the physicians would still be violating the moral rule against causing pain, their having Mr. L's consent would make their actions strongly justified. Indeed, it would be morally unacceptable for them not to treat Mr. L. However, Mr. L. ranks the harms differently: he prefers death to months of daily pain and months or years of multiple surgical procedures, all of which will result in his being a severely disabled person. His ranking, like the opposing one of his physicians, is rational.

The kind of violation being engaged in by the physicians involves their causing a great amount of pain by imposing their rational ranking of harms on a person whose own rational ranking is different. No rational person would publicly allow this kind of violation because of the terrible consequences of living in a world where great pain could be inflicted on persons against their rational desires whenever some other person could do so by appealing to his own different rational ranking of harms. Thus, consideration of the consequences of publicly allowing the kind of violation in which the physicians are engaged leads to the conclusion that their paternalistic act is unjustified. Note how similar the reasoning and conclusion of this analysis are to the cases of paternalism discussed in chapter 10. The advantage of using the moral framework we provide is that it facilitates seeing the similarity in superficially dissimilar cases.

We mentioned above that if Mr. L agreed with the ranking of his physicians, it would be morally unacceptable not to treat him. A change in moral judgment would also occur if the case were varied in another way. Suppose Mr. L had to undergo only one week of painful treatment and then had a high probability of resuming an essentially normal life, one in which he could resume all of his former activities. If he claimed to prefer death over one week of treatment, we would deny that his ranking of harms was rational, if fact, we would regard it as seriously irrational. We would now describe the kind of violation being engaged in by the physicians as involving their preventing death by causing a great amount of pain for a short time for a person whose contrary ranking of harms is irrational. A rational person could publicly allow this kind of violation. We believe that considering the consequences of publicly allowing this kind of violation yields the conclusion that the paternalistic intervention of the physicians in this kind of case would be at least weakly justified.

Killing Versus Allowing to Die

Having shown that a physician does not have a duty to prolong the lives of competent patients who rationally prefer to die, the next issue to be settled is whether not treating such patients counts as killing them. If it does count as killing them, then the conclusions of the previous section may have to be revised. In the previous section we showed that physicians do not and cannot have a duty to overrule the rational refusal of a competent, informed patient. We also showed that even if prolonging life is following a moral ideal, in the circumstances of a competent patient's rational refusal, following this moral ideal does not justify breaking the moral rule against depriving of freedom. However, if not treating is killing, then not treating must itself be justified, for it would involve killing, perhaps the most serious violation of a moral rule.

Not treating is sometimes correctly regarded as killing. If a physician turns off the respirator of a competent patient who does not want to die, with the result that the patient dies, the physician has killed him. The same is true if the physician discontinues antibiotics or food and fluids, and it may sometimes count as killing if the physician refuses to start any of these treatments for his patient, when the patient wants the treatment and there is no medical reason for not starting it. Just as parents whose children die because of not being fed can be regarded as having killed their children, physicians who have a duty to provide life-saving treatment for their patients can be regarded as killing them if they do not provide that treatment. However, we have shown that a physician does not have a duty to provide life-saving treatment when a competent patient rationally refuses such treatment. Not treating counts as killing only when there is a duty to treat; in the absence of such a duty, not treating does not count as killing.[15]

When a competent, informed patient rationally refuses treatment, there is no duty to treat; thus, it does not make any moral difference whether the physician stops treating by an act, for example, turning off the respirator, or an omission, for example, not giving antibiotics. It also makes no moral difference whether the physician stops some treatment that has already started, for example, turning off the respirator or discontinuing antibiotics, or simply does not start such treatment. Granted that it may be psychologically easier to omit rather than act, and not to start than to stop, nevertheless, there is no moral difference between these different ways of abiding by a patient's refusal. Similarly, it makes no moral difference whether the treatment is extraordinary (e.g., involving some elaborate technology), is quite ordinary (e.g., simply providing food and fluids), or whether the death is due to natural causes. If there is no duty to treat, not treating is not killing. If a competent informed patient rationally refuses treatment, there is no duty to treat. Therefore, if a competent patient rationally refuses treatment, abiding by that refusal is not killing. Further, since the refusal is rational, it is, in fact, morally prohibited to override the patient's refusal by treating, and to do so is an unjustified deprivation of the patient's freedom.

Stopping Food and Fluids

One might object that the analysis given above does not apply to providing food and fluids because providing food and fluids, especially if they are not provided intravenously, is not a treatment, and so failing to provide food and fluids is not merely not treating, it is killing. As we noted before, children who die because their parents did not feed them are correctly regarded as having been killed by their parents. Similarly, one may object, patients who die because their physicians do not provide them with food and fluids are killed by them. This objection is based on the mistaken view that anything in our analysis depends upon the concept of treatment. Parents have a duty to feed their children, which is why it counts as killing if they do not feed them. Physicians have no duty to overrule rational refusals by competent patients, so their not doing anything to prolong the life of these patients, including providing them with food and fluids, does not count as killing. When a patient wants not to be kept alive and it is rational to want not to be kept alive, then it is morally required that his physician not force him to keep living. Further, it is a justified following of a moral ideal for his physician to continue to provide comfort and palliative care.

Since the point of dying sooner is to avoid the pain and suffering of a terminal illness, stopping only food and continuing fluids is not a good method of dying because it takes a much longer time, often several months. However, when fluids are also stopped, dying is much quicker; usually unconsciousness occurs within a week, and death about a week later. Further, contrary to what is widely assumed, dying because of lack of food and fluids is not painful, as long as there is even minimal nursing care.[16] When there is no medical treatment that is keeping the patient alive, stopping food and fluids may sometimes be the only way of allowing a patient to die. Again, stopping food and fluids rarely results in pain, and can always be made painless; the time it takes is long enough so that the patient has the opportunity to change his mind, but is short enough that significant relief from pain and suffering is gained. Indeed, death usually occurs as soon as or sooner than it would under all proposed physician-assisted suicide laws. Recognizing that abiding by the rational refusal of treatment, and of food and fluids, is not killing, but, at most, allowing to die, solves most of the practical problems with passive euthanasia that have led many to recommend legalizing physician-assisted suicide or active euthanasia.

Analysis of Killing

It may be thought that, if abiding by a patient's refusal of treatment requires the physician to perform some identifiable act (e.g., turning off a respirator), which is the act that causes the patient's death, then regardless of what was said before, the doctor has killed the patient. This may seem to have the support of the *Oxford English Dictionary*, which says that to kill is simply to deprive of life. However, this depends on what is meant by "deprive." And as we saw in the discussion of prohibiting the violation of the rule against depriving of freedom, it is not a simple matter to say what counts as "depriving" someone of something. It is not clear that the physician is "depriving" the refusing patient of anything. If one admitted that the physician is depriving the patient of his life, one could claim that she is justified in doing so because she is morally and legally required to turn off the respirator. However, this seems to entail that she is killing him. Even those who accept the death penalty, and hold that some prison official is morally and legally required to execute the prisoner, do not deny that the official has killed the prisoner. Killing in self-defense is both morally and legally allowed, yet no one denies that it is still killing. Similarly, one could agree that the doctor is doing nothing morally or legally unacceptable by turning off the respirator, even that the doctor is morally and legally required to turn off the respirator, yet claim that in doing so the doctor is killing the patient.

Accepting this analysis makes it seem plausible to say that an identifiable decision to omit a life-prolonging treatment, even if such an omission is morally and legally required, also counts as killing the patient. Why not simply stipulate that doctors are sometimes morally and legally required to kill their patients, namely, when their action or omission is the result of a competent patient rationally refusing to start or to continue a life-prolonging treatment? Isn't the important point that the doctor is morally and legally required to act as she does, not whether what she does is appropriately called killing? However, having a too simple account of killing may cause numerous problems. Although whether a doctor's abiding by a rational refusal counts as killing is not as important as whether she is morally and legally required to so abide, it is still significant whether such an action should be regarded as killing.

Many doctors do not want to regard what they do as killing their patients, even justifiably killing them. More important, all killing requires a justification or an excuse and, if all the morally relevant features are the same, the justification or excuse that is adequate for one method of killing should be adequate for all other methods of killing.[17] Thus, because some would not publicly allow other ways of killing, for example, injecting a lethal dose of morphine, then they would not publicly allow this way of killing, for example, disconnecting the patient from the respirator. If abiding by a competent patient's rational refusal of treatment is killing, then it might be justifiable to prohibit physicians from abiding by them when it is known that doing so will result in the patient's death. Since even advocates of active euthanasia do not propose that doctors should ever be morally and legally required to kill their patients, even justifiably, doctors would no longer be required to abide by rational refusals of treatment by competent patients that are known to result in death. Unless one favors such restrictions on patients' ability to hasten their death by refusing, changing the way killing is understood, that is, counting abiding by a patient's rational refusal as killing him, would have significant risks.

Those who favor legalizing active euthanasia do not want to require doctors to kill their patients; they merely want to allow those doctors who are willing to kill to do so. Similarly for physician-assisted suicide, no one suggests that a doctor be required to comply with a patient's request for a prescription for lethal pills. Since doctors are morally and legally required to abide by a competent patient's rational refusal of life-sustaining treatment, abiding by such a refusal is not only not regarded as killing but also not even regarded as assisting suicide. Providing a patient who refuses life-sustaining treatment with palliative care is not controversial either. Although some physicians feel uncomfortable doing so, no one wants to prohibit providing such palliative care. Neither killing a competent patient on his rational request, nor assisting him to commit suicide is morally uncontroversial. Nor does anyone claim that doctors are, or should be morally and legally required to do either. Thus, it is clear that abiding by a competent patient's rational refusal of treatment is not normally regarded as killing, or as assisting suicide, even when accompanied by palliative care.

Part of the problem is that insufficient attention is paid to the way in which the term "kill" is actually used. Killing is not as simple a concept as it is often taken to be. Killing is causing death, but what counts as causing any harm is a complex matter.[18] If the harm that results from a person's action, or omission, needs to be justified or excused, then he is regarded as having caused that harm. Of course, causing harm often can be completely justified or excused, so that a person can cause a harm and be completely free of any unfavorable moral judgment, for example, killing in self-defense. So killing, taken as causing death, may be completely justified, perhaps even morally required. Nonetheless, it is important to distinguish these morally justifiable acts of killing from those acts that need no justification or excuse although they result in a person's death, that is, they are not acts that killed the person or caused his death.

An action (or omission) intended to result in the death of a patient, which does result in his death, counts as killing, for such acts need justification. Furthermore, if the act that results in death is also a violation of one of the second five moral rules, knowingly performing the act (or omission) needs justification and so counts as killing. That is why a child who dies because her parents did not feed her means they have killed her, for parents have a duty to feed their children. This is also why it was important to make clear that doctors have no duty to treat, or even feed, patients who refuse treatment or food and fluids. However, if one does not intend, but only knows, that one's act will result in someone's death, and the act is not a violation of one of the other moral rules, then performing the act that has this result may not be done to cause the person's death or to kill him.[19]

When a doctor abides by the rational refusal of a competent patient, she is normally not violating any of the second five moral rules, or any moral rule at all. In fact, she is avoiding violating the moral rule prohibiting depriving a person of freedom, and may also be avoiding violating the rule prohibiting causing pain. The doctor's intention is to abide by the patient's refusal even though she knows that the result of her doing so will be that the patient dies. Even if the doctor agrees that it is best for the patient to die, her abiding by that refusal does not count as intentionally causing his death. Of course, an individual doctor can want the patient to die, but her intention in these circumstances is not determined by what is going on in her head. Rather, the intention is determined by what facts account for her action. If she would cease treatment even if she did not want the patient to die, and would not cease it if the patient had not refused such treatment, then her intention is not to kill the patient but to abide by the patient's refusal. Most doctors do not want to kill their patients even if such an action were morally and legally justified, and so their intention is clearly not to kill the patient, but simply to abide by their patients' rational refusals.[20]

Whether an act or omission that not intentionally but only knowingly results in someone's death, and does not involve a violation of one of the second five moral rules, counts as killing depends on whether those in the society regard such acts as needing a justification or an excuse.[21] In our society at the present time, doctors do not need a justification or excuse to abide by a competent patient's rational refusal even if everyone knows that such an act will result in the patient's death. Even when abiding by a competent patient's rational refusal results in death, it is not considered killing for a doctor to abide by such a refusal.[22] In our society at the present time, it is considered killing for a doctor to grant a competent patient's rational request to do something that will immediately result in the patient's death. Few who favor active euthanasia argue that such actions are not killings; rather, many argue that passive euthanasia, that is, abiding by patients' refusals, is also killing, and since it is allowed, active euthanasia should also be allowed.

Thus, as philosophers are wont to do, they accuse people of being inconsistent in allowing, or even requiring, passive euthanasia but not allowing active euthanasia or even assisting suicide.[23]

That our society does not regard the death resulting from abiding by a competent patient's rational refusal, even a refusal of food and fluids, as killing, is shown by the fact that almost all states have advance directives that explicitly require a physician to stop treatment, even food and fluids, if the patient has the appropriate advance directive. All of them also allow a presently competent patient to refuse treatment and food and fluids. None of these states allow a physician to kill a patient, no matter what. All but one of these states do not even allow physicians to assist suicide, which strongly suggests that turning off a respirator is not regarded even as assisting suicide when doing so is required by the rational refusal of a competent patient.

Abiding by a competent patient's rational refusal of treatment is not killing or assisting suicide, and it may even be misleading to say that the physician allows the patient to die. To talk of the physician allowing the patient to die suggests that the physician has a choice, that it is up to her to decide whether to prolong the patient's life. When a competent patient has rationally refused treatment, however, the physician has no choice. She is morally and legally prohibited from overruling the patient's refusal. She allows the patient to die only in the sense that it is physically possible for her to prolong the patient's life and she does not. Abiding by the rational refusal of life-saving treatment by a competent patient does not violate any moral rule. Overruling such a refusal is itself an unjustified violation of the moral rule against depriving of freedom. Thus, it is not merely morally acceptable to abide by such a refusal, it is morally required. It does not make any moral difference whether abiding by that refusal involves an act or an omission, stopping treatment or not starting it, whether the treatment is ordinary or extraordinary, or whether it results in a death from natural causes. If abiding by a competent patient's rational refusal of treatment or of food and fluids were all that was involved, there would be no further problems to resolve. However, it is normally the case that the doctor must also provide palliative care at the same time, and this creates a new problem.

Physician-Assisted Suicide (PAS)

Showing that it is morally and legally prohibited to overrule competent patients' rational refusals of treatment and of food and fluids does not solve the practical problem that doctors often face. For almost always, the disease that has led the patient to refuse treatment or to refuse food and fluids continues to involve some pain and suffering if there is no appropriate palliative care. Doctors are not morally and legally required to provide that palliative care to a patient who has refused life-prolonging treatment. This distinction between doctors being required to abide by a competent patient's refusal, but not being required to provide palliative care, was made quite clearly in the Elizabeth Bouvia case. This woman, who was suffering from a severe case of cerebral palsy and very crippling degenerative arthritis, wanted to stay in the hospital and be given palliative treatment while she was refusing food and fluids. Her doctors wanted to force her to take food and fluids. The court decided, correctly, that her doctors could not force her to take food and fluids, but that she could not force her doctors to keep her in the hospital and provide palliative care.

However, if a patient is competent and the request is rational, it would be justifiably acting on a moral ideal to help relieve the preventable pain and suffering of a patient who is refusing life-prolonging treatment. Providing such palliative care is neither killing nor even assisting suicide, but acting on one of the primary goals of medicine: to relieve pain and suffering. Thus, we strongly support doctors providing psychological support and appropriate palliative care to competent patients who have made rational decisions to discontinue life-prolonging treatment, including refusing food and fluids. Providing palliative care to competent patients who are rationally refusing treatment or food and fluids does not count as assisting suicide. However, if the patients' refusals of treatment, especially refusal of food and fluids, do count as suicide, then it seems, at least initially, that providing palliative care to these patients should count as assisting suicide.

There are two questions here. The first is whether a patient's refusal of treatment, including refusing food and fluids, counts as suicide. The second is whether a physician who provides palliative care for such a patient is assisting suicide. Indeed, usually a patient will not refuse treatment if the doctor will not provide the appropriate palliative care. If the answer to the first question is that the patient's refusal does not count as suicide, then there is no need to be concerned with the second question, for providing palliative care to such a patient cannot be assisting suicide. However, if the answer to the first question is that a patient's refusal does count as suicide, then it is still an open question whether providing palliative care to such a patient counts as assisting suicide.

Does the Refusal of Life-Sustaining Treatment Count as Suicide?

That patients' refusals are rational does not show that their actions do not count as suicide, for there can be rational suicide. However, if the refusal is irrational, it is more likely to be regarded as suicide. If suicide is regarded simply as killing oneself, then the analysis of killing should apply to it in a fairly straightforward fashion. An action or omission intended to result in the death of a patient, and which does result in his death, counts as killing. Therefore, one might argue that the refusal of treatment or food and fluids that is intended by the patient to result in his own death and which does result in his death, should count as suicide. And if "assisting suicide" is not an idiomatic phrase, but simply means doing those acts that help the person commit suicide, then physicians who provide palliative care to patients who are refusing life-sustaining treatments are assisting suicide. Accepting this analysis would make providing palliative care to a patient refusing life-preserving treatment a kind of assisted suicide.

This conclusion would place physician-assisted suicide much closer to passive euthanasia than to active euthanasia, and so allowing physician-assisted suicide, one could argue, need not lead to allowing active euthanasia. We agree with this aspect of the conclusion, for we believe that physician-assisted suicide does not violate the rule against killing, as active euthanasia does. We believe that the major argument against physician-assisted suicide is that legalizing it will have worse consequences than not legalizing it. Many also hold that doctors should not participate in that practice, that it is inconsistent with their role as physicians, and that it will adversely affect the way in which they are viewed by the public. But unless this change in the view of physicians has harmful consequences, it is not clear that it is a morally significant point.

It is compatible with our analyses so far that one can either be for or against legalizing physician-assisted suicide. We agree that one's view on this matter should be determined by the consequences of publicly allowing physician-assisted suicide. But we are also aware that different people can rank these consequences differently. How much additional unwanted pressure to commit suicide would legalizing physician-assisted suicide result in? How much pain and anxiety would be relieved by legalizing physician-assisted suicide? Even if one could answer these questions with any precision, which is extremely unlikely, it is still unlikely that everyone would agree whether the amount of pain and anxiety relieved outweighs the increase in the number of unwanted deaths, or vice versa.

However, it is not clear that the view held by some that suicide is simply killing oneself should be accepted. Partly, this may be because "killing oneself" does not seem to need a justification or excuse as much as does killing another person. This may be because our society, with some limitations, regards each person as allowed to do anything he wants to himself, as long as no one else is harmed. Indeed, it seems that any act that one does that is not intended to be immediately harmful but that one knows will result in one's own death does not count as suicide (except in the extended sense that someone who continues to smoke, drink, or eat too much, when she knows that it may result in her death, is said to be committing [slow] suicide).[24] It also seems that our society does not count as suicide any death that results from omissions—at least rational decisions to omit or to stop treatment—but only counts as suicide those positive acts that are done in order to bring about one's own death immediately, for these acts so closely resemble the paradigms of killing. The act-omission distinction that was incorrectly applied to killing may be correctly applied when talking about suicide. Patients who take some pills to bring about their own deaths are committing suicide, but those who have the respirator removed, or who refuse food and fluids are not regarded as committing suicide.[25]

This more complex analysis of suicide explains why the law has never regarded providing palliative care to those who are refusing treatment as assisting suicide. Even those states that explicitly forbid assisting suicide do not prohibit providing palliative care to those who are refusing treatment or food and fluids. Of course, as with killing, those who favor physician-assisted suicide favor the simpler account of suicide, claiming that some physician-assisted suicide is already allowed, so it is simply inconsistent not to legally allow more active physician-assisted suicide, which they regard as quicker and less painful than what they consider suicide by refusal of treatment, or food and fluids. That our society does not count refusals of treatment as suicide, and, hence, does not count palliative care for patients who refuse treatment as assisting suicide, is not intended as an argument against allowing physician-assisted suicide. However, it does show that one argument for physician-assisted suicide, namely, that physician-assisted suicide is already allowed by the act of providing palliative care for those who are refusing life-prolonging treatment, is based on a misunderstanding of how our society regards providing such palliative care.

Although our argument against physician-assisted suicide is not based on the use of the term "suicide," we are aware that calling a death a suicide has a negative connotation, even though suicide is no longer illegal. Whether one uses the term "suicide" depends, in part, on one's attitude toward the kind of act or omission taken by the person that results in his own death. Further, "assisting suicide" also has a negative connotation, and many physicians would refuse to carry out an act so named. We are concerned that describing the act of providing palliative care to those who refuse life-sustaining treatment as assisting suicide may discourage some physicians from providing that palliative care. We want to encourage physicians to provide palliative care; we are against any terminology that may discourage them from doing so. Thus, we are against counting as suicide any rational refusal of treatment, or food and fluids, and so do not count providing palliative care to patients who are refusing such treatment or food and fluids as assisting suicide.

We believe that the major argument against physician-assisted suicide is that, given the alternatives available, it does not provide sufficient benefit to patients to justify the risks that it poses. Patients already have the alternative of refusing treatment or food and fluids, and of being provided with palliative care while they are refusing that treatment. If physicians were to educate patients about these matters, and to make clear that physicians will support their choice and continue to care for patients if they choose to refuse treatment, there would be little, if any, call for physician-assisted suicide. Patients are far less likely to be pressured into refusing treatment than they are to avail themselves of physician-assisted suicide. There are also far fewer opportunities for abuse. Physician-assisted suicide provides less incentive to be concerned with palliative care. And finally, given the bureaucratic safeguards that most regard as necessary with physician-assisted suicide, death that resulted from refusal of food and fluids would come just as soon as or sooner than it would with physician-assisted suicide.[26]

In order to clarify this point and to provide a preferable alternative to physician-assisted suicide as a method for allowing seriously ill patients to determine the timing of their deaths, we think that states should consider passing legislation such as the following.

If a competent patient is terminally ill or suffering from a condition involving severe chronic pain or serious permanent disability, that patient's refusal of treatment, including refusal of food and fluids, shall not count as suicide, even though the patient knows that death will result from not starting or from stopping that treatment. All physicians and other health care workers shall be informed that they are legally prohibited from overruling any rational refusal of a competent patient, including refusal of food and fluids, even though it is known that death will result. All patients will be informed that they are allowed to refuse any treatment, including food and fluids, even though it is known that death will result, and that physicians and other health care workers are legally prohibited from overruling any such rational refusal by a competent patient.

Further, there shall be no prohibition placed upon any physician who provides pain relief in any form, in order to relieve the pain and suffering of the patient who has refused treatment, including food and fluids. In particular, providing pain medication shall not be considered as assisting suicide, and there shall be no liability for the physician who provides such pain medication for the purpose of relieving pain and suffering. The physician shall not provide such medication for the purpose of hastening the time of death, but is not prohibited from providing medication that is consistent with adequate pain relief even if he knows that such medication will hasten the time of death. Physicians are required to follow rigorously the accepted standards of medical practice in determining the competence of patients who refuse any treatment, including food and fluids, when physicians know that death will result from abiding by that refusal.

The Supreme Court Decision on Physician-Assisted Suicide

We are pleased that the United States Supreme Court reversed the rulings of the United States Court of Appeals for the Second Circuit and the Ninth Circuit, rulings that invalidated the New York and Washington State laws banning assisted suicide. However, we are troubled by some of the Supreme Court's arguments. The majority opinion by Chief Justice William Rehnquist is correct in denying the claim of the United States Court of Appeals for the Second Circuit "that ending or refusing lifesaving medical treatment 'is nothing more than assisted suicide.' Unlike the Court of Appeals, we [the Supreme Court] think the distinction between assisting suicide and withdrawing life sustaining treatment, a distinction widely recognized and endorsed in the medical profession and in our legal traditions, is both important and logical; it is certainly rational."

The Supreme Court is also correct in claiming that none of the following are constitutionally established rights: "a right to 'determin[e] the time and manner of one's death,' the 'right to die,' a 'liberty to choose how to die,' a right to 'control one's final days,' 'the right to choose a humane, dignified death,' and 'the liberty to shape death.'" According to the opinion of the Court, "the constitutionally protected right to refuse lifesaving nutrition and hydration that was discussed in *Cruzan* . . . was not simply deduced from abstract concepts of personal autonomy, but was instead grounded in the Nation's history and traditions, given the common law rule that forced medication was a battery, and the long legal tradition protecting the decision to refuse unwanted medical treatment." The Court was also correct in pointing out the interests that support a law prohibiting PAS, including "protecting the poor, the elderly, disabled persons, the terminally ill, and persons in other vulnerable groups from indifference, prejudice, and psychological and financial pressure to end their lives; and avoiding a possible slide towards voluntary and perhaps even involuntary euthanasia."

However, some claims that are made in the course of these decisions are quite misleading. For example, Rehnquist says, "When a patient refuses life sustaining medical treatment, he dies from an underlying fatal disease or pathology, but if a patient ingests lethal medication prescribed by a physician, he is killed by that medication . . . (when the feeding tube is removed, death 'result[s] . . . from [the patient's] underlying medical condition')." By putting the matter in this way, Rehnquist, like too many other jurists and philosophers before him, simply overlooks those cases in which a patient's refusal of food and fluids is not being administered intravenously. Someone who is able to eat and drink in the normal way and refuses food and fluids may not even be suffering from a terminal disease, but rather from severe chronic pain or serious permanent disability. In such a case, the patient does not die from "an underlying fatal disease or pathology," but from an electrolyte imbalance caused by the lack of fluids.

Rehnquist is closer to the mark when he says, "A physician who withdraws, or honors a patient's refusal to begin, life sustaining medical treatment purposefully intends, or may so intend, only to respect his patient's wishes and 'to cease doing useless and futile or degrading things to a patient when [the patient] no longer stands to benefit from them.' The same is true when a doctor provides aggressive palliative care; in some cases, painkilling drugs may hasten a patient's death, but the physician's purpose or intent is, or may be, only to ease his patient's pain. A doctor who assists a suicide, however, 'must necessarily and indubitably, intend primarily that the patient be made dead.'" But this way of putting it is misleading. It does not make clear that if the doctor intends the patient be made dead because that is required in order to respect the patient's refusal, he is not assisting suicide.

Although, in his concurring opinion, Justice John Paul Stevens gets this point about the intention of the doctor partly right, saying that a doctor who assists a suicide may only intend to respect his patient's wishes to commit suicide, he also makes a number of mistakes. He seems to equate refusing life-prolonging treatment with committing suicide and by using the phrase, "his patient's wishes," Stevens obscures the crucial distinction between requests and refusals. The crucial feature is that a physician is morally and legally required to comply with a patient's refusal of treatment, for not doing so is violating the patient's freedom. There is, however, no similar moral and legal requirement to grant a patient's request for lethal medication, nor does any proponent of legalizing physician-assisted suicide even propose that physicians be required to grant such requests. By failing to note the morally crucial distinction between refusals and requests, neither Rehnquist nor Stevens is able to explain why the right to refuse life-sustaining medication cannot be glossed simply as the right to die, and so forth. Nor is Stevens able to support as well as he could his claim that "the distinction between assisting suicide and withdrawing life sustaining treatment . . . is certainly rational."

Further, by using the phrase "medical treatment," Rehnquist continues the misleading view that a person only has the right to refuse *artificial* life support, rather than a more general right to refuse even *natural* life support, such as food and fluids. The court notes "nearly all states expressly disapprove of suicide and assisted suicide either in statutes dealing with durable powers of attorney in health care situations or in 'living will' statutes." Almost all state statutes make clear that a person has the right to refuse food and fluids. It is absurd to claim that providing nutrition and hydration to those who cannot eat in the normal way can be refused only because it is a medical treatment. As the Bouvia case and other cases have consistently decided, patients have the right to refuse food and fluids whether they are capable of taking food and fluids in the normal way or only intravenously.[27] Any competent patient is permitted to refuse food and fluids and physicians are more than permitted—they are encouraged—to provide her with palliative care while she is refusing, regardless of whether she is on life support. Consider the consequences of someone not being permitted to refuse taking food and fluids in the normal way while being permitted to refuse taking them intravenously. Imagine a patient who has a condition such that her refusal of intravenous food and fluids would be considered rational and thus must be respected. Now imagine that this same patient can eat and drink in the normal way, but refuses to do so. If this refusal is not respected, will she be force-fed intravenously? If so, this creates a serious problem, for by hypothesis, her refusal of intravenous food and fluids must be respected.

Stevens, in his concurring opinion, claims "that there are situations in which an interest in hastening death is legitimate," and even "that there are times when it is entitled to constitutional protection." But Stevens seems unaware that no one is even proposing a law that allows physician-assisted suicide without at least a two-week waiting period, so that legalizing physician-assisted suicide would not result in death coming earlier than by the refusal of food and fluids. Furthermore, the right to refuse food and fluids is already constitutionally protected. However, in other places Stevens is clear that he is not talking primarily about the hastening of death, but of how one dies. Stevens is correct that a person may have an interest in how she dies, for example, "in determining the character of the memories that will survive long after her death." However, given that the time involved in dying by refusing food and fluids is as short as or shorter than that provided by physician-assisted suicide, and that this way of dying can be as pain free as physician-assisted suicide, the state interest in preventing suicide would not have to be very great in order to allow states to continue prohibiting physician-assisted suicide.

Stevens also agrees with Rehnquist's mistaken view "that the distinction between permitting death to ensue from an underlying fatal disease and causing it to occur by the administration of medication or other means provides a constitutionally sufficient basis for the State's classification." Our point in this context is that it is not what causes death that justifies the distinction between refusing treatment and physician-assisted suicide. Rather, it is that refusing treatment is a constitutionally protected liberty interest that involves preventing unauthorized touching or forcing anything into a person, and there is no similarly strong liberty interest that involves preventing someone from assisting with a suicide. A patient who is suffering from severe chronic pain or serious permanent disability may refuse food and fluids and this refusal must be honored even though the patient will not die from an underlying fatal malady. It is the refusal, not the cause of death, that is important.

Other justices who concurred with Rehnquist's decisions also failed to take into account the option of refusing food and fluids. Justice Sandra Day O'Connor agrees that "a patient who is suffering from a terminal illness and who is experiencing great pain has no legal barriers to obtaining medication, from qualified physicians, to alleviate that suffering, even to the point of causing unconsciousness and hastening death." But O'Connor does not mention that all patients have the right to refuse food and fluids, taken normally or intravenously. Not only is it morally acceptable for physicians to provide patients with appropriate pain medication for the week or less that they remain conscious, present standards of medical practice encourage them to do so.

Knowledge of the facts is crucial in making any moral or legal decision, and unfortunately it seems that the Supreme Court, like both of the court of appeals cases that it overruled, did not know all of the relevant facts about the refusal of food and fluids. We are pleased that the Supreme Court rejected many of the court of appeals arguments and that it makes some of the same distinctions that we provide in our discussion of these decisions earlier in this chapter. However, we believe that by failing to uncover the real basis for the distinction between physician-assisted suicide and passive euthanasia, that is, that between *refusing* treatment or food and fluids, and *requesting* physician assistance in suicide, the Court perpetuates the confusion that permeates this issue.

Is Killing Patients Ever Justified?

Stopping food and fluids is often the very best way of allowing a patient to die, but one may claim that killing is sometimes better. Given present knowledge and technology, one can kill a patient absolutely painlessly within a matter of minutes. If patients have a rational desire to die, why wait several days or weeks for them to die? Why not kill them quickly and painlessly in a matter of minutes? We have provided no argument against killing patients who want to die that applies to an ideal world where there are never any misunderstandings between people and everyone is completely moral and trustworthy. In such a world, if one can inject the appropriate drugs and kill the patient painlessly and almost instantaneously, there is no need to worry about the distinction between killing and allowing to die, or between active and passive euthanasia. But in the real world, there are misunderstandings and not everyone is completely moral and trustworthy, so that in this world no one even proposes that killing patients be allowed without elaborate procedural safeguards, which almost always require waiting at least two weeks. So, on a practical level, legalizing physician-assisted suicide or killing would not result in a quicker death than stopping food and fluids.[28]

On our account, passive euthanasia is abiding by the rational refusal of life-saving treatment or food and fluids by a competent patient. Since there is no duty to overrule a rational refusal by a competent patient, abiding by this refusal does not count as killing. Further, failing to abide by such a refusal is itself morally prohibited, for it is an unjustified deprivation of the freedom of the patient. Also, in some newer codes of medical ethics, for example, that of the American College of Physicians, respecting patients' refusals is now listed as a duty. Physicians are not merely morally allowed to practice passive euthanasia, they are morally required to do so. Active euthanasia is killing; it is complying with the rational request of a competent patient to be killed. It involves active intervention by the physician that is more than merely stopping treatment. It is not simply abiding by the patient's desire to be left alone, it is, for example, injecting some substance that causes his death, when one has no duty to do so.

Since active euthanasia is killing, it is a violation of a moral rule and so needs to be justified. This contrasts quite sharply with passive euthanasia, and even physician-assisted suicide, which need not violate any moral rule, and hence may not even need to be morally justified. It is prolonging a patient's life by overruling that patient's refusal that involves the violation of a moral rule and hence needs to be justified. But, as we noted earlier, physicians often break the moral rule against causing pain with regard to their patients and are completely justified, because they do so at their patients' request, or at least with their consent, and do it in order to prevent what the patient takes to be a greater harm, for example, greater future pain or death. Why should active euthanasia be regarded as anything different from any other instance of a doctor breaking a moral rule with regard to a patient, at the patient's request or with his valid consent, in order to prevent what the patient takes to be a greater harm? In active euthanasia, the patient takes death to be a lesser harm than suffering pain and requests that the moral rule prohibiting killing be violated with regard to himself.

If causing pain can be justified, why is killing not justified when all of the other morally relevant features are the same? Because of a special feature of death that distinguishes it from all of the other serious harms, killing needs a stronger justification than violations of the other moral rules. The special feature is that after death, the person killed no longer exists, and so cannot protest that he did not want to be killed. All impartial rational persons would advocate that violations against causing pain be publicly allowed when the person toward whom the rule is being violated rationally prefers to suffer that pain rather than suffer some other harm, for example, greater pain or death. It is uncertain how many impartial, rational persons would advocate that killing be publicly allowed when the person being killed rationally prefers to be killed rather than to continue to suffer pain. This uncertainty stems from taking seriously the two features that make moral rules central to morality: the public character of morality and the fallibility of persons.

Violations of the rule against causing pain with valid consent can be publicly allowed without any significant anxiety being caused thereby. Patients need have no anxiety that the rule will be mistakenly violated and that they will suffer serious unwanted pain for a prolonged period, for they can usually correct the mistake rather quickly by ordering a stop to the painful treatment. Also, physicians have a strong incentive to be careful not to violate the rule by mistake, for patients will complain if they did not really want the rule violated. Violations of the rule against killing, even with valid consent, being publicly allowed may create significant anxiety. Patients may fear that the rule will be mistakenly violated and that they will have no opportunity to correct that mistake. That a patient will not be around to complain if the rule is mistakenly violated removes a strong safeguard against mistaken violations. It is not merely mistakes about which a patient would not be able to complain. If a physician tries to take advantage of this kind of violation being publicly allowed and intentionally kills a patient who has not requested to be killed, the patient would not be around to complain. Taking advantage of violations of the rule against causing pain being publicly allowed does not pose similar problems.

Although active euthanasia—killing a patient painlessly and quickly—when requested to do so by that patient, might, if publicly allowed, prevent a significant amount of pain and suffering, it would also be likely to create significant anxiety and some unwanted deaths. Impartial, rational persons can therefore disagree about advocating that such violations of the rule against killing be publicly allowed. There should be no disagreement among impartial, rational persons about passive euthanasia, for no moral rule is even being violated. Further, once it is recognized that withholding food and fluids (1) can be painless, (2) usually results in unconsciousness in one week and death in two weeks, (3) allows for patients to change their minds, and (4) is not killing at all, the need for active euthanasia or killing of patients, and even for physician-assisted suicide, significantly diminishes, even if it is not completely eliminated.

Unlike others who argue against active euthanasia, we do not claim that physician-assisted suicide and active euthanasia are morally unjustified, only that they are not strongly justified. Since they are only weakly justified, they are controversial. If the goal is to allow a patient to choose her own time of dying and also to allow dying to be accomplished relatively painlessly, there seems to be little need for active euthanasia or physician-assisted suicide. If patient refusal of treatment, including refusal of food and fluids, were not sufficient for a relatively quick and painless death for terminally ill patients, then we would favor physician-assisted suicide, although we would still have serious reservations about active euthanasia. However, since passive euthanasia, especially when this includes refusing food and fluids, is available together with appropriate palliative care, it seems far more difficult to justify controversial methods like physician-assisted suicide or active euthanasia. The harms prevented by physician-assisted suicide or active euthanasia are no longer the long-term suffering of patients who have no other way to die; they are only the one week of suffering that may be present while the patient is refusing food and fluids, and this suffering can be completely controlled by appropriate palliative care. This is an excellent example of why the presence of an alternative is a morally relevant feature (see chapter 2).

Given the alternative of refusing food and fluids, very little harm seems to be prevented by physician-assisted suicide or active euthanasia. The presence of an alternative that does not violate any moral rule is a morally relevant feature and makes it far more difficult to justify violating a moral rule. Thus, it seems far more difficult to justify active euthanasia. Physician-assisted suicide, if legalized, would not violate a moral rule, but it is questionable whether it provides sufficient benefits to justify the risks involved in legalizing it.[29] There are good reasons for believing that the advantages of refusing food and fluids, together with adequate palliative care, make it preferable to legalizing physician-assisted suicide. This is especially true in a multicultural society where doctors and patients sometimes do not even speak the same language. Even if there were a small number of cases in which refusal of food and fluids might be difficult, it is not clear how to weigh the benefit to this relatively small number of people to the harm that might be suffered by a great number of people by the legalizing of physician-assisted suicide.[30] However, given that the Supreme Court has approved terminal sedation for a terminally ill patient whose pain cannot be controlled in other ways, no pain need be suffered by anyone refusing treatment or food and fluids.

There are several morally significant disadvantages that are shared by physician-assisted suicide and active euthanasia that are not shared by refusing food and fluids. Physician-assisted suicide and active euthanasia, although they would usually require a two-week waiting period, allow for almost instantaneous death. This makes it less likely that their legalization will support the use of palliative care. The refusal of food and fluids takes a week before the patient is unconscious, thus, it is clear that palliative care must be practiced. The relative speed and ease with which physician-assisted suicide and active euthanasia can bring about death makes it more likely that patients will be pressured to hasten their deaths when they would prefer not to do so. Because of the time it takes, it is much less likely that patients will be pressured to refuse food and fluids. This time also permits patients to change their minds, and for friends and families to know that the patients were firm in their decision to die. Indeed, for patients not on life-sustaining treatments, refusing food and fluids seems to have more overall benefits than any other method of hastening death.[31] Major drawbacks are public and physician ignorance of the fact that it is not painful for terminal patients to do without food and fluids, the association of feeding with caring, and some patients' dislike of the idea of refusing food and fluids.

Both physician-assisted suicide and active euthanasia are morally controversial, and so physicians would not be required to practice them. This means that physicians would always have to take full personal responsibility for assisting suicide or performing active euthanasia. Like physicians performing abortions, they are likely to be subject to criticism from those opposed to such practices. Physicians are morally and legally required to practice passive euthanasia, that is, they are not allowed to overrule a competent patient's refusal of treatment, so that they do not have to bear this burden. Patients cannot require someone to kill them; they can require others to leave them alone, even if that requires physicians to discontinue their treatment. Thus, from the point of view of physicians, providing their terminally ill patients with adequate palliative care and informing them that they can refuse any life-preserving treatment— including food and fluids—together with assuring them that palliative care will continue for as long as necessary during their refusal, seems, on balance, a safer and more desirable option than the legalization of physician-assisted suicide.[32]

Advance Directives

Since a person often loses competence in the latter stages of a terminal illness, all that has been said above may seem to be of limited practical value. However, abiding by the advance directives of a formerly competent patient after that patient becomes incompetent is similar in all moral respects to abiding by the directives of a currently competent patient. This means that if competent patients explicitly state in an advance directive (either a living will or durable power of attorney for health care) that if they reach some specified gravely ill stage, they would want food and fluids to be withheld, then the physician is morally required to abide by that refusal. Advance directives avoid the very troubling matter of dealing with gravely ill, permanently incompetent patients who have not expressed their wishes about whether they would wish life-prolonging treatment to be discontinued. Patients should be told the facts about the withholding of food and fluids, including the fact that it is not a painful way to die, and should be asked to explicitly state whether they want food and fluids withdrawn or withheld.

We have not discussed the questions of nonvoluntary euthanasia, as common morality does not provide as clear an answer to the questions this issue raises as it does to the questions raised by voluntary euthanasia. Recognizing that voluntary, passive euthanasia is not merely morally allowed, but is morally required, whereas nonvoluntary passive euthanasia is, at most, morally allowed, and that some impartial rational persons would not publicly allow it is itself of moral significance. Physicians should make every effort to have patients, when competent, express their desires about what they would want to be done if they should become permanently incompetent, and also have patients appoint someone to determine when it is appropriate to have those desires acted on. As long ago as March 31, 1976, the New Jersey Supreme Court handed down its decision in the Karen Ann Quinlan case that a feeding tube could be removed from a permanently comatose person even though she had not filled out an advance directive. However, the Terri Schiavo case in Florida shows that even in 2005, although one family member has the legal authority to have the feeding tube removed, if there is disagreement among family members, it is still a very controversial matter. This makes evident the need for a patient to fill out an advance directive with clear and reasonably precise instructions, and to explicitly appoint the person she wants who will decide when to act on those instructions.[33]

If competent patients explicitly state in an advance directive that, if they become permanently incompetent, they want life-prolonging treatments, including food and fluids, to be discontinued, then physicians are morally required to abide by those refusals. This view has been challenged by those claiming that the views of the competent person who filled out the advance directive are not always the same as the views of the incompetent person to whom they are being applied.[34] They hold that advance directives need not be followed if the physician believes that the incompetent person would not now choose to have life-prolonging treatment withdrawn. One must judge a public policy, however, in terms of the effects that this policy would have on all of the people involved, if all of them knew about the policy. Competent persons who fill out advance directives refusing life-prolonging treatment if they become permanently incompetent consider it very distasteful and devoid of dignity to live as a permanently incompetent person. The now incompetent person, however, having no sense of dignity, does not view her life with distaste.

If everyone knew that advance directives need not be honored in these cases, some permanently incompetent persons would live longer than they would if such advance directives were honored. This might be viewed by some as a positive result, but it is not clear how the incompetent person views it. It is clear, however, that another result of everyone knowing that their advance directives might not be honored would be anxiety, anger, and other unpleasant feelings by those competent persons who had made out such advance directives. This could result in an increase in such competent persons taking their own lives while they were competent (e.g., Janet Adkins, the first client of Dr. Jack Kevorkian), in order to avoid the unwanted prolongation of their lives as incompetent persons. The consequences of a public policy of not honoring such advance directives seem likely to have worse consequences than the present policy of honoring advance directives.

Hospitals are now required to ask patients if they have filled out an advance directive. It would be even better if they made filling out an advance directive a standard part of their admitting procedure. Persuading patients to express their desires on these matters and to appoint someone to determine how best to satisfy their desires when they become incompetent, could, if properly implemented, give patients a genuine sense of being able to control their own deaths. We realize, however, that presently, advance directives seem to have little or no effect on the treatment of seriously ill patients entering the hospital. (See the support studies by Joanne Lynne and Joan Teno.) We regard this lack of effect as unfortunate and know that much more work must be done in order for physicians and patients to see advance directives as an appropriate and desirable opportunity to allow patients greater control over the times of their deaths.

One of the problems with the advance directive forms currently completed (by the small number of people who do fill them out) is that the "directives" they allow the person to choose have only a remote resemblance to the kinds of decisions that actually need to be made about treating gravely ill patients. For example, many of the standard forms allow the person to say that she would not want treatment that was "extraordinary," or "futile," or "heroic." Almost never is such a directive of any usefulness in making decisions at the bedside of a now incompetent patient. Other directives (like the "medical directive") are needlessly lengthy, complex, and confusing. Few directives take into account the probabilistic nature of prognoses in gravely ill patients and allow a person to say whether or not she would want life-support to be discontinued if her chance of recovery or partial recovery were extremely slight but not non-existent, a situation that underlies a large number of the ethics consultation requests fielded by ethics consultants and committees.[35]

Gravely Ill Patients without Advance Directives

Even with aggressive attempts to have large numbers of persons fill out advance directives, there will inevitably be, in the foreseeable future, many incompetent and gravely ill patients who have not done so. How should such patients be treated? The current procedure frequently seems to be to continue treatment and life support until the patient dies or until the probability that the patient will die very soon becomes essentially 100%. One reason this is done is because it is assumed that, unless otherwise stated, persons would want to be treated until their situation became hopeless. This assumption is mistaken in most cases.

Our experience, for example, suggests that essentially no one would want to be kept alive if he were in a persistent vegetative state or any other state in which there was almost no chance of his becoming conscious again. Our experience also suggests that almost no one would want to be kept alive even if there were a significant chance of their becoming conscious, if there were not also a chance of significant interaction with others. Almost no one wants to be kept alive while in a coma when the best they can expect if they come out of the coma does not include recognizing family and friends. In fact, we believe that only a small minority of gravely ill patients would want to be kept alive if their chances of completely recovering from a coma were less than 5%, and they would still be gravely ill after their recovery.[36]

Our experience is limited, however, and we would not want to base any policy upon it. Rather, we propose that over a several-year period there be a very large survey of suitably constructed advance directives. If the overwhelming majority (at least 90%) of those advance directives state that they would not want treatment to be continued in a particular clinical state, we propose that, in the absence of an advance directive requesting treatment in that clinical state, treatment be discontinued. These data would rebut the presumption that most persons want to be kept alive in that situation. Of course, if a patient had completed an advance directive requesting that treatment be continued, this should be honored. Further, this policy should not be implemented until it had been given such sufficiently wide publicity that essentially everyone had heard of it, so that those who did not wish treatment to be stopped would have had an opportunity to fill out a suitable advance directive.

We do not propose that people vote on whether people without advance directives should be kept alive or allowed to die. We are not concerned with whether other people want a patient in a particular clinical state to be kept alive or allowed to die. This is not a decision that people should make for others. Rather, we want to know what people choose for themselves when they fill out their own advance directives. It is what people choose for themselves that is the best guide for determining what would be chosen by someone who has not made an explicit choice. That is why we want a very large survey of actual advance directives, not a vote, to determine what should be done in particular clinical situations.

Another reason sometimes given for continued treatment is that since death is irreversible; doctors who err should err on the side of life. We agree that doctors normally should err on the side of life and that is why we state that treatment should be discontinued only when the overwhelming majority (at least 90%, and not a mere majority of 51%) would choose to have treatment and life support stopped in particular circumstances. Given the great costs—emotional as well as financial—as well as the minimal benefits of any kind that are involved in continuing treatment in situations where the overwhelming majority of persons would want it discontinued, we believe it is harder to justify continuing treatment than to justify discontinuing it.

Summary

The examination of four standard ways of making the distinction between active and passive euthanasia—acts versus omissions, stopping treatment versus not starting treatment, ordinary care versus extraordinary care, and whether death is due to natural causes—shows that they cannot provide a way of making a morally relevant distinction between killing and allowing to die. Using the distinction between patient requests and patient refusals, however, does provide such a way. Our moral analysis of the distinction between active and passive euthanasia reaches some different conclusions than all of the ad hoc ways of making the distinction. Of the four standard ways of making the distinction, active euthanasia is morally prohibited whereas doctors are morally allowed to practice passive euthanasia. We do not claim that active euthanasia is morally prohibited, only that it is morally controversial. On our view, doctors are not merely morally allowed to practice voluntary passive euthanasia; they are morally required to practice passive euthanasia.

Physician-assisted suicide was seen to be neither active euthanasia nor passive euthanasia. It resembles active euthanasia in that it is a request by a patient for an action by the physician (e.g., prescribing lethal drugs that will result in the patient's death), but it does not violate the rule against killing as active euthanasia does. It is not passive euthanasia, for it is not based on a refusal of treatment that a physician is morally required to abide by. However, it partly resembles providing palliative care to those who are refusing life-prolonging treatment or food and fluids. It differs from providing such palliative care in that those who refuse life-prolonging treatment or food and fluids are not committing suicide, and those for whom the lethal drugs are prescribed are committing suicide. Since physician-assisted suicide does not violate the rule against killing, the only moral argument against legalizing it is that it will lead to overall worse consequences. But whether this is true is an empirical matter. Since physician-assisted suicide does not violate the rule against killing, its legalization does not provide a reason for legalizing active euthanasia, which does violate this rule.

The moral system thus makes clear the moral significance of the distinction between refusals and requests and allows for a meaningful distinction between active and passive euthanasia. There is no need to make an ad hoc distinction that applies only to dying patients, as the standard discussions do; rather, the moral significance of a commonly used distinction in medical practice, between requests and refusals, is acknowledged and applied to the question of euthanasia. The medical facts about the consequences of refusing food and fluids (i.e., that it normally causes no additional suffering) makes clear that there is a viable alternative open to all patients—regardless of whether they are on life support—to hasten the time of their death. Our explicit account of morality is not only helpful in showing the inadequacy of accepting the standard ad hoc and unsystematic attempts to distinguish between active and passive euthanasia, it also shows how common morality, together with a commonly applied medical distinction between requests and refusals, clarifies and justifies this distinction.

Notes

1. As will be apparent later, this seemingly innocent way of expressing way of the has some serious problems.
2. See Foley (1991).
3. See Clouser (1977).
4. See Rachels (1975), and Brock (1992).
5. See U.S. Court of Appeals for the Ninth Circuit, no. 94–35534, March 6, 1966.
6. Ibid.
7. Ibid.
8. "Hydration and nutrition" are the terms normally used when food and fluids are being supplied by medical means; it is considered a medical treatment. Since patients can refuse any medical treatment, "hydration and nutrition" are the terms used by those who hold that a patient can refuse food and fluids. Since we hold that patients are not limited to refusing medical treatments, we generally use the simpler phrase "food and fluids."
9. Ibid., U.S. Court of Appeals for the Ninth Circuit.
10. This is true not only of a "natural death" but also of "natural ingredients," "natural behavior," and so forth.
11. See Gert, Bernat, and Mogielnicki (1994).
12. Sometimes the patient has a rationally allowed belief, for example, a religious belief, that is not shared by the doctor, and this difference in belief accounts for the patient's refusal to consent to the suggested treatment.

13. Of course, sometimes it is rational because they have not been provided with adequate palliative care and do not know that such care is available. That this happens so often is another reason that many people are reluctant to make physician-assisted suicide or active euthanasia legal.

14. This case is adapted from Case No. 228, "A Demand to Die" in *Hastings Center Report*, published in White and Engelhardt (1975), and refers to Dax's case, one of the most famous cases in the medical ethics literature. It is also available in two different videotape formats. A test of the adequacy of our description is whether one would find other morally relevant features in the more detailed descriptions and also whether these would affect the decision one would make. We realize that our description lacks detail, for we have provided only the morally relevant features. Real cases presented in full detail are often the best kinds of cases to present, because one has to search for the morally relevant features. Learning how to find the morally relevant features amid the complexities of real life is one of the most important skills in moral reasoning. It is indispensable in the process of ethics consultation. In making real-life decisions, often only limited precision and certainty is possible. These are factors that make coming to decisions in real cases sometimes so difficult. See Aristotle, *Nichomachean Ethics*, 1.3.1094b.

15. See Clouser (1977).

16. See Foley (1991). A reply to that line of reasoning is found in Kasting (1994). See also Bernat, Gert, and Mogielnicki (1993).

17. One may claim that killing that is the result of abiding by a refusal never has the same morally relevant features as killing that is done at the request of a patient, but if both count as killing, there is no morally important distinction between requests and refusals. Both have the consent of the victim, and so both can have the same morally relevant features. Furthermore, killing is such a serious violation of a moral rule that the morally relevant features would have to be dramatically different for one method of killing to be justified and the other not.

18. Contrary to one's initial inclination, what counts as "causing harm" is not determined by some scientific analysis, but rather by whether it is held that a justification or excuse is needed for such behavior. See Gert (2005, 175–176).

19. But you can also kill a person unintentionally, even when you are not negligent, as when your car skids on some black ice and hits a person, resulting in his death. Such a killing may be completely excusable, but it is still killing.

20. Given that it is not only morally but also legally required to abide by a patient's rational refusal of treatment, legally abiding by such refusals cannot be treated as intentionally killing.

21. Some who are involved in cognitive science suggest that people do not operate on the basis of rules, but rather on paradigms or prototypes. But as this discussion makes clear, there is no conflict between using both rules and prototypes in moral reasoning. Indeed, the proper role of paradigms or prototypes is to determine whether an act should be considered as an act of a certain kind, for example, killing, and hence needs a justification or excuse. See May, Friedman, and Clark (1996), especially chapter 5, "The Neural Representation of the Social World" by Paul M. Churchland, and chapter 6, "Connectionism, Moral Cognition, and Collaborative Problem Solving" by Andy Clark.

22. In our society not everyone uses or extends the paradigms or prototypes in the same way, and so there will be disagreements on whether a given act counts as killing. Nonetheless, there is usually substantial agreement on most cases. However, in trying to change a long-standing practice, it is not uncommon for people, especially philosophers, to try to change the ways of extending the paradigms, so as to justify the change they are

promoting. And sometime these efforts are successful and what counts as killing does change.

23. See Brock (1992). People would be inconsistent if such concepts as "killing" were as simple as some philosophers claim them to be. However, some philosophers confuse complexity with inconsistency.

24. That this is an extended sense is shown by the fact that life insurance policies that exclude payment if death is due to suicide cannot refuse to pay if death is due to these kinds of causes.

25. This view is not held by all. Some, especially those with religious views, regard refusing treatment, and especially refusing food and fluids, as committing suicide. They may not regard such refusals as suicide if death is imminent with or without treatment, but they would regard all refusals of treatment as suicide when treatment would sustain life for any appreciable time.

26. See Clouser (1991). See also Bernat, Gert, and Mogielnicki (1993).

27. See David Eddy (1994) in an article about his mother refusing food and fluids.

28. This is not an argument against killing someone in an emergency situation, for example, someone who has been captured by a sadistic enemy, or an unrescuable person in an accident who is about to be burned to death. This shows the importance of the morally relevant feature concerning emergency situations. (See chapter 2 for further discussion of morally relevant features.)

29. Many people claim to prefer physician-assisted suicide, or even active euthanasia, to discontinuing food and fluids. However, this may be due to their focus on their own particular cases, namely, they see only the ease and quickness of the former two methods, and fail to appreciate their far greater potential for abuse. Also, there is so much misinformation about the pain and suffering involved in discontinuing food and fluids that it is unlikely that their preferences count as informed preferences. However, even with accurate information and the support of their physicians, some patients may still prefer physician-assisted suicide to discontinuing food and fluids. How much importance should be given to these preferences is a matter of dispute, even among the authors of this book.

30. This is an argument against legalizing physician-assisted suicide. It is not an argument against using it if it were legalized.

31. However, for some the personal benefits of knowing that they can die quickly and painlessly may outweigh all of the benefits of discontinuing food and fluids. This is not an irrational ranking.

32. However, legalizing physician-assisted suicide may have some benefits not directly related to the patients knowing that they can die quickly and painlessly. It may be that legalizing physician-assisted suicide will promote discussion of end-of-life decisions and encourage more people to fill out living wills and durable powers of attorney for health care. Some health care workers in Oregon have made this claim.

33. See Culver (1998).

34. See Dresser and Robertson (1989).

35. For a critique of current advance directive forms and suggestions about how they might be improved, see Culver (1998).

36. See Culver and Gert (1990b).

Bibliography

American Psychiatric Association. 2000. *Diagnostic and Statistical Manual of Mental Disorders. DSM-IV-TR.* American Psychiatric Association: Washington, D.C. Earlier volumes: *DSM-III* (1980), *DSM-III-R* (1987), *DSM-IV* (1994).

Bailey, Alan, David Robinson, and A. M. Dawson. 1977. "Does Gilbert's disease exist?" *Lancet* 1, 931–933.

Bayles, Michael D. 1974. "Criminal paternalism." In *The Limits of Law-Nomos XV*, ed. J. Roland Pennock, and John W. Chapman. New York: Lieber-Atherton, 174–188.

Beauchamp, Thomas. 2003. "A defense of common morality." *Kennedy Institute of Ethics Journal* 13, 259–274.

Beauchamp, Thomas, and James Childress. 2001. *Principles of Biomedical Ethics*, 5th ed. New York: Oxford University Press. Earlier editions: 1 [1979], 2 [1983], 3 [1989], 4 [1994].

Begg, Colin B., Laura D. Cramer, William J. Hoskins, and Murray Brennan. 1998. "Impact of hospital volume on operative mortality for major cancer surgery." *Journal of the American Medical Association* 280, 1747–1751.

Bernat, James L., Charles M. Culver, and Bernard Gert. 1981. "On the definition and criterion of death." *Annals of Internal Medicine* 94, 389–394.

Bernat, James L., Bernard Gert, and R. P. Mogielnicki. 1993. "Patient refusal of hydration and nutrition. An alternative to physician assisted suicide or voluntary euthanasia." *Archives of Internal Medicine* 153, 2723–2728.

Birkmeyer, J. D., T. Stukel, Siewers, A., Goodney, P., Wennberg, D. E., and Lucas, F. L. 2003. "Surgeon volume and operative mortality in the United States. *New England Journal of Medicine* 349, 2117–2127.

Birkmeyer, J. D., Warshaw, A. L., Finlayson, S. R., Grove, M. R., and Tosteson, A. N. 1999. "Relationship between hospital volume and late survival after pancreaticoduodenectomy." *Surgery* 126, 178–183.

Boorse, Christopher. 2004. "On the distinction between disease and illness." In *Health, Disease, and Illness*, ed. Arthur L. Caplan, James J. McCartney, and Dominic A. Sisti. Washington, D.C.: Georgetown University Press, 77–89.

Braddock, Clarence A., Kelly A. Edwards, Hasenberg, N. M., Laidley, T. L., and Levinson, W. 1999. "Informed decision making in outpatient practice." *Journal of the American Medical Association* 282, 2313–2320.

Brand-Ballard, Jeffrey. 2003. "Consistency, common morality, and reflective equilibrium." *Kennedy Institute of Ethics Journal* 13, 231–258.

Brock, Dan W. 1983. "Paternalism and promoting the good." In *Paternalism*, ed. Rolf Sartorius. Minneapolis: University of Minnesota Press, 237–260.

———. 1992. "Voluntary active euthanasia." *Hastings Center Report* 22, 10–22.

Buchanan, Allan B., and Dan W. Brock. 1986. "Deciding for others." *Milbank Quarterly* 64, 17–94.

———. 1990. *Deciding for Others: The Ethics of Surrogate Decision-Making*. New York: Cambridge University Press.

Butler-Sloss, Dame Elizabeth. 2002. "Ms B and an NHS Hospital Trust." EWHC 429 (Fam) in the High Court of Justice, Family Division.

Cabana, Michael D., Cynthia S. Rand, Powe, W. R., Wu, A. W., Wilson, M. H., Abboud, P. A., and Rubin, H. R. 1999. "Why don't physicians follow clinical practice guidelines?" *Journal of the American Medical Association* 282, 1458–1465.

Center for Evaluative Clinical Sciences. 1999. *The Dartmouth Atlas of Health Care*. Hanover, N.H.: Dartmouth College.

Chell, Byron. 1998. "Competency: What it is, what it isn't, and why it matters." In *Health Care Ethics: Critical issues for the 21st Century*, ed. John F. Monagle, and David C. Thomasma. Gaithersburg, Md.: Aspen, 117–127.

Childress, James F. 1979. "Paternalism and health care." In *Medical Responsibility*, ed. Wade L. Robison, and Michael S. Pritchard Clifton, N.J.: Humana, 15–27.

———. 1982. *Who Should Decide? Paternalism in Health Care*. New York: Oxford University Press.

Clarke, S. G., and Evan Simpson. 1989. *Anti-Theory in Ethics and Moral Conservatism*. Albany: State University of New York Press.

Clouser, K. Danner. 1977. "Allowing or causing: Another look." *Annals of Internal Medicine* 87, 622–624.

———. 1991. "The challenge for future debate on euthanasia." *The Journal of Pain and Symptom Management* 6, 306–311.

———. 1995. "Common morality as an alternative to principlism." *Kennedy Institute of Ethics Journal* 5, 219–236.

Clouser, K. Danner, Charles M. Culver, and Bernard Gert. 1981. "Malady: A new treatment of disease." *Hastings Center Report* 11, 29–37.

Clouser, K. Danner, and Bernard Gert, ed. 1986. "Rationality and Medicine." *The Journal of Medicine and Philosophy* 11, (May).

———. 1990. "A critique of principlism." *The Journal of Medicine and Philosophy* 15, 219–236

———. 1994. "Morality vs. principlism." In *Principles of Health Care Ethics*, ed. Raamon Gillon. Baltimore: Wiley, 251–266.

———. 2004. "Common morality." In *Bioethics: A Philosophical Overview*, ed. George Kushf. Boston: Kluwer Academic Publishers.

Cohen, Bruce. 2003. *Theory and Practice of Psychiatry*. New York: Oxford University Press.

Conrad, P., and J. W. Schneider. 1980. *Deviance and Medicalization.* St. Louis: Mosby.

Culver, Charles M. 1998. "Advance directives." *Psychology, Public Policy and Law* 3, 676–687.

———. 2004. "Commitment to mental institutions." In *Encyclopedia of Bioethics*, ed. Stephen G. Post. 3rd ed. New York: Macmillan, 1815–1820.

Culver, Charles M., and Bernard Gert. 1980. "Regionalization of surgical services." Letter to the editor, *New England Journal of Medicine* 302, 1034–1035.

———. 1982. *Philosophy in Medicine.* New York: Oxford University Press; Japanese ed., trans. Masakatsu Okada and eight others. Tokyo: Hokuju Shuppan, 1984.

———. 1990a. "The inadequacy of incompetence." *Milbank Quarterly* 68, 619–643.

———. 1990b. "Beyond the living will: Making advance directives more useful." *Omega* 21, 253–258.

Daniels, Norman. 1994. "The genome project, individual differences, and just health care." In *Justice and the Human Genome Project*, ed. Timothy F. Murphy and Marc A. Lappe. Berkeley and Los Angeles: University of California Press, 110–132.

DeGrazia, David. 1992. "Moving forward in bioethical theory: Theories, cases, and specified principlism." *The Journal of Medicine and Philosophy* 17, 511–539.

Drane, James. 1985. "The many faces of competency." *Hastings Center Report* 15, 17–21.

Dresser, Rebecca, and John A. Robertson. 1989. "Quality of life and non-treatment decisions for incompetent patients." *Law, Medicine and Health Care* 17, 234–244.

Duggan, Timothy J., and Bernard Gert. 1967. "Voluntary abilities." *American Philosophical Quarterly* 4, 127–135.

Dworkin, Gerald. 1972. "Paternalism." *The Monist* 56, 64–84.

———. 1983. "Paternalism: Some second thoughts." In *Paternalism*, ed. Rolf Sartorious Minneapolis: University of Minnesota Press, 105–111.

Eddy, David. 1994. "A conversation with my mother." *Journal of the American Medical Association* 272, 179–181.

Emanuel, Ezekiel J. 1995. "The beginning of the end of principlism." *Hastings Center Report* 25, 37–38.

Emanuel, Linda L. 1995. "Reexamining death: The asymptotic model and a bounded zone definition." *Hastings Center Report* 25, 27–35.

Federal Register, 1979, 44, no. 76, 23192–23197.

Feinberg, Joel. 1985. *Offense to Others: The Moral Limits of the Criminal Law.* New York: Oxford University Press.

Feinberg, Joel, and Susan Dwyer, ed. 1997. *The Problem of Abortion.* 3rd ed. Belmont, Calif.: Wadsworth.

Foley, Kathleen M. 1991. "The relationship of pain and symptom management to patient requests for physician-assisted suicide." *Journal of Pain and Symptom Management* 6, 289–297.

Geddes, John R., Stuart M. Carney, Davies, C., Fukukawa, T. A., Kupfer, D. J., Frank, E., and Goodwin, G. M. 2003. "Relapse prevention with antidepressant drug treatment in depressive disorders: A systematic review." *Lancet* 361, 653–661.

Gert, Bernard. 1967. "Can the brain have a pain?" *Philosophy and Phenomenological Research* 27, 432–436.

———. 1971. "Personal identity and the body." *Dialogue* 10, 458–478.

———. 1972. "Coercion and freedom." In *Coercion*, ed. J. Roland Pennock, and John W. Chapman Nomos XIV. New York: Lieber-Atherton, 189–210.

———. 1988. *Morality: A New Justification of the Moral Rules.* New York: Oxford University Press.

————. 1989. "Morality versus slogans." *Western Michigan University Center for the Study of Ethics in Society* 3, no. 2 (December).

————. 1990a. "Rationality, human nature, and lists." *Ethics* 100, 279–300.

————. 1990b. "Irrationality and the DSM-III-R definition of mental disorder." *Analyze & Kritik*, Jahrgang 12, Heft 1, 34–46.

————. 1992. "A sex caused inconsistency in DSM-III-R: The definition of mental disorder and the definition of paraphilias." *The Journal of Medicine and Philosophy* 17, 155–171.

————. 1993. "Defending irrationality and lists." *Ethics* 103, 329–336.

————. 1996. "Moral impartiality." *Midwest Studies in Philosophy*, Vol. XX., 102–127.

————. 2004. *Common Morality.* New York: Oxford University Press.

————. 2005. *Morality: Its Nature and Justification.* Rev. ed. New York: Oxford University Press.

Gert, Bernard, Edward M. Berger, George F. Cahill Jr., K. Danner Clouser, Charles M. Culver, John B. Moeschler, and George H. S. Singer. 1996. *Morality and the New Genetics.* Boston: Jones & Bartlett.

Gert, Bernard, James L. Bernat, and R. Peter Mogielnicki. Distinguishing between patients' refusals and requests." *The Hastings Center Report* 24, 13–15.

Gert, Bernard, and Charles M. Culver. 2004. "Defining mental disorder," in *The Philosophy of Psychiatry*, ed. Jennifer Radden. New York: Oxford University Press, 415–425.

Gert, Bernard, Charles M. Culver, and K. Danner Clouser. 2000. "Common morality versus specified principlism: Reply to Richardson." *Journal of Medicine and Philosophy* 25, 308–322.

Gert, Bernard, and Timothy J. Duggan. 1979. "Free will as the ability to will." *Nous* 13, 197–217.

Gert, Heather. 1997. "Viability." In *The Problem of Abortion*, ed. Joel Feinberg and Susan Dwyer 3rd ed. Belmont, Calif.: Wadsworth, 24–39.

————. 2002. "Avoiding surprises: A model for informing patients." *Hastings Center Report* 32, 23–32.

Giardiello, Francis M., Jill D. Breninger, Gloria M. Petersen, Luce, M. C., Hylind, L. M., Bacon, J. A., Booker, S. V., Parker, R. D., and Hamilton, S. R. 2003. "The use and interpretation of commercial APC testing for familial adenomatous polyposis. *New England Journal of Medicine* 336, 823–827.

Gigerenzer, Gerd. 2002. *Calculated Risks.* New York: Simon & Schuster.

Goldman, Howard H. 2000. *Review of General Psychiatry.* 5th ed. New York: Lange.

Goodwin, Donald W., and Samuel B. Guze. 1979. *Psychiatric Diagnosis.* 2nd ed. New York: Oxford University Press.

Gordon, Toby A., Burleyson, G. P., Tielsch, J. M., and Cameron, J. L. 1995. "The effects of regionalization on cost and outcome for one general high-risk surgical procedure." *Annals of Surgery* 221, 43–49.

Grisso, Thomas, and Paul S. Appelbaum. 1998. *Assessing Competence to Consent to Treatment.* New York: Oxford University Press.

Hales, Robert E., and Stuart F. Yudofsky. 2004. *Essentials of Clinical Psychiatry.* 2nd ed. Washington, DC: American Psychiatric Publishing.

Hannan, E. L., M. Racz, Ryan, T. J., McCallister, B. D., Johnson, L. W., Arani, D. T., Guercie, A. D., Sosa, J., and Topol, E. J. 1997. "Coronary angioplasty volume-outcome relationships for hospitals and cardiologists." *Journal of the American Medical Association* 277, 892–898.

Hurst, J. Willis. 1992. "Practicing Medicine." In *Medicine for the Practicing Physician*, ed. J. Willis Hurst, and Samuel S. Ambrose. Boston: Buttersworth.

Jennett, B., and F. Plum. 1972. "Persistent vegetative state after brain damage: A syndrome in search of a name." *Lancet* 1, 734–737.

Jonas, Hans. 1974. *Philosophical Essays: From Ancient Creed to Technological Man.* Englewood Cliffs, NJ. Prentice Hall, pp. 134–140.

Jonsen, Al, and Stephen Toulmin. 1988. *The Abuse of Casuistry.* Berkeley and Los Angeles: University of California Press.

Juengst, Eric T. 1998. "What does enhancement mean?" In *Enhancing Human Traits*, ed. Eric Parens. Washington, D.C.: Georgetown University Press, 29–47.

Kant, Emmanuel. 1785. *Grounding for the Metaphysics of Morals*, First Section, 395. Both Kant and Mill are available from Hackett Publishing Company. Indianapolis, Indiana.

Kasting, Gregg A. 1994. "The non-necessity of euthanasia." In *Physician-Assisted Death*, ed. J. D. Humber, R. F. Almeder, and G. A. Kasting. Totowa, N.J.: Humana Press, 25–43.

Kendell, R. E. 1986. "What are mental disorders?" In *Science, Practice and Social Policy*, ed. A. M. Freedman, R. Brotman, I. Silverman, and D. Hutson. New York: Human Sciences Press.

Kizer, Kenneth. 2003. "The volume-outcome conundrum." *New England Journal of Medicine* 349, 2159–2161.

Lamont, Elizabeth B., and Nicholas A. Christakis. 2003. "Complexities in prognostication of advanced cancer." *Journal of the American Medical Association* 290, 98–104.

Lavernia, C. J., and Guzman, J. F. 1995. "Relationship of surgical volume to short-term mortality, morbidity, and hospital charges in arthroplasty." *Journal of Arthroplasty* 10, 133–140.

Law Reform Commission of Canada. 1979. "Criteria for the determination of death." Ottawa: Law Reform Commission of Canada.

Luft, Harold S., John P. Bunker, and Alain C. Enthoven. 1979. "Should operations be regionalized? The empirical relation between surgical volume and mortality." *New England Journal of Medicine* 302, 1364–1369.

Mallary, Steven D., Bernard Gert, and Charles M. Culver. 1986. "Family coercion and valid consent." *Theoretical Medicine* 7, 123–126.

Malm, H. H. 1999. "Medical screening and the value of early detection: When unwarranted faith leads to unethical recommendations." *Hastings Center Report* 29, 26–38.

May, Larry, Marilyn Friedman, and Andy Clark. 1996. *Mind and Morals.* Cambridge: MIT Press.

Mill, John Stuart. 1863. *Utilitarianism.* Both Kant and Mill are available from Hackett Publishing Company. Indianapolis, Indiana.

Morison, Robert S. 1971. "Death: Process or Event?" *Science* 173, 694–698.

Multi-Society Task Force on PVS. 1994. "Medical aspects of the persistent vegetative state." Parts I and II. *New England Journal of Medicine*, Vol. 30, 1499–1508, 1572–1579.

Murphy, Michael J., Ronald L. Cowan, and Lloyd I. Sederer. 2001. *Blueprints in Psychiatry.* 2nd ed. Malden, Mass.: Blackwell.

Nicoll, Diana, and Michael Pignone. 2004. "Chapter 1. Basic principles of diagnostic test use and interpretation." In *Pocket Guide to Diagnostic Tests*, ed. Diana Nicoll, Stephen J. McPhee, and Michael Pignone. 4th ed. New York: McGraw Hill, 1–20.

O'Connor, Gerald T., Hebe Quinton, Traven, N. D., Rammunno, L. D., Dodds, T. A., Marciniak, T. A., and Wennberg, J. E. 1999. "Geographical variation in the treatment of acute myocardial infarction." *Journal of the American Medical Association* 281, 627–633.

Orwell, George. *Animal Farm* and *1984*.

O'Shea, B. 1990. "Brain transplants: Myth or monster?" *British Journal of Psychiatry* 156, 645–653.

Parens, Erik. 1998. "Is better always good? The enhancement project." In *Enhancing Human Traits*, ed. Erik Parens. Washington, D.C.: Georgetown University Press, 25.

Peery, Thomas M. and Frank Miller. 1971. *Pathology*. 2nd ed. Boston: Little, Brown.

President's Commission for the Study of Ethical Problems in Medicine and Biomedical and Behavorial Research. 1981. *Defining Death, A Report on the Medical, Legal, and Ethical Issues in the Determination of Death*. Washington, D.C.

Rachels, James. 1975. "Active and passive euthanasia." *New England Journal of Medicine* 292, 78–80.

Rawls, John. 1971. *A Theory of Justice*. Cambridge: Harvard University Press.

Regan, Donald H. 1974. "Justifications for paternalism." In *The Limits of Law—Nomos XV*, ed. J. Roland Pennock, and John W. Chapman. New York: Lieber-Atherton, 189–210.

Report of the Medical Consultants on the Diagnoses of Death to the President's Commission for the Study of Ethical Problems in Medicine and Biomedical and Behavioral Research. 1981. "Guidelines for the determination of death." *Journal of the American Medical Association* 246, 2184–2186.

Roth, Loren H., Alan Meisel, and Charles W. Lidz. 1977. "Tests of competency to consent to treatment." *American Journal of Psychiatry* 134, 279–284.

Sadock, Benjamin J., and Virginia A. Sadock. 2000. *Comprehensive Textbook of Psychiatry*. 7th ed. Vol. 1. Philadelphia: Lippincott Williams & Wilkins.

Simunovic, M., T. To, M. Theriault, and B. Langer. 1999. "Relation between hospital surgical volume and outcome for pancreatic resection for neoplasm in a publicly funded health care system." *Canadian Medical Association Journal* 160, 643–649.

Singer, Peter. 1993. *Practical Ethics*. 2nd ed. Cambridge: Cambridge University Press.

Soble, Alan G. 2004. "Desire: Paraphilia and distress in DSM-IV." In *The Philosophy of Psychiatry*, ed. Jennifer Radden. New York: Oxford University Press, 54–63.

Spitzer, Robert L., and Jean Endicott. 1978. "Medical and mental disorder: Proposed definition and criteria." In *Critical Issues in Psychiatric Diagnosis*, ed. Robert L. Spitzer and Donald F. Klein. New York: Raven, 15–39.

Stone, Alan A. 1975. *Mental Health and Law: A System in Transition*. Rockville, Md.: U.S. Department of Health, Education and Welfare.

Talso, Peter J., and Alexander P. Remenchik. 1968. *Internal Medicine*. St. Louis: Mosby.

Teno, J., J. Lynn, N. Wenger, R. S. Phillips, D. P. Murphy, A. F. Connors, Jr., N. Desbiens, W. Fulkerson, P. Bellainy, and W. A. Khaus. 1997. "Advance Directives for seriously ill hospitalized patients." *Journal of the American Geriatric Society* 45, 519–520.

Thomson, Judith Jarvis. 1997. "A defense of abortion." In *The Problem of Abortion*, ed. Joel Feinberg and Susan Dwyer. 3rd ed. Belmont, Calif.: Wadsworth, 59–74.

Tomb, David A. *Psychiatry*. 1999. 6th ed. Philadelphia: Lippincott Williams & Wilkins.

Tu, Jack V., Peter C. Austin, and Benjamin T. B. Chan. 2001. "Relationship between annual volume of patients treated by admitting physicians and mortality after acute myocardial infarction." *Journal of the American Medical Association* 285, 3116–3122.

Turner, Leigh. 2003. "Zones of consensus and zones of conflict: Questioning the 'Common Morality' presumption in bioethics." *Kennedy Institute of Ethics Journal* 13, 193–218.

Veatch, Robert M. 1976. *Death, Dying and the Biological Revolution: Our Last Quest for Responsibility*. New Haven: Yale University Press.

Wakefield, Jerome. 1992a. "The concept of mental disorder: On the boundary between biological facts and social values." *American Psychologist* 47, 373.

———. 1992b. "Disorder as harmful dysfunction: A conceptual critique of DSM-III-R's definition of mental disorder." *Psychological Review* 99, 233, 239.

Welch, H. Gilbert. 2004. *Should I Be Tested for Cancer? Maybe Not and Here's Why*. Berkeley and Los Angeles: University of California Press.

Wennberg, John E. 1999. "Understanding geographic variations in health care delivery." *New England Journal of Medicine* 340, 52–53.

White, R. B., and H. T. Engelhardt Jr. 1975. Vol. 5. "A demand to die." *The Hastings Center Report*, 9–10.

White, R. J., L. R. Wolin, Massopust, L. C., Taslitz, N., and Verdura, J. 1971. "Cephalic exchange transplantation in the monkey." *Surgery* 70, 135–139.

White, William A. 1926. *The Meaning of Disease*. Baltimore: Williams & Wilkins.

Wikler, Daniel. 1979. "Paternalism and the mildly retarded." *Philosophy and Public Affairs* 8, 377–392.

Index